Muscles

And Their

Exercises

A Pictorial Reference Guide:

Highlighted Major Muscles of the Body and the Exercises that Work Them.

Mark Meissner CPT

Fit Anatomy™

Copyright Information

Published by Fit Anatomy™
Published in the United States of America

ISBN: 978-0-692-47084-8

1. Health and Fitness 2. Exercise 3. Weight Training and Bodybuilding

Consult With Your Physician

Before beginning any exercise routine a person should consult with their physician to determne if there are any underlying health issues that they should be aware of, and to determine if they are cleared to exercise. This is especially of importance if a person beginning exercise is 40 years old and older or has previously led a significantly sedentary lifestyle.

Discontinue Exercise if Experiencing:

- Chest discomfort (Unusual pressure, tightness, shortness of breath, heart burn, and aching in the neck radiating down the left arm)
- Sudden onset of headache
- Sudden onset of "No Energy" or light headedness
- Severe joint or muscle pain
- Flu symptoms
- Any other unusual symtoms of concern

(If necessary consult with a medical professional)

During Exercise Focus on Proper Breathing

During exercise a person should breathe naturally and comfortably while avoiding holding their and putting pressure on their cardio-vascular system, where it can be felt as throbbing in the head or stress on the heart.

Introduction

My name is Mark Meissner. I am a personal fitness trainer who has been certified for 13 years through the American Council on Exercise, and I am the owner of Fit Anatomy™.

I developed "Muscles And Their Exercises" for sports/fitness trainers, fitness enthusiasts, as well as men and women from all walks of life who have never been into exercise, to use as a quick reference guide to learn which base exercises work specific muscles. This pictorial guide will assist those looking to develop personal workout routines for getting into shape with a collection of my own hand sketched highlighted anatomy images of most of the individual major muscles and muscle groups of the body. Following each color highlighted muscle image, I have included beginning and finishing movement demo pictures of most of the base exercises that work each specific muscle and muscle group. I demonstrate the primary isolation exercises that work each muscle and include other non-isolation exercises in which the muscles participate, while also providing recommended set and repitiion ranges for each exercise. This is not a complete reference of all exercises, but it provides each reader with a good example of how each muscle is involved with movement in the various exercises. Each person can then, through practice and experience, make exercise adjustments to better isolate the specific muscles on which they want to focus. On page 191 I provide a good beginning full body exercise routine for people to perform at home.

I am in my ealy 50's and have experienced the many health, cardiovascular conditioning, weight management, muscle development and redevelopment, shaping and toning benefits that my bodybuilding routine has produced in my life. I have learned first hand how to develop, shape, tone, and maintain lean muscle mass with the right workout routine and with a meal plan consisting of the right protein, carbohydrate and good fat intake. Over the past 13 years I have had the opportunity to witness the excellent health benefits of lower blood pressure, lower cholesterol, lower blood sugar levels and improved thyroid function that many of my 120-plus clients have experienced. Several of my client's physicians have reduced and/or eliminated their medications for each of the conditions. I have also witnessed the weight loss, muscle development, shaping and toning results that many experienced while consistently performing my natural body building and body-toning routines. Many of my clients have now trained with me anywhere from three to ten years, working out two to three days per week. Because I have been able to monitor their progress and watch how they have maintained their results over time, I know first hand the benefits exercise can produce in a person's life.

Introduction (Continued)

After age 25 a person can lose half of a pound of muscle per year through atrophy or shrinking of the muscles, which is largely due to a sedentary lifestyle. Training all of the major muscle groups of the body with the right resistance routine and getting the recommended protein intake, the right carbohydrate intake timing, and good fat intake is what I have found to be necessary to develop, redevelop and maintain lean muscle. Full range of motion resistance exercise promotes good circulation to the muscles, connective tissues and joints, and facilitates the lymph system flow to help boost and maintain the immune system. Many of the degenerative conditions associated with aging are related to muscle shrinking. Resistance exercise is one of the best ways to counter the degenerative conditions associated with aging and keep the biological clock younger, as muscle is redeveloped and the cardiovascular system is strengthened. People in their fifties, sixties and seventies can begin to see the body rebound and progressively get into better shape as they begin and consistently stick with a good balanced resistance routine, at an intensisty level that is comfortable for them. The results can be experienced by just going through the exercise motions with the right weight, at a comfortable pace that the person can enjoy. This needs to be performed on a consistent scheduled basis, workout after workout, week after week.

Cardio exercise (walking, running, biking, swimming, and aerobic exercise) 3-6 days per week strengthens the cardio-vascular and respiritory system, and can be performed for metabolizing body fat stores and achieving weight loss. It is recommended that a person start moderately 3 days per week of 10-15 minutes per day. As the body conditions, a person can then increase it to 3-5 days per week of 20-50 minutes per day. For weight loss it may be necessary to increase the cardio exercise to 6 days per week of 50 minutes per day, and once they reach their goal weight they can back it down to 3 days per week of 20-40 minutes per day for maintainance. This is what has really played a part in several of my clients experiencing significant weight loss of 2 lbs per week or a total of 30-70 lbs over a 4-9 month period, and reaching their goal weight.

"Muscles And Their Exercises" is one of what I hope are several books and videos to come that will educate men and women on the many health benefits of an exercise lifestyle, as well as how to workout for their desired muscle development and redevelopment, shaping and toning goals. My desire is to help people achieve optimum fitness and experience the muscle firming, shaping and toning they desire. I hope this reference guide proves to be a useful tool for everyone!

Contents

Contents (Continued)

Contents (Continued)

Major Muscles (Anterior) - Male

Superficial / Intermediate **Intermediate / Deep**

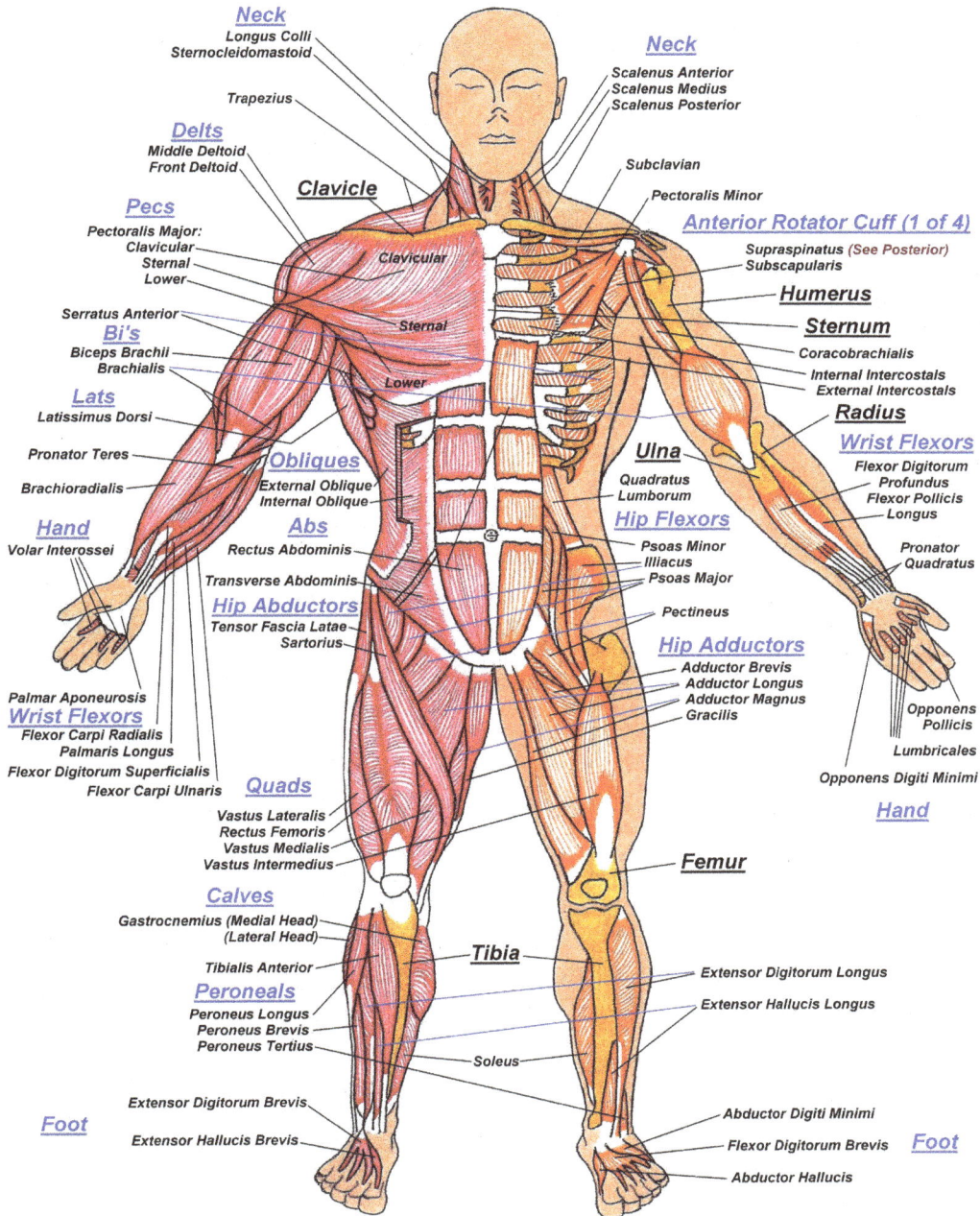

Neck
Longus Colli
Sternocleidomastoid

Trapezius

Delts
Middle Deltoid
Front Deltoid

Clavicle

Pecs
Pectoralis Major:
Clavicular
Sternal
Lower

Serratus Anterior

Bi's
Biceps Brachii
Brachialis

Lats
Latissimus Dorsi

Pronator Teres

Brachioradialis

Hand
Volar Interossei

Obliques
External Oblique
Internal Oblique

Abs
Rectus Abdominis

Transverse Abdominis

Hip Abductors
Tensor Fascia Latae
Sartorius

Palmar Aponeurosis
Wrist Flexors
Flexor Carpi Radialis
Palmaris Longus
Flexor Digitorum Superficialis
Flexor Carpi Ulnaris

Quads
Vastus Lateralis
Rectus Femoris
Vastus Medialis
Vastus Intermedius

Calves
Gastrocnemius (Medial Head)
(Lateral Head)

Tibialis Anterior

Peroneals
Peroneus Longus
Peroneus Brevis
Peroneus Tertius

Foot

Extensor Digitorum Brevis

Extensor Hallucis Brevis

Clavicular

Sternal

Lower

Neck
Scalenus Anterior
Scalenus Medius
Scalenus Posterior

Subclavian

Pectoralis Minor

Anterior Rotator Cuff (1 of 4)
Supraspinatus (See Posterior)
Subscapularis

Humerus

Sternum
Coracobrachialis
Internal Intercostals
External Intercostals

Radius

Wrist Flexors
Flexor Digitorum
Profundus
Flexor Pollicis
Longus

Ulna

Quadratus
Lumborum

Hip Flexors
Psoas Minor
Illiacus
Psoas Major

Pronator
Quadratus

Pectineus

Hip Adductors
Adductor Brevis
Adductor Longus
Adductor Magnus
Gracilis

Opponens
Pollicis

Lumbricales

Opponens Digiti Minimi

Hand

Femur

Tibia

Extensor Digitorum Longus

Extensor Hallucis Longus

Soleus

Abductor Digiti Minimi

Flexor Digitorum Brevis

Foot

Abductor Hallucis

Pectoralis Major (Pecs)

Pecs

Pectoralis Major:
Clavicular
Sternal
Lower

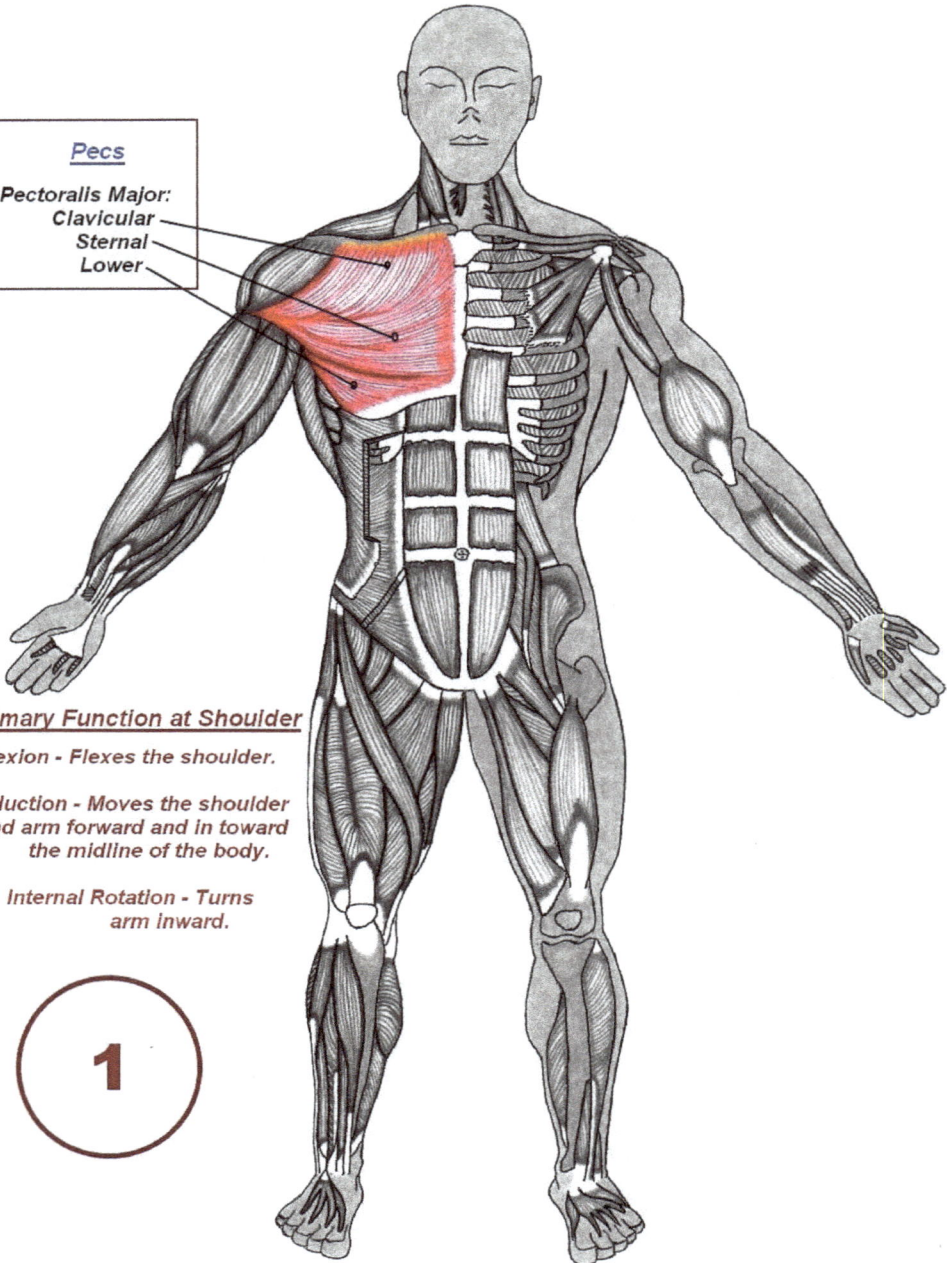

Primary Function at Shoulder

Flexion - Flexes the shoulder.

Adduction - Moves the shoulder and arm forward and in toward the midline of the body.

Internal Rotation - Turns arm inward.

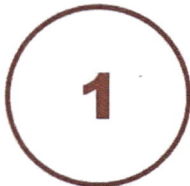

1

Pecs - Pectoralis Major (Sternal Region)

Pecs

Pectoralis Major:
Clavicular
Sternal
Lower

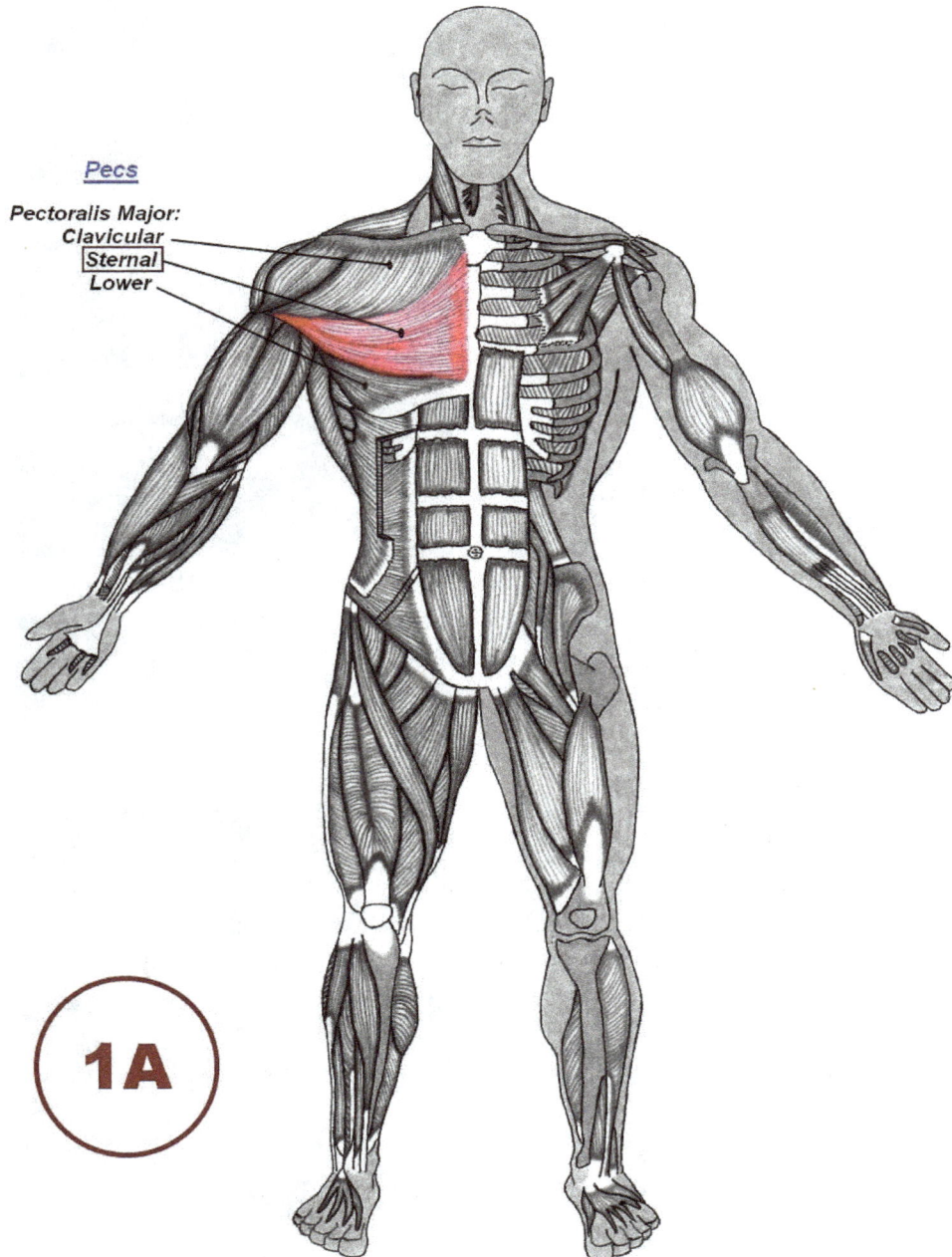

1A

1A - Exercises

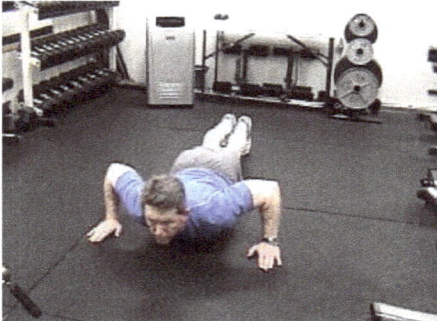

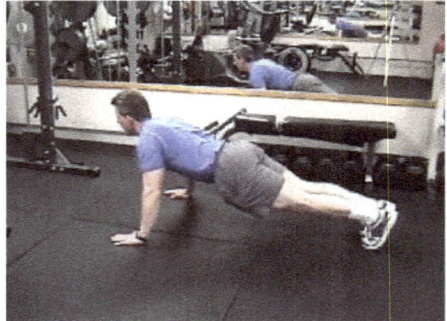

Push Ups (1-3 Sets 10-50 Reps)

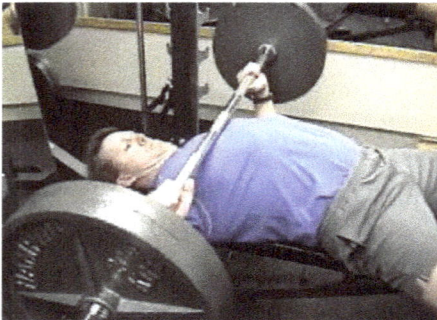

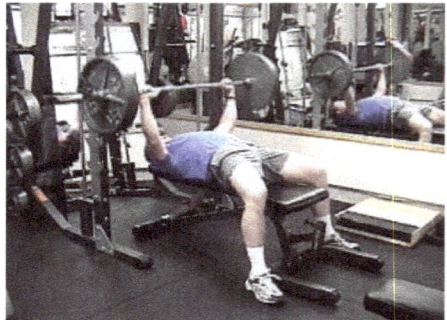

Chest Flat Bar Press "Bench Press" (1-5 Sets 7-15 Reps)

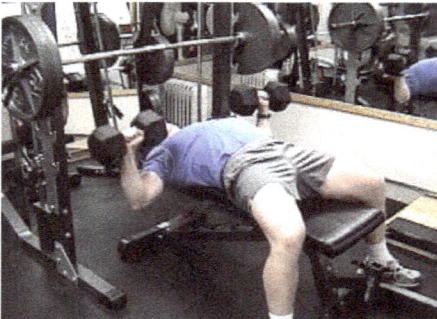

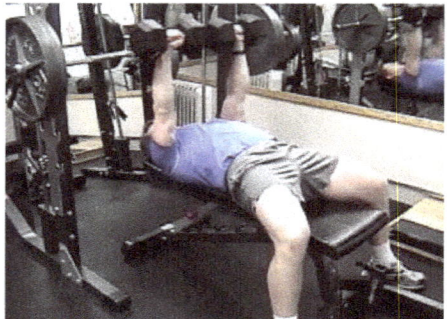

Chest Flat Dumbbel Press (1-5 Sets 7-15 Reps)

Chest Flat Rotate Dumbbell Press (1-5 Sets 7-15 Reps)

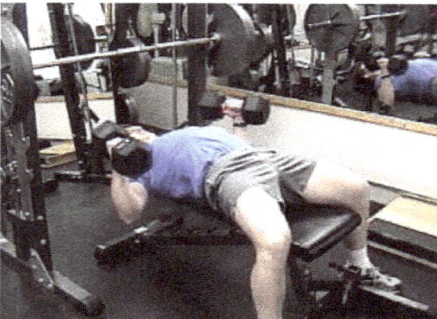

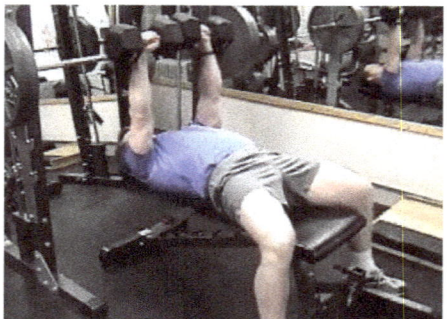

1A - Exercises

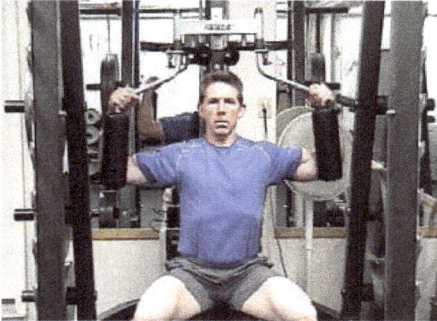

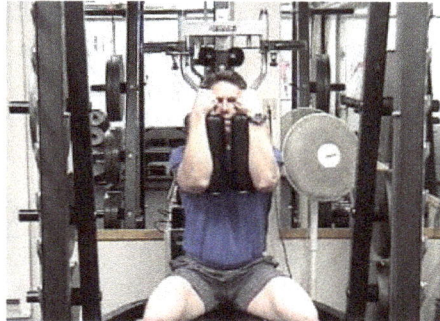

Pec Dec (1-3 Sets 7-15 Reps)

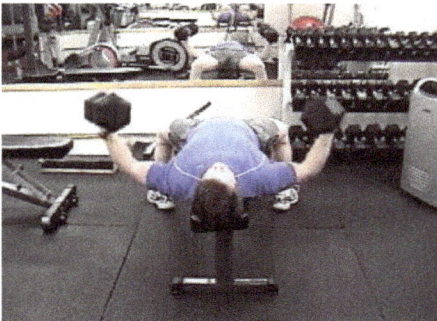

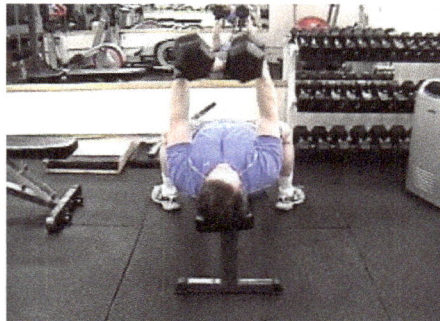

Chest Flat Flye (1-3 Sets 7-15 Reps)

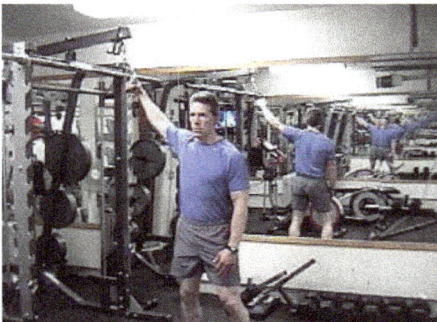

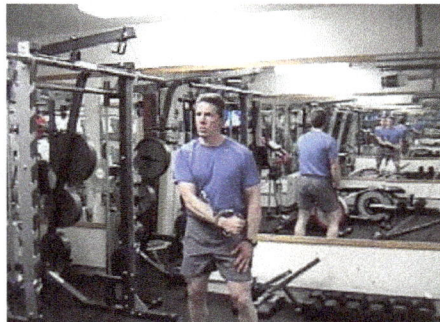

Cable Cross-Over (1-3 Sets 7-15 Reps)

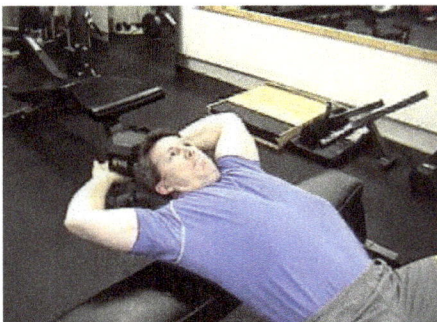

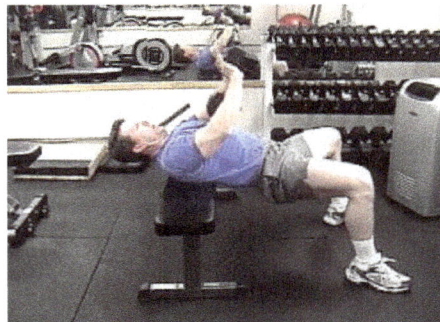

Lying Dumbbell Pull-Over "Bridge Position" (1-3 Sets 7-15 Reps)

Pecs - Pectoralis Major (Clavicular Region)

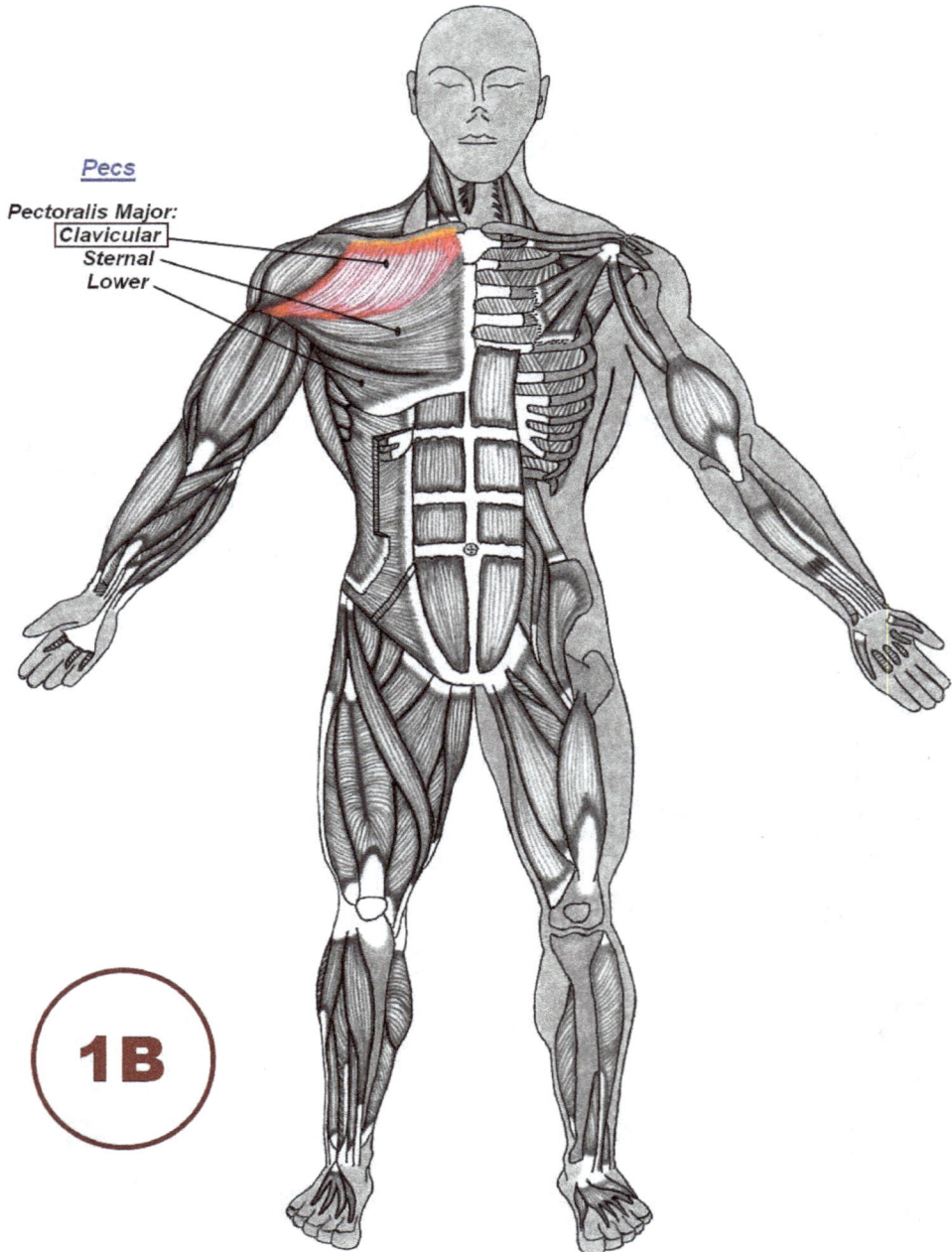

Pecs

Pectoralis Major:
Clavicular
Sternal
Lower

1B

1B - Exercises

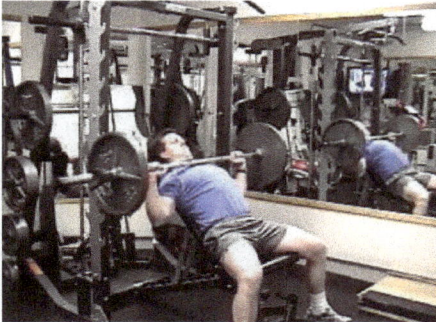

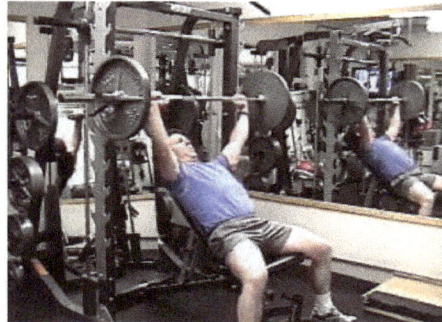

Chest Incline Bar Press (1-3 Sets 7-10 Reps)

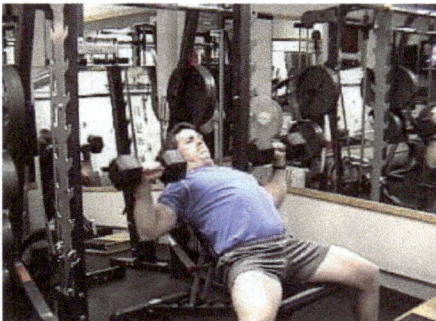

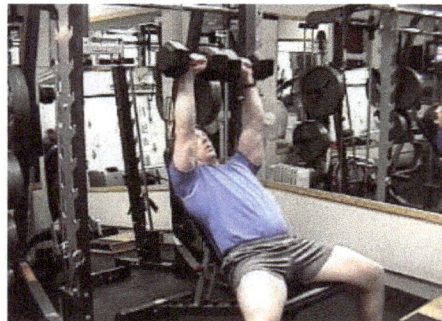

Chest Incline Dumbbell Press (1-3 Sets 7-10 Reps)

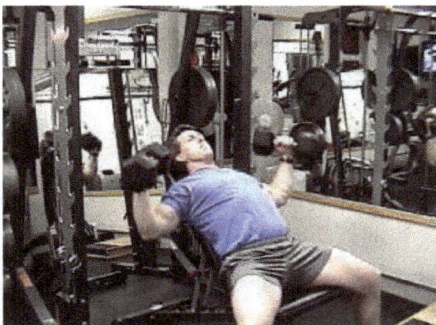

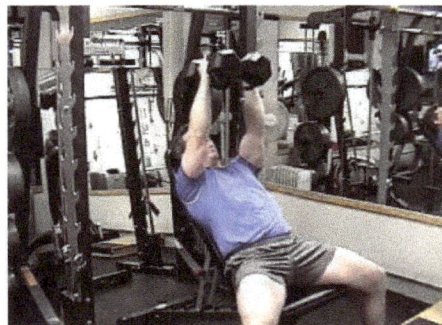

Chest Incline Flye (1-3 Sets 7-10 Reps)

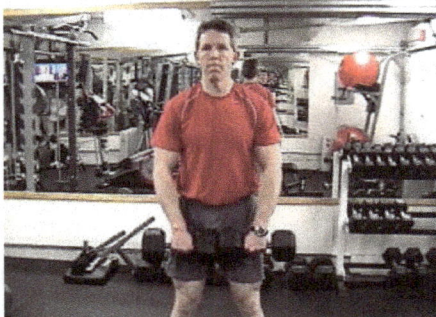

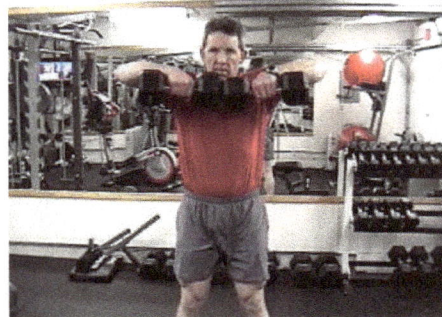

Standing Upright Dumbbell Row (1-3 Sets 7-10 Reps)

1B - Exercises

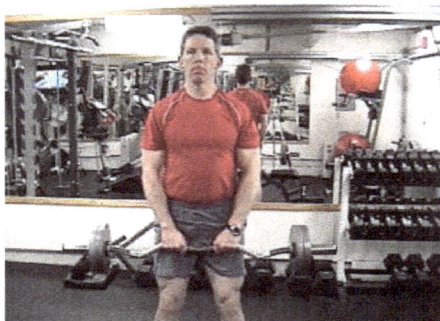

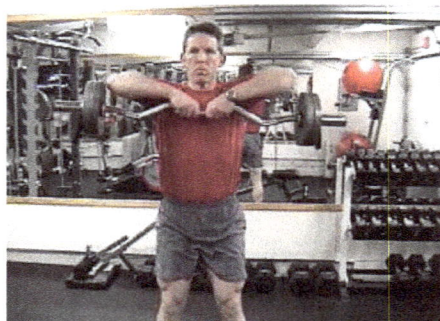

Standing Upright EZ-Bar Row (1-3 Sets 7-10 Reps)

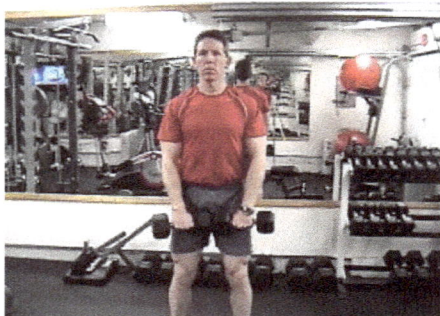

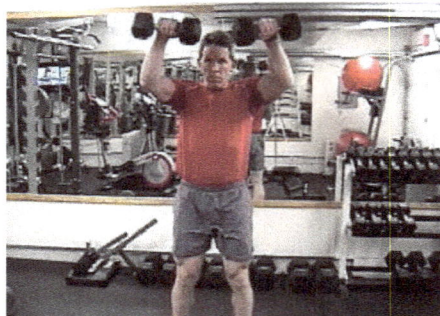

Shoulder Front Double Dumbbell Raise (1-3 Sets 7-10 Reps)

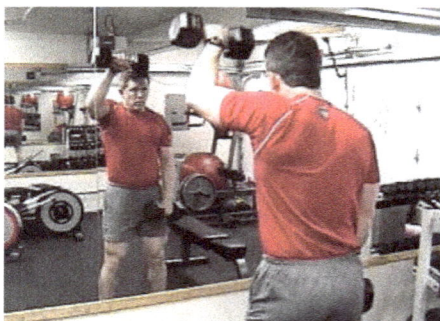

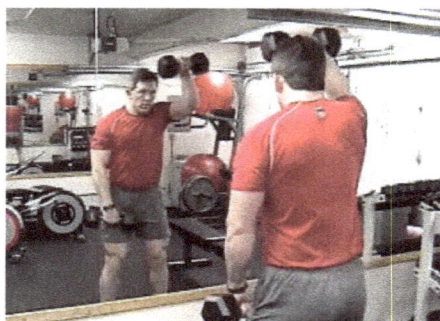

Shoulder Alternating Front Dumbbell Raise (1-3 Sets 7-10 Reps)

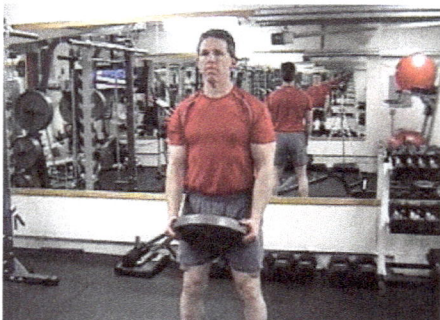

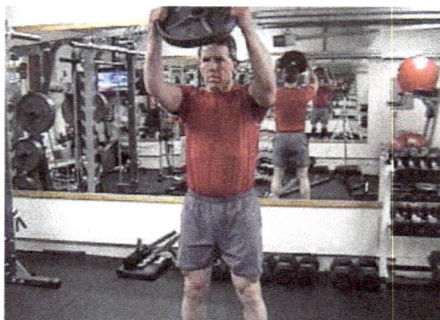

Shoulder Front Plate Raise (1-3 Sets 7-10 Reps)

Pecs - Pectoralis Major (Lower Region)

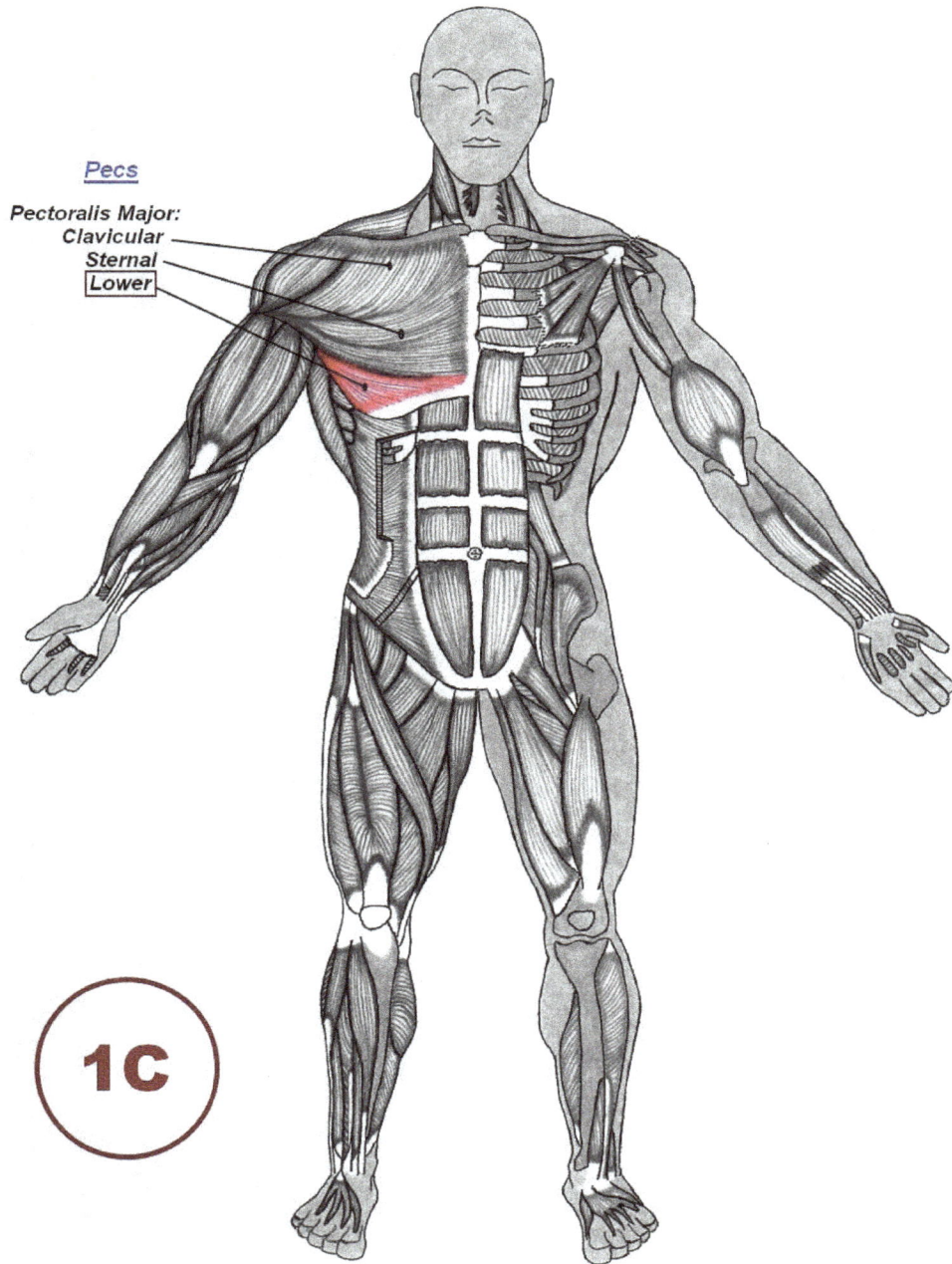

Pecs

Pectoralis Major:
Clavicular
Sternal
Lower

1C

1C - Exercises

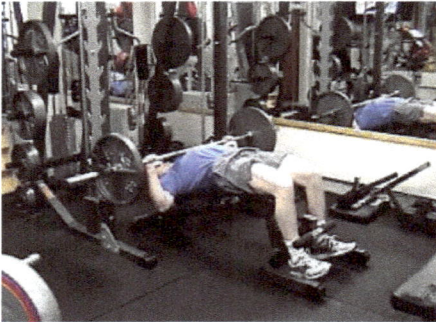

Chest Decline Bar Press (1-3 Sets 7-10 Reps)

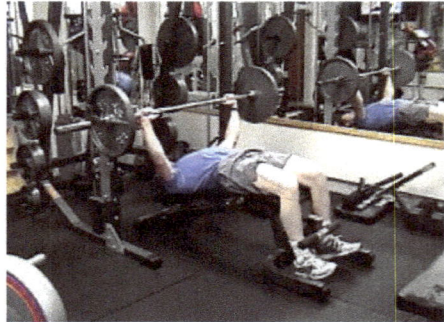

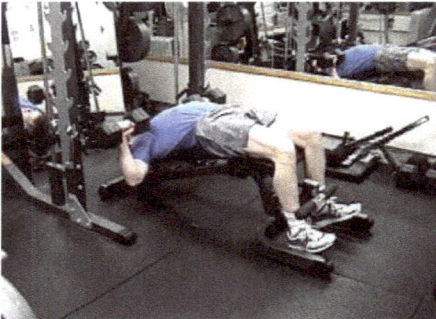

Chest Decline Dumbbell Press (1-3 Sets 7-10 Reps)

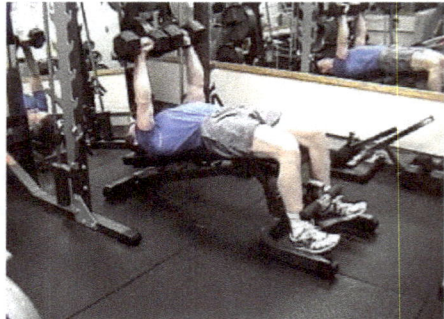

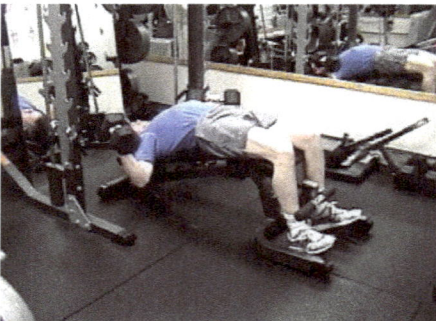

Chest Decline Flye (1-3 Sets 7-10 Reps)

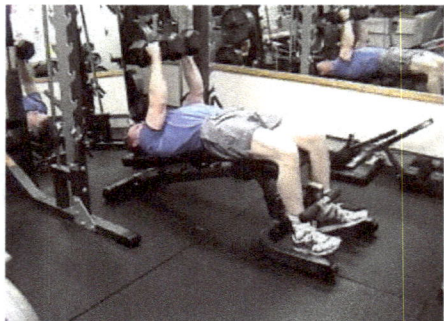

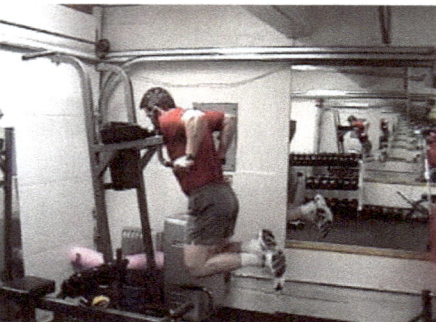

Parallel Bar Dips (1-3 Sets 7-15 Reps)

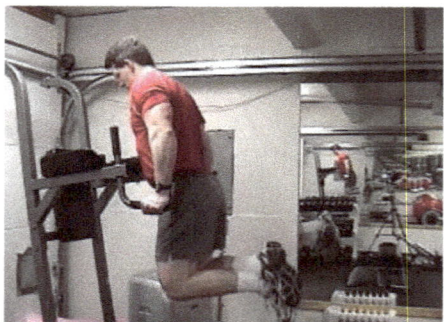

Pectoralis Minor

2

Pectoralis Minor

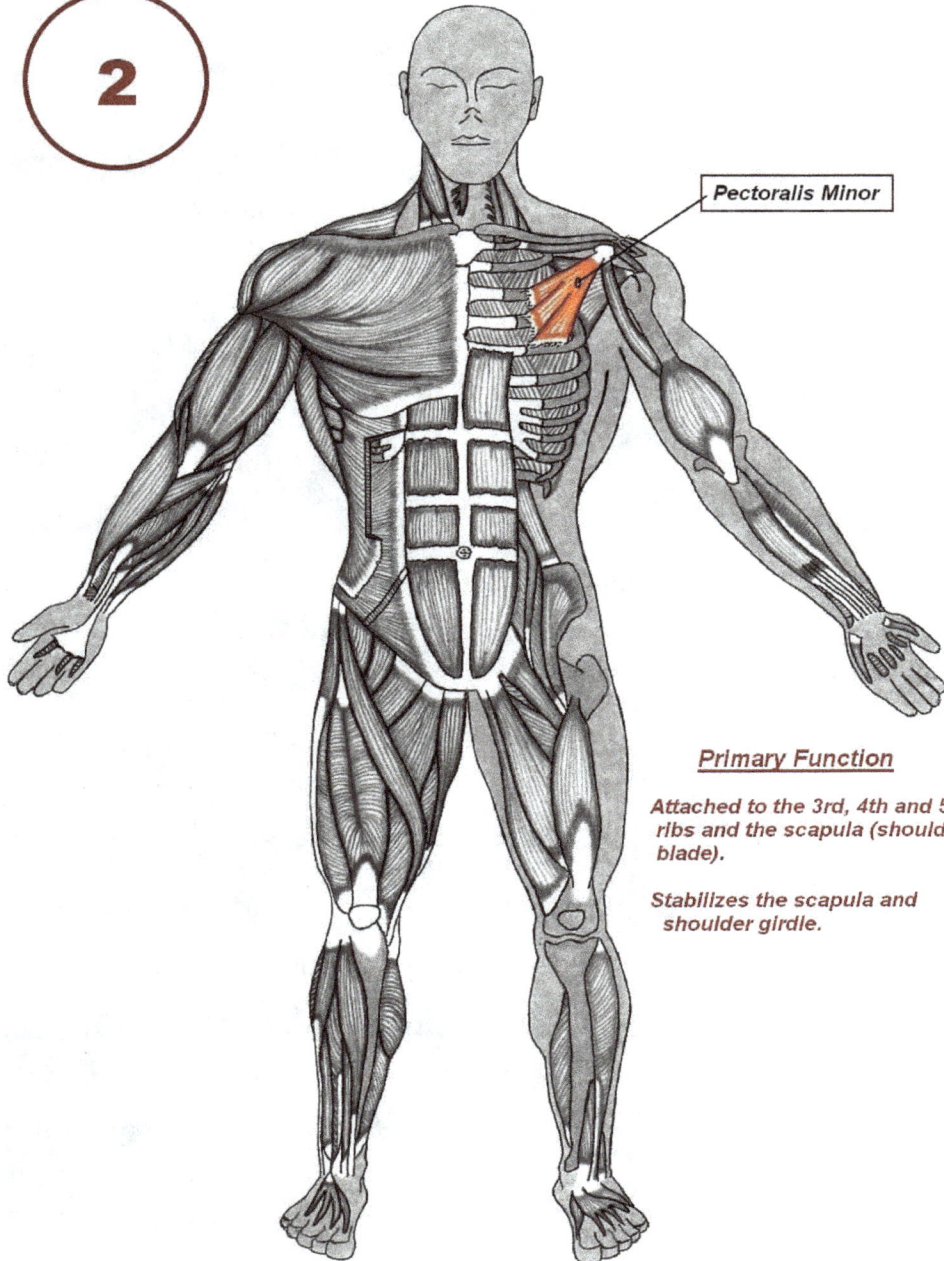

Primary Function

Attached to the 3rd, 4th and 5th ribs and the scapula (shoulder blade).

Stabilizes the scapula and shoulder girdle.

2 - Exercises

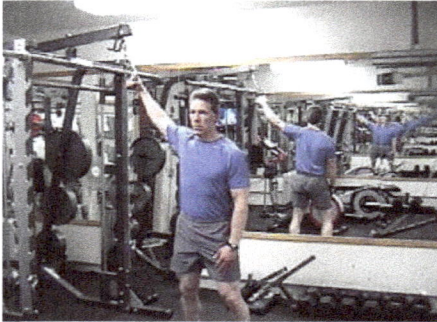

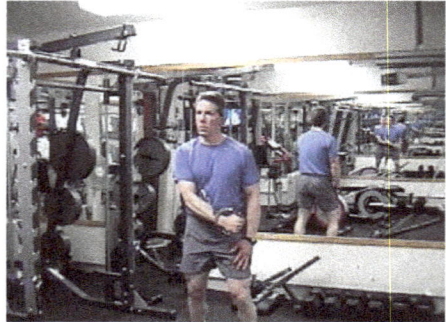

Cable Cross-Over (Stabilize Shoulder: 1-3 Sets 7-15 Reps)

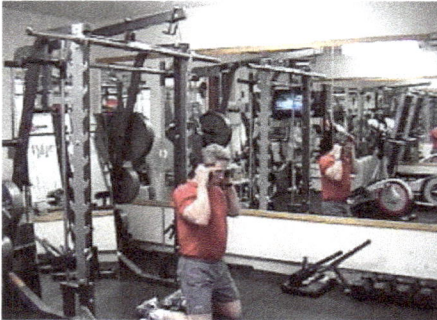

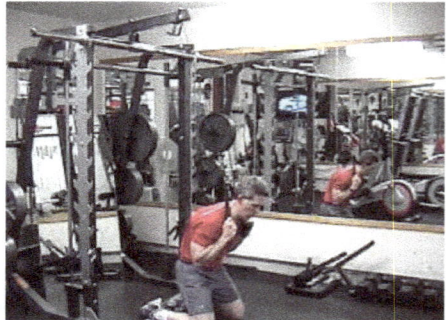

Kneeling Cable Crunch (Stabilize Shoulder: 1-3 Sets 10-30 Reps)

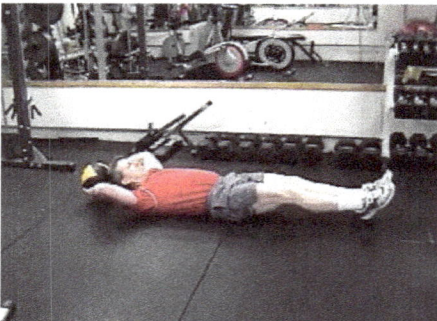

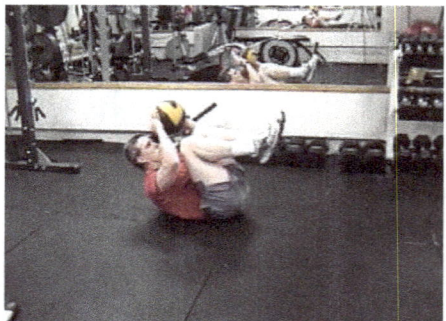

Medicine Ball Full Crunch on Floor (Stabilize Shoulder: 1-3 Sets 10-30 Reps)

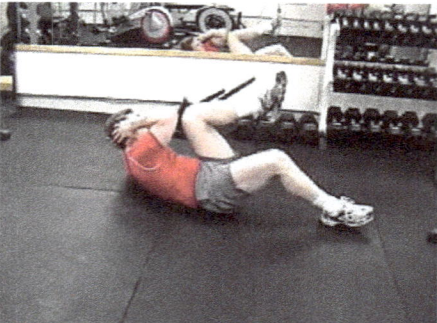

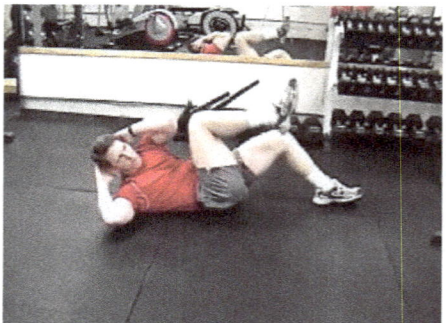

Lying Floor Twist "Bicycles" (Stabilize Shoulder: 1-3 Sets 10-15 Reps Each Side)

Serratus Anterior

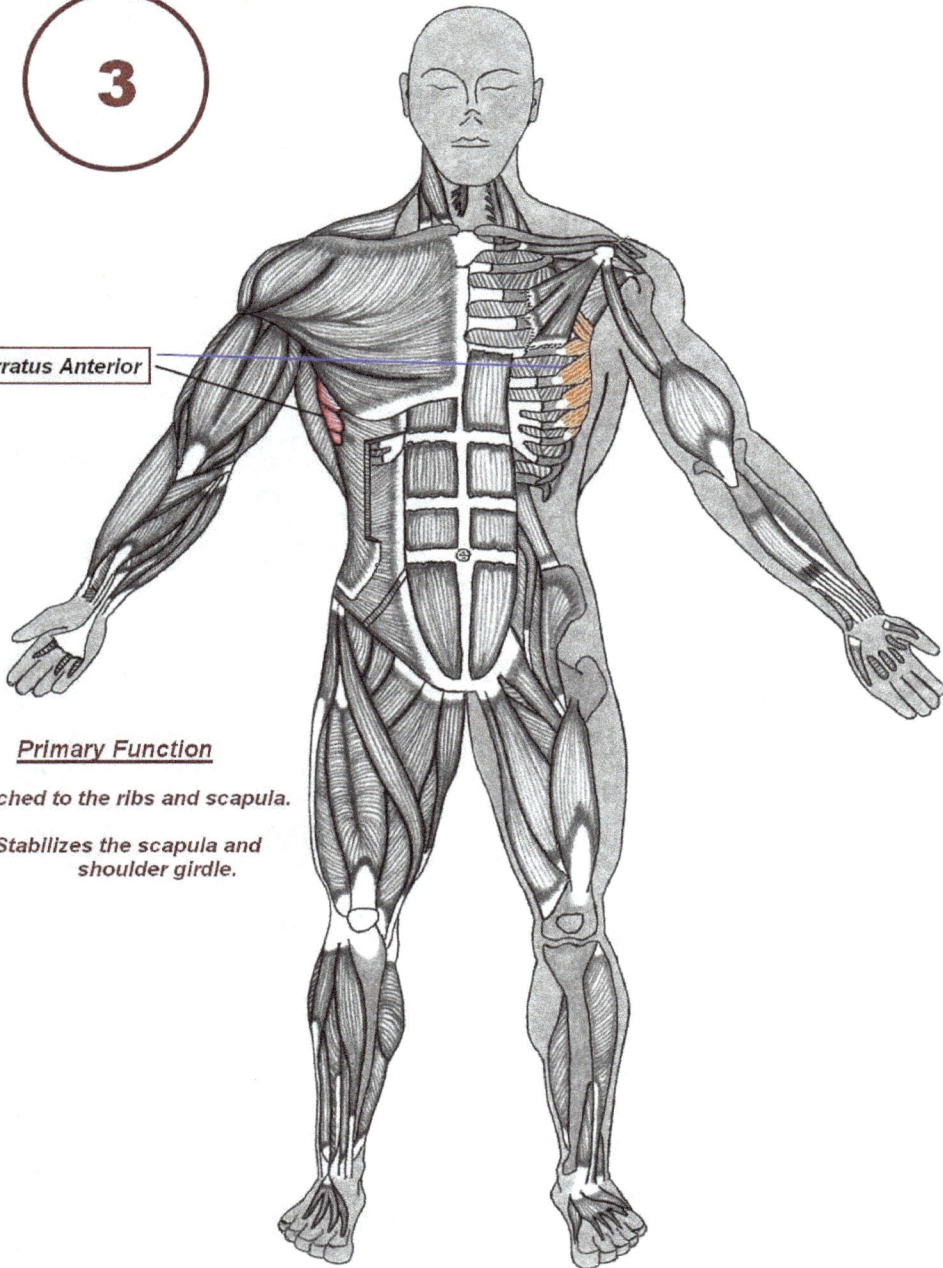

3

Serratus Anterior

Primary Function

Attached to the ribs and scapula.

Stabilizes the scapula and shoulder girdle.

3 - Exercises

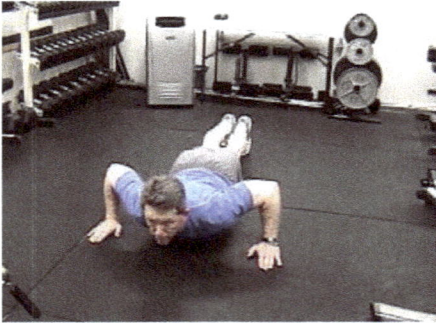

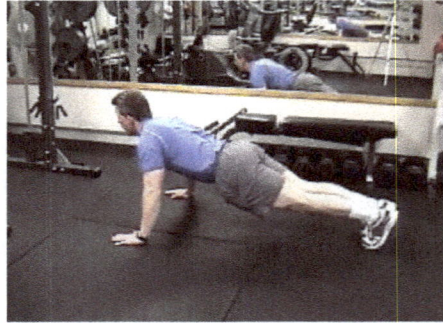

Push Ups (1-3 Sets 10-50 Reps)

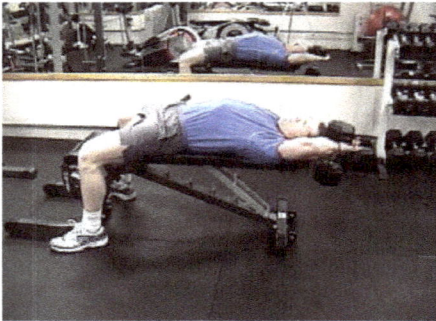

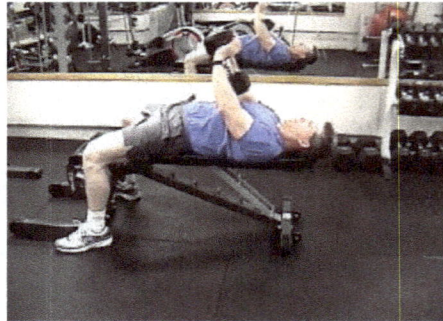

Lying Dumbbell Pull-Over (1-3 Sets 7-15 Reps)

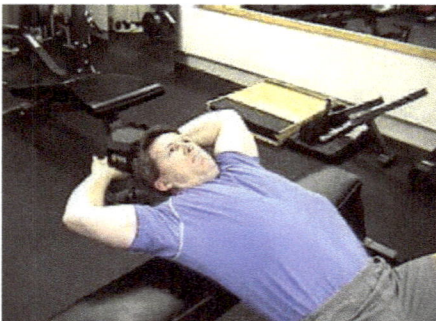

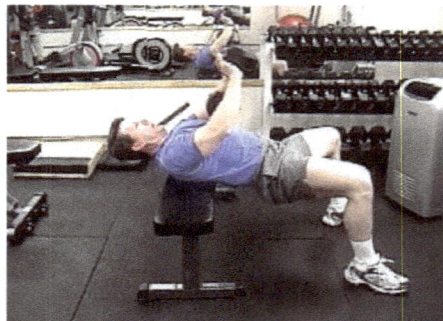

Lying Dumbbell Pull-Over "Bridge Position" (1-3 Sets 7-15 Reps)

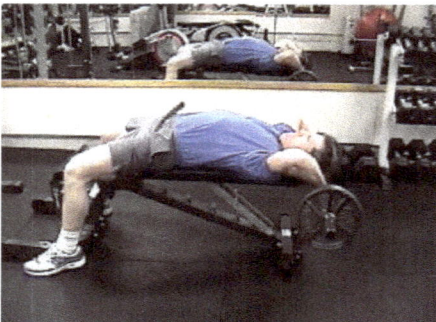

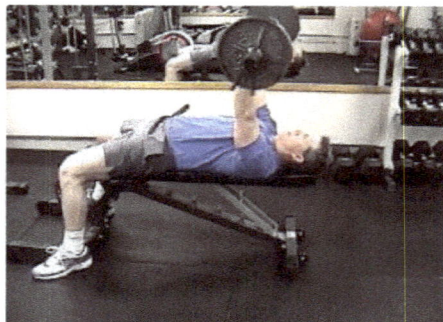

Lying EZ-Bar Pull-Over (1-3 Sets 7-15 Reps)

3 - Exercises

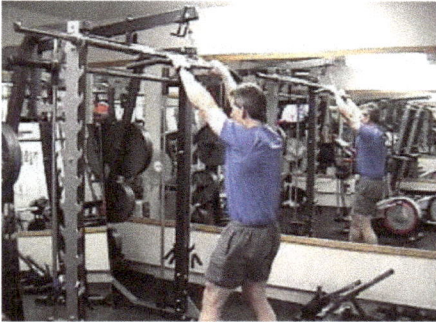

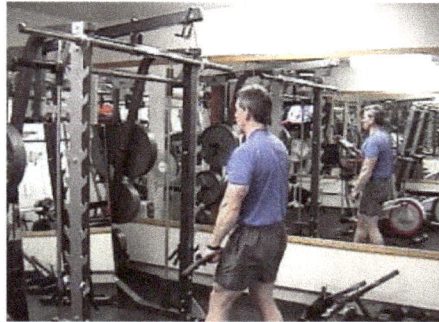

Straight Arm Narrow Grip Cable Pull Down (1-3 Sets 7-15 Reps)

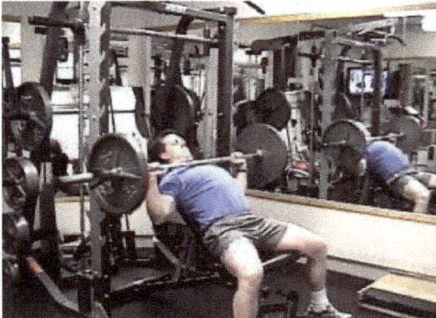

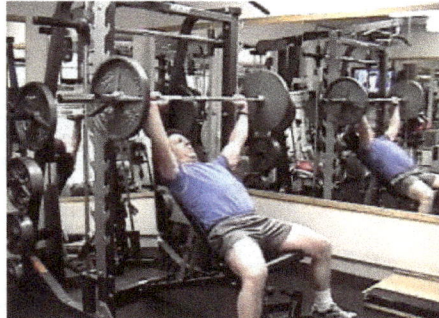

Chest Incline Bar Press (1-3 Sets 7-10 Reps)

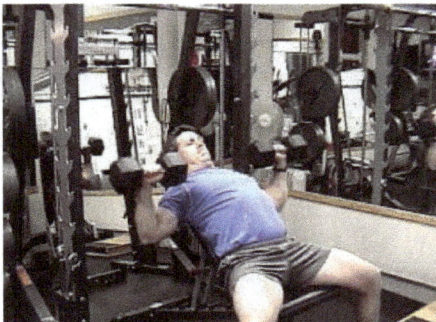

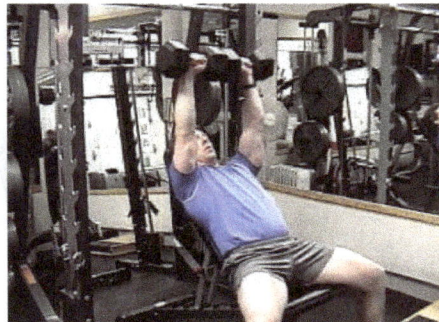

Chest Incline Dumbbell Press (1-3 Sets 7-10 Reps)

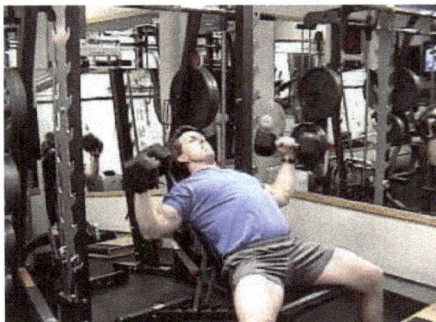

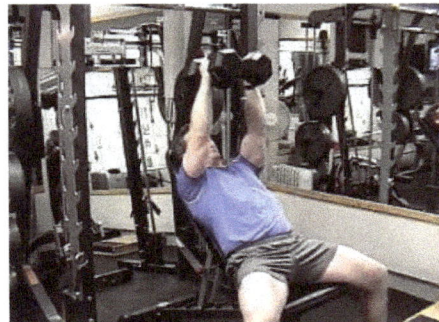

Chest Incline Flye (1-3 Sets 7-10 Reps)

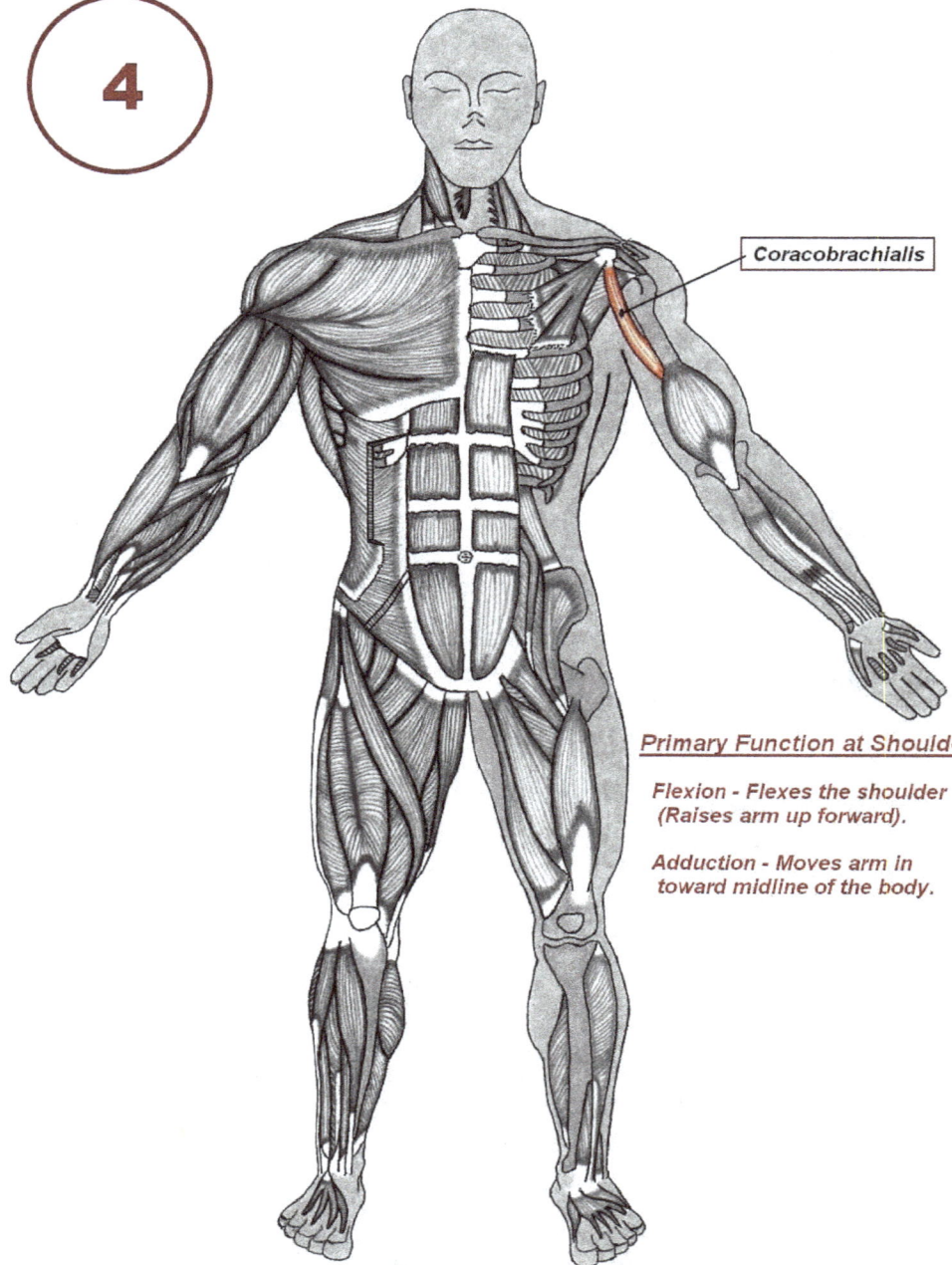

Coracobrachialis

4

Coracobrachialis

Primary Function at Shoulder

*Flexion - Flexes the shoulder
(Raises arm up forward).*

*Adduction - Moves arm in
toward midline of the body.*

4 - Exercises

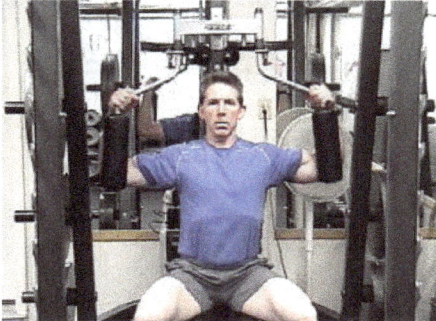

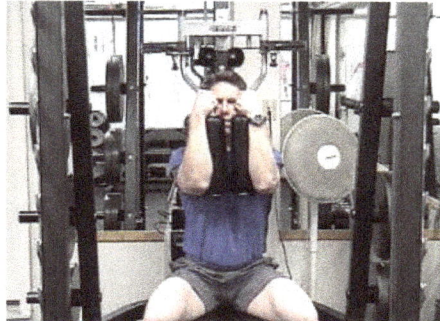

Pec Dec (1-3 Sets 7-15 Reps)

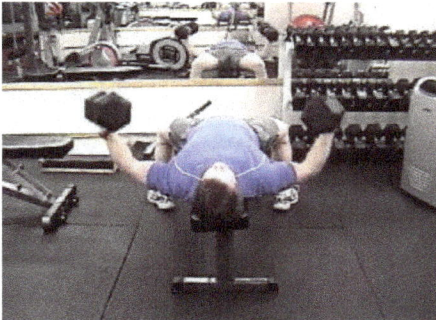

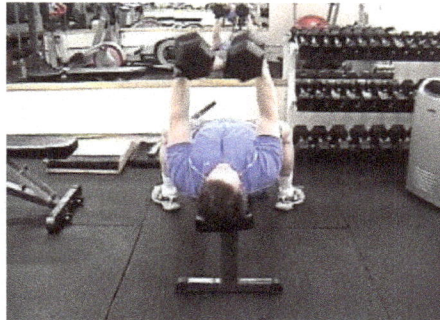

Chest Flat Flye (1-3 Sets 7-15 Reps)

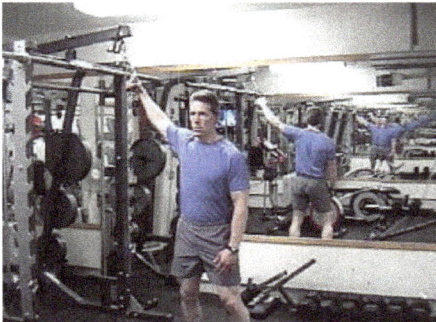

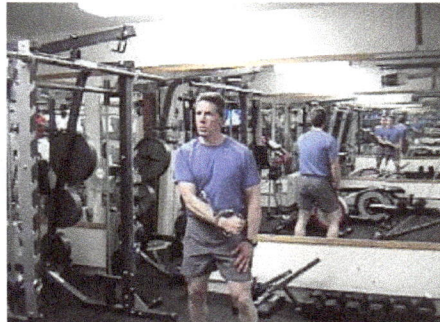

Cable Cross-Over (1-3 Sets 7-15 Reps)

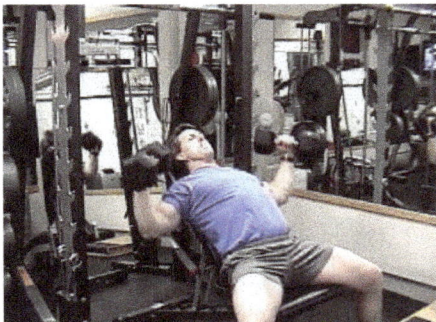

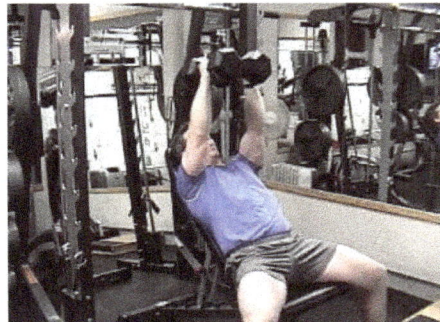

Chest Incline Flye (1-3 Sets 7-10 Reps)

Intercostals - Internal and External

5

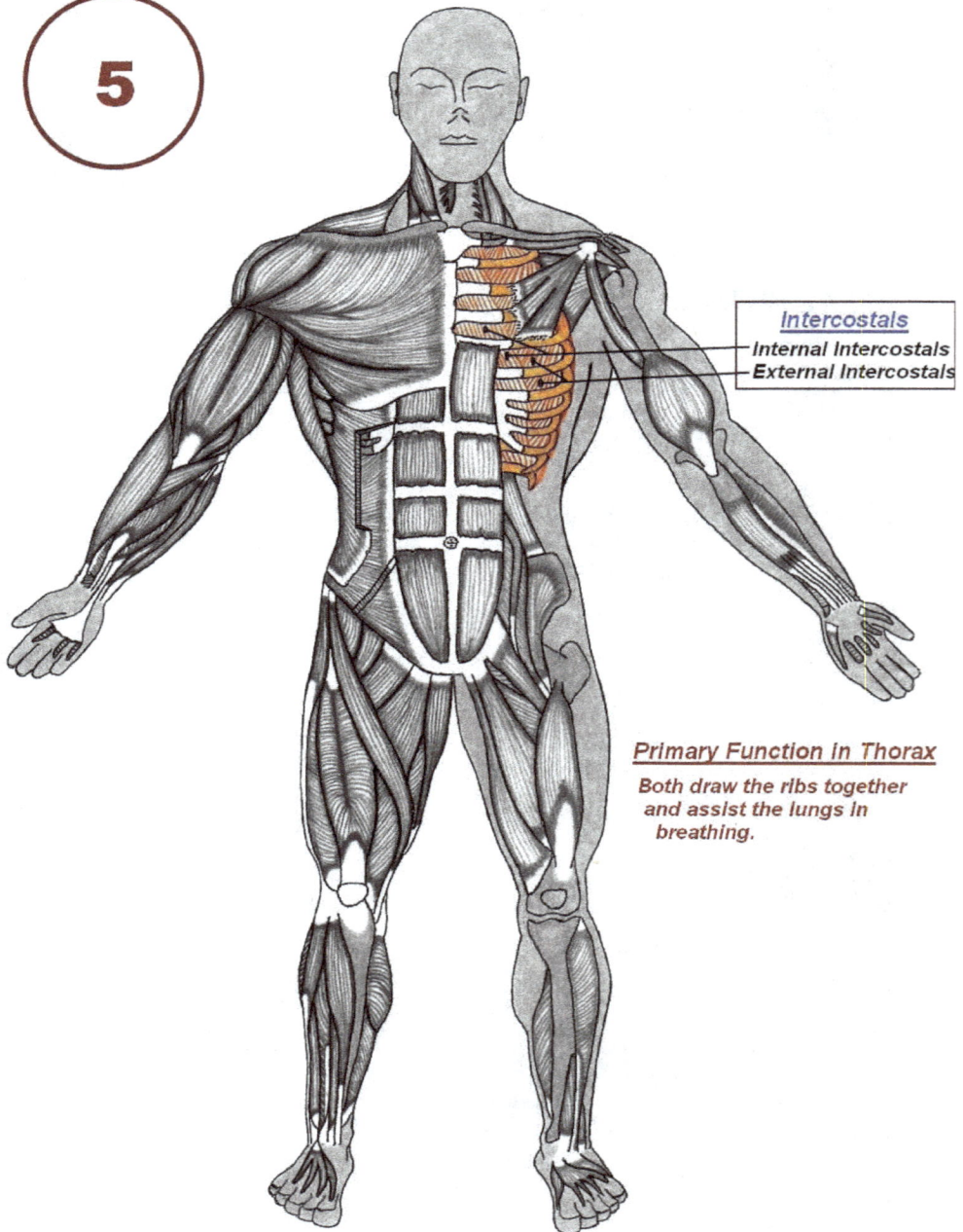

Intercostals
- Internal Intercostals
- External Intercostals

Primary Function in Thorax

Both draw the ribs together and assist the lungs in breathing.

Delts - Front Deltoid

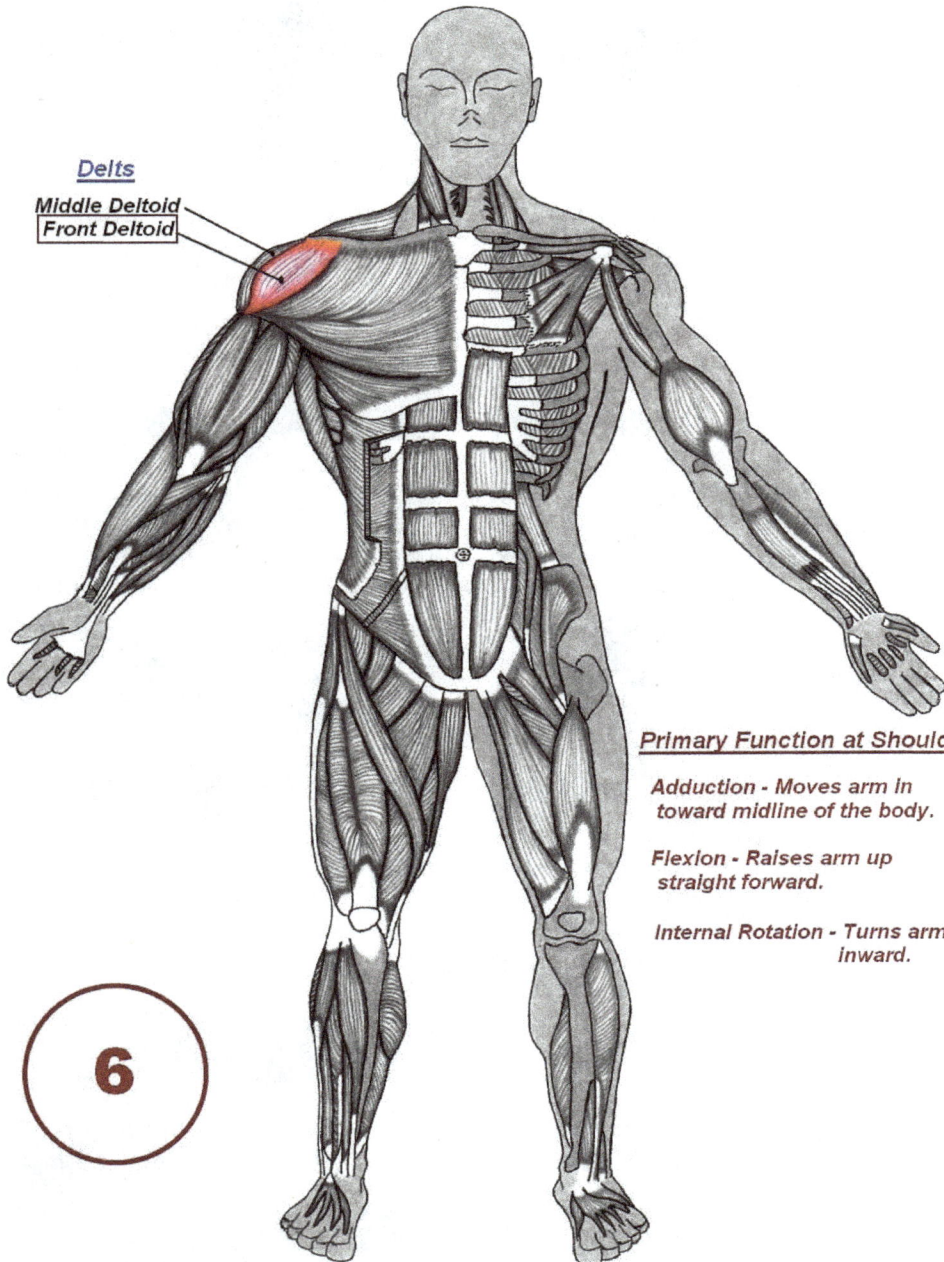

Delts

Middle Deltoid
Front Deltoid

Primary Function at Shoulder

Adduction - Moves arm in toward midline of the body.

Flexion - Raises arm up straight forward.

Internal Rotation - Turns arm inward.

6

6 - Exercises

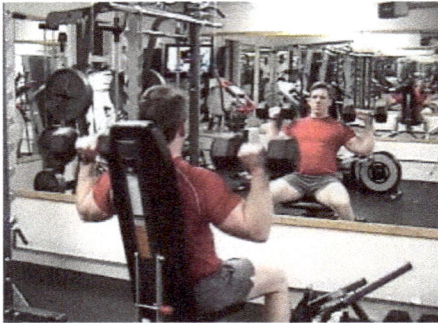

Shoulder Seated Dumbbell Press (1-5 Sets 7-10 Reps)

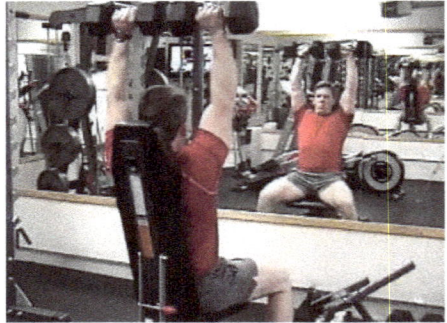

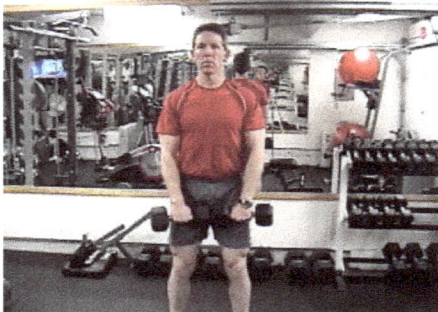

Shoulder Front Double Dumbbell Raise (1-3 Sets 7-10 Reps)

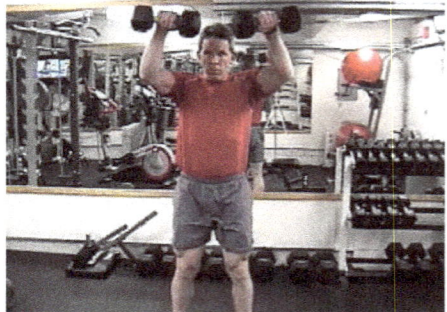

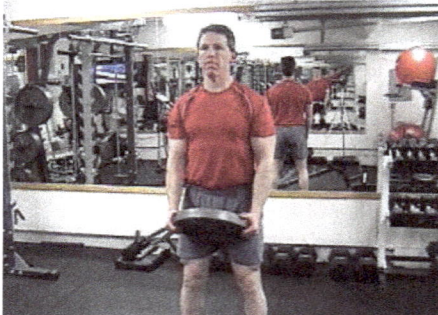

Shoulder Front Plate Raise (1-3 Sets 7-10 Reps)

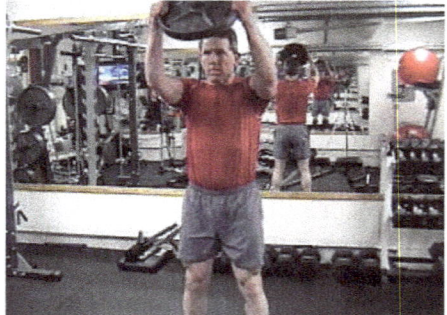

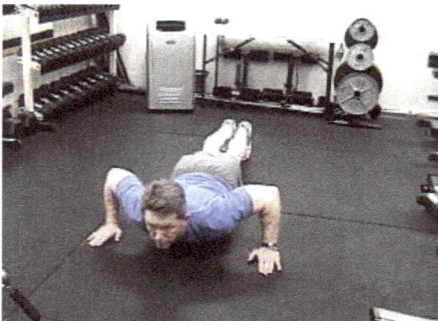

Push Ups (1-3 Sets 10-50 Reps)

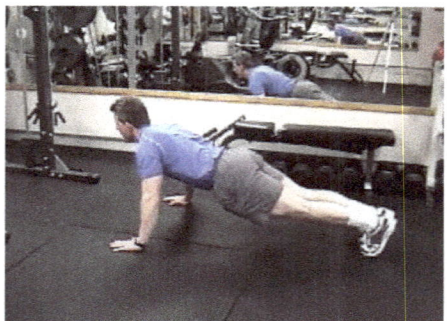

6 - Exercises

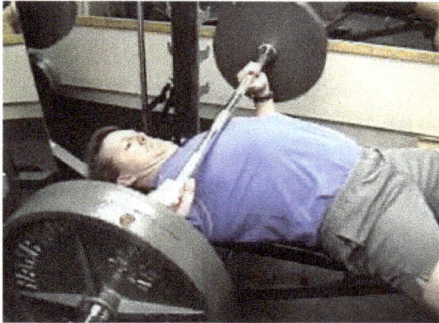

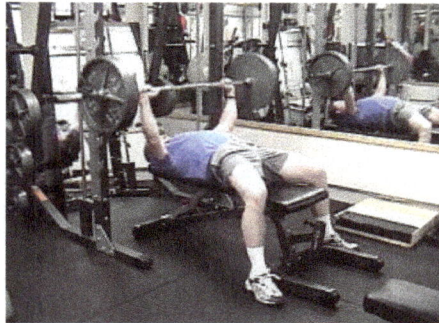

Chest Flat Bar Press "Bench Press" (1-5 Sets 7-15 Reps)

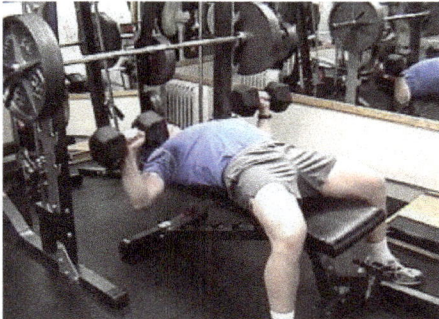

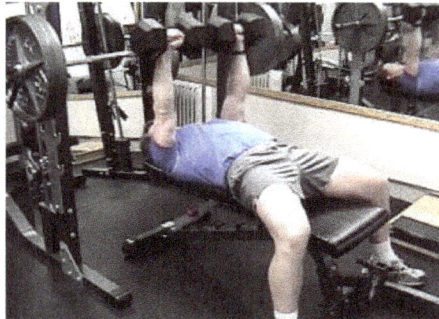

Chest Flat Dumbbell Press (1-5 Sets 7-15 Reps)

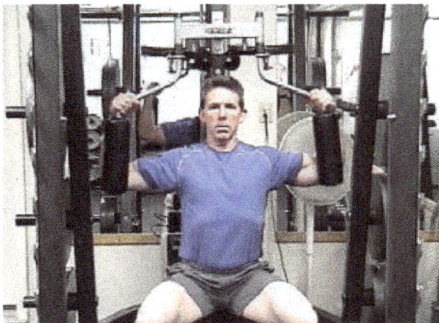

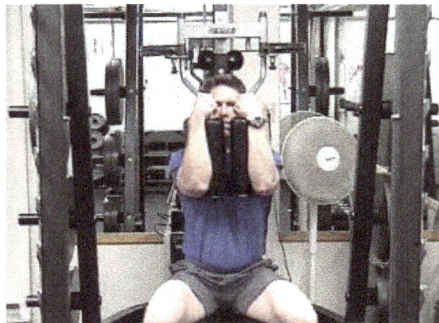

Pec Dec (1-3 Sets 7-15 Reps)

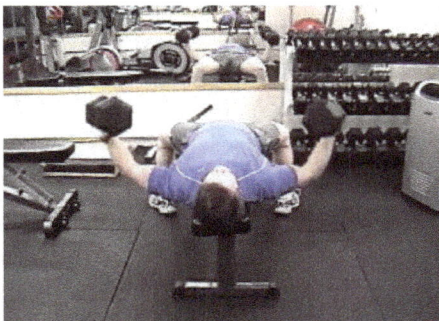

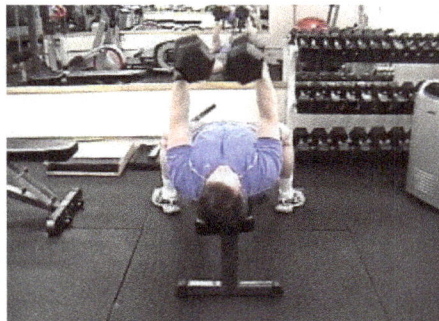

Chest Flat Flye (1-3 Sets 7-15 Reps)

6 - Exercises

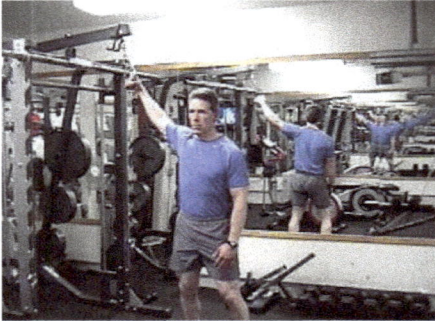

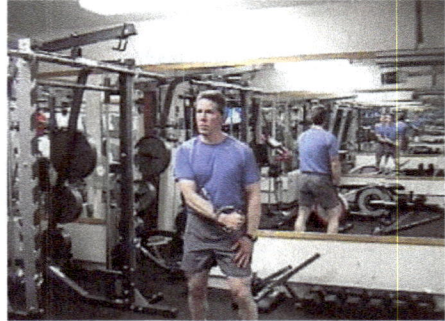

Cable Cross-Over (1-3 Sets 7-15 Reps)

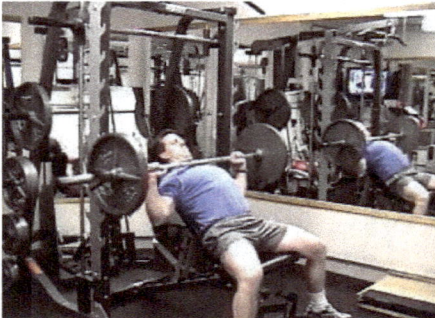

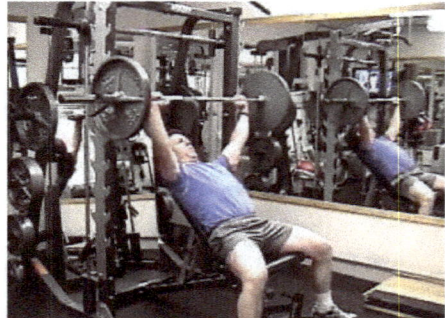

Chest Incline Bar Press (1-3 Sets 7-10 Reps)

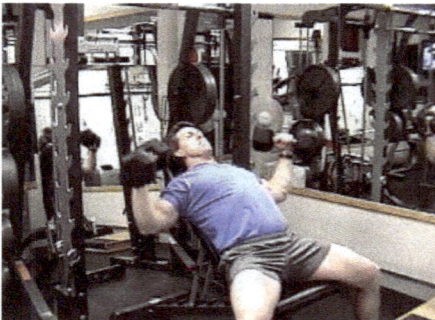

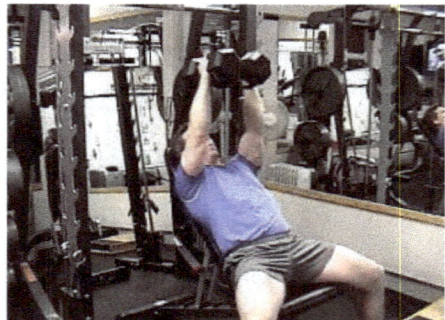

Chest Incline Flye (1-3 Sets 7-10 Reps)

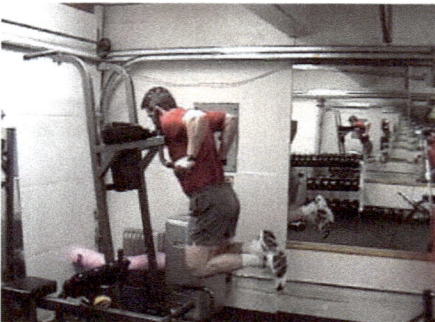

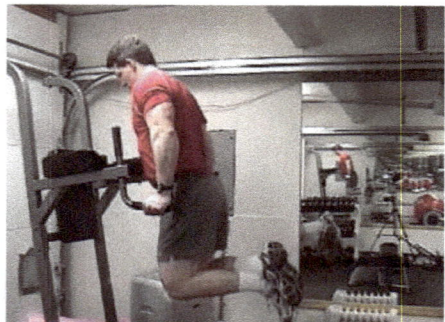

Parallel Bar Dips (1-3 Sets 7-15 Reps)

Delts - Middle Deltoid

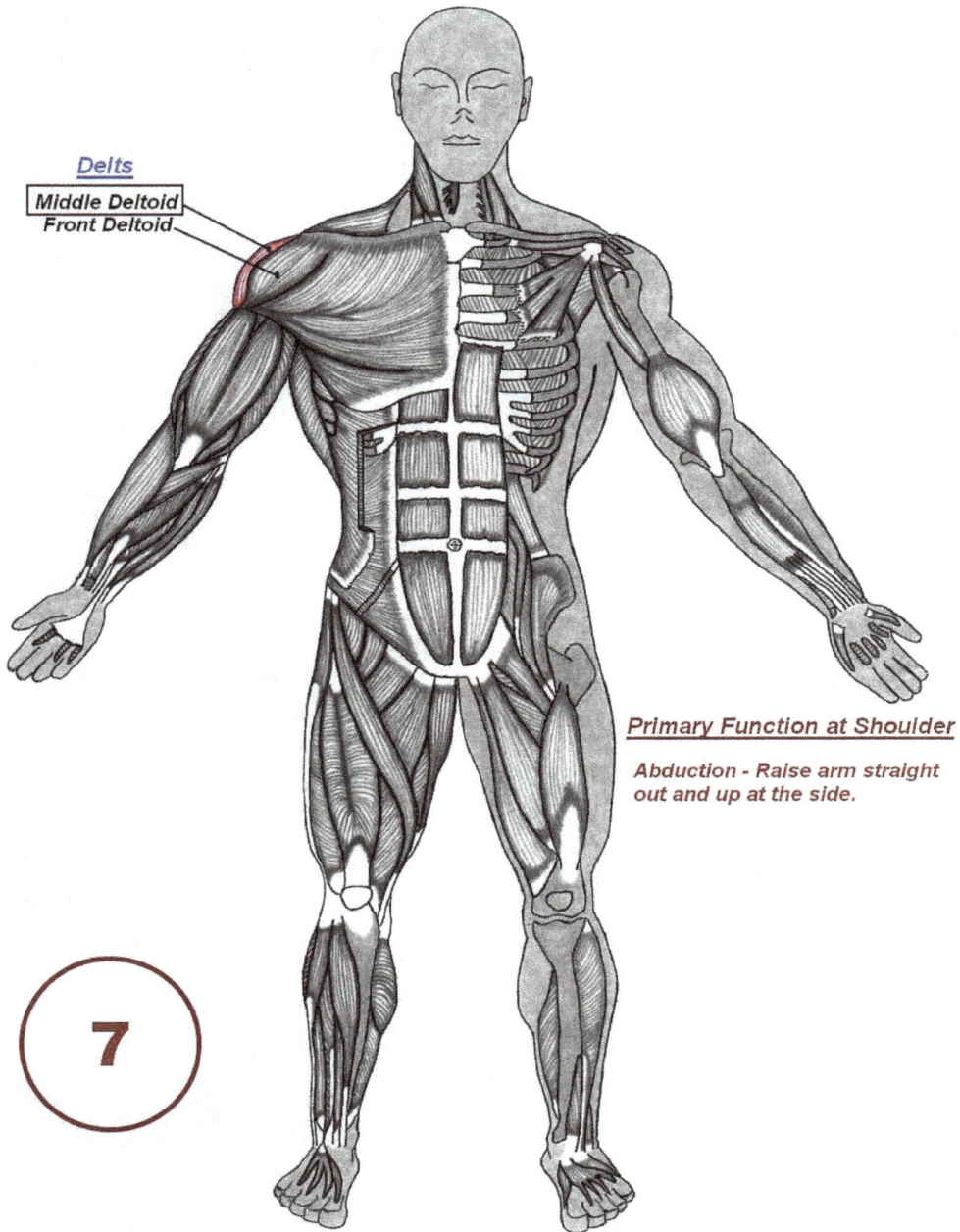

Delts
Middle Deltoid
Front Deltoid

Primary Function at Shoulder

Abduction - Raise arm straight
out and up at the side.

7

7 - Exercises

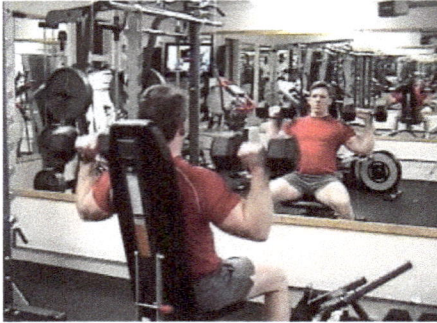

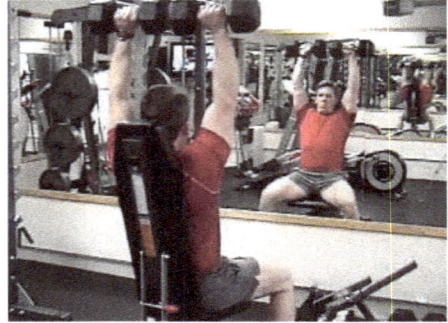

Shoulder Seated Dumbbell Press (1-5 Sets 7-10 Reps)

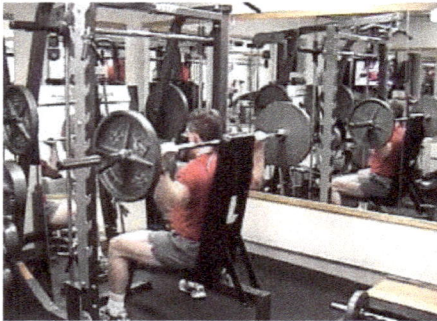

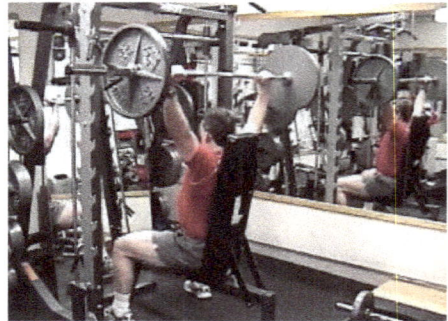

Shoulder Seated Bar Press "Military Press" (1-5 Sets 7-10 Reps)

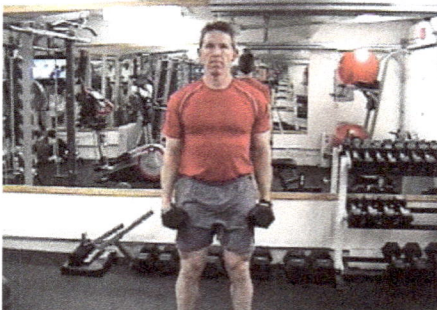

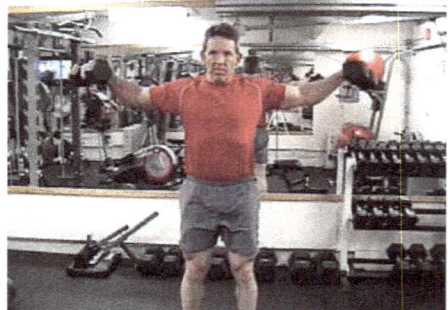

Shoulder Upright Lateral Raise - Side Start Position (1-3 Sets 7-10 Reps)

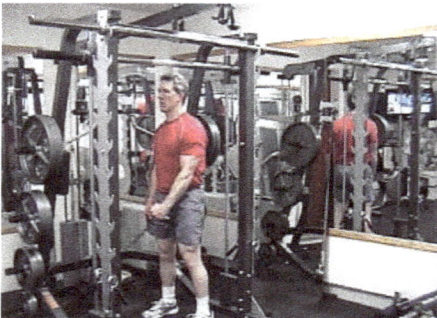

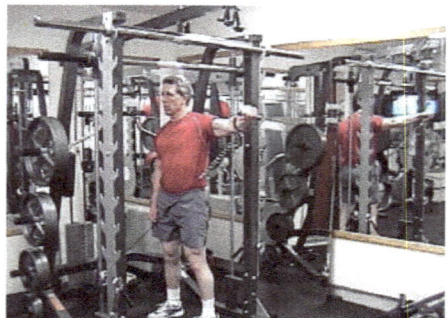

Shoulder Standing Cable Lateral Raise (1-3 Sets 7-10 Reps)

7 - Exercises

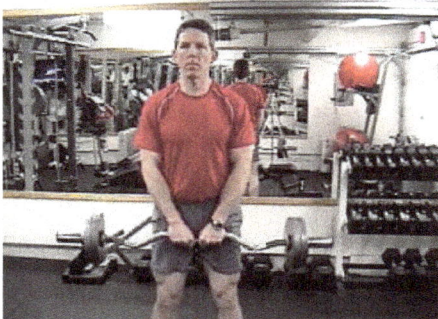

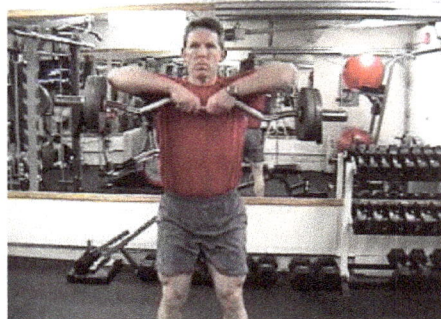

Standing Upright EZ-Bar Row (1-3 Sets 7-10 Reps)

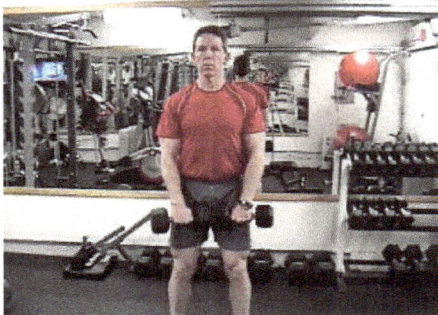

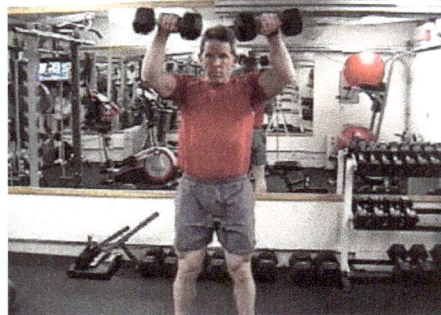

Shoulder Front Double Dumbbell Raise (1-3 Sets 7-10 Reps)

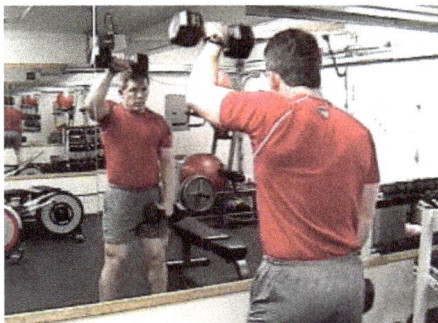

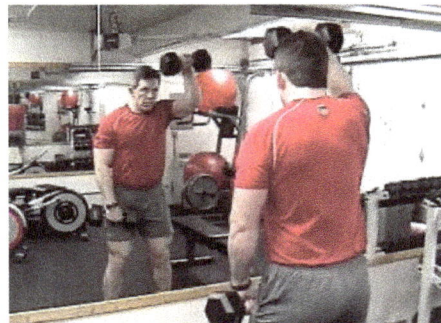

Shoulder Alternating Front Dumbbell Raise (1-3 Sets 7-10 Reps)

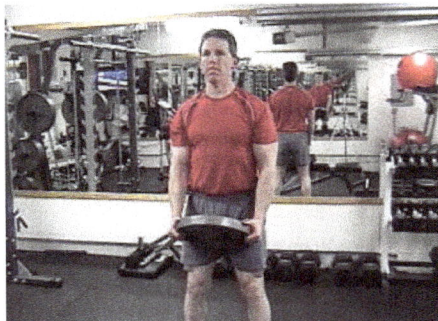

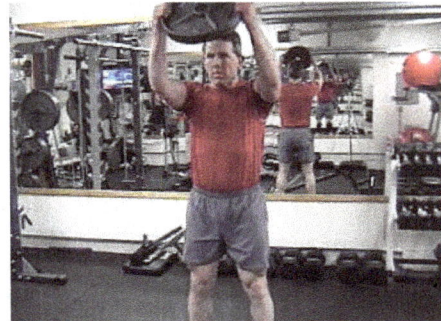

Shoulder Front Plate Raise (1-3 Sets 7-10 Reps)

Anterior Rotator Cuff - Subscapularis

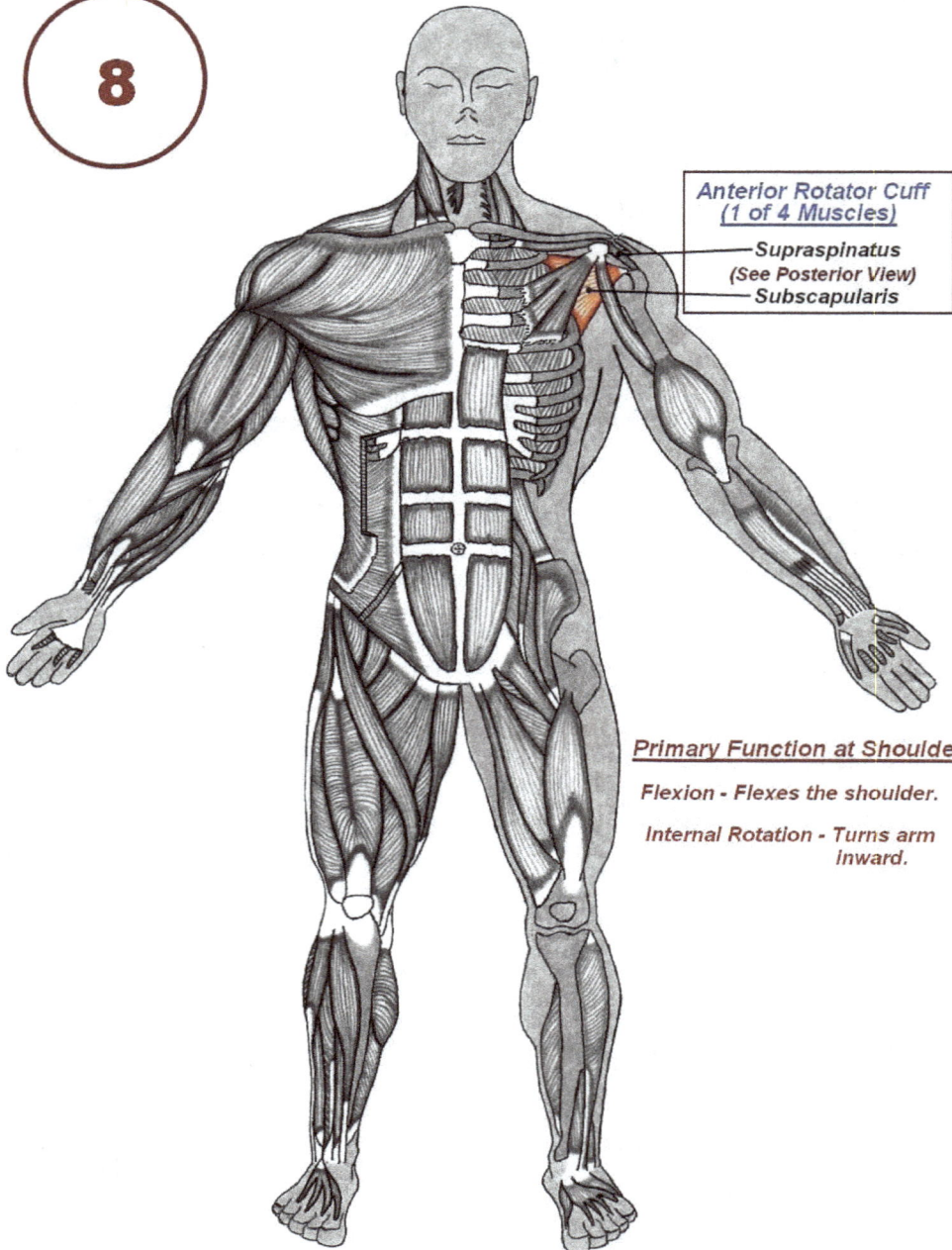

8

Anterior Rotator Cuff
(1 of 4 Muscles)
— *Supraspinatus*
(See Posterior View)
— *Subscapularis*

Primary Function at Shoulder

Flexion - Flexes the shoulder.

Internal Rotation - Turns arm inward.

8 - Exercises

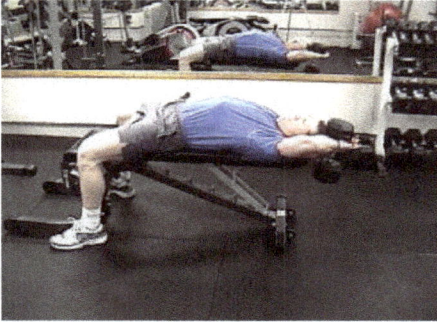

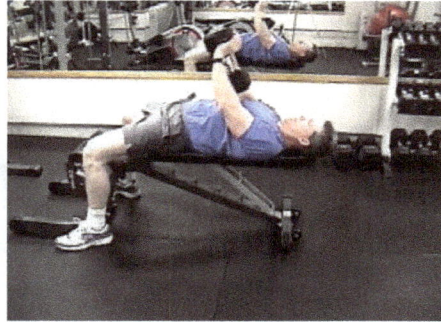

Lying Dumbbell Pull-Over (1-3 Sets 7-15 Reps)

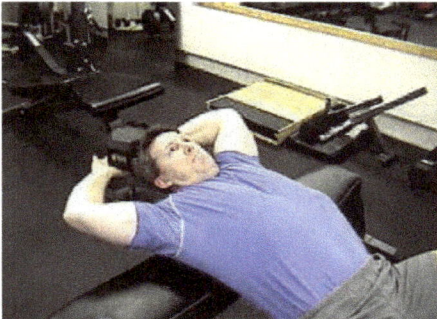

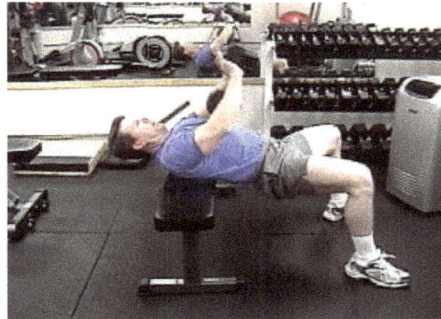

Lying Dumbbell Pull-Over "Bridge Position" (1-3 Sets 7-15 Reps)

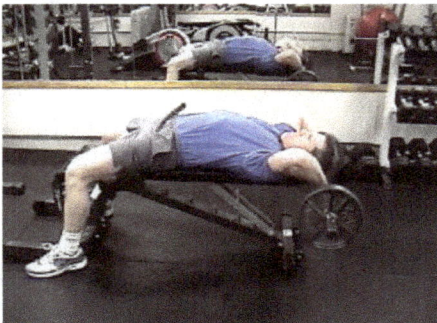

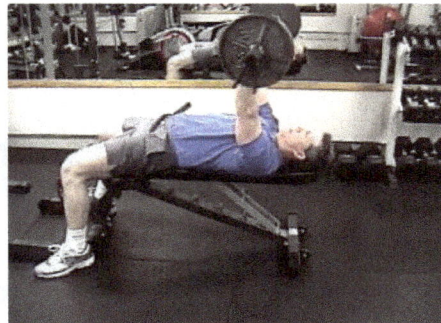

Lying EZ-Bar Pull-Over (1-3 Sets 7-15 Reps)

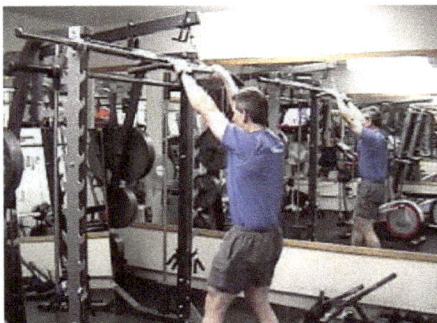

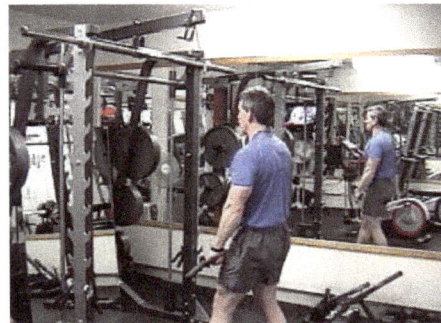

Straight Arm Narrow Grip Cable Pull Down (1-3 Sets 7-15 Reps)

Biceps - Biceps Brachii

9A

Biceps (Bi's)
Biceps Brachii
Bracialis

Primary Function at Shoulder

Long Head (Left Side):
Flexion - Raises arm straight
up forward.

Abduction - Raises arm straight
out to side and up away from
midline of the body.

Short Head (Right Side):
Flexion - Raises arm straight
up forward.

Adduction - Raises arm up and
in toward midline of the body.

Internal Rotation - Turns arm
inward.

Primary Function at Elbow

Flexion - Flexes the elbow.

Supination - Supines the
forearm (Turns the hand palm
forward while down at side,
palm up while elbows are bent
90 degrees, and palm back
while arms are above
the head during a
reverse chin up).

28

Brachialis

9B

Biceps Brachii
Bracialis

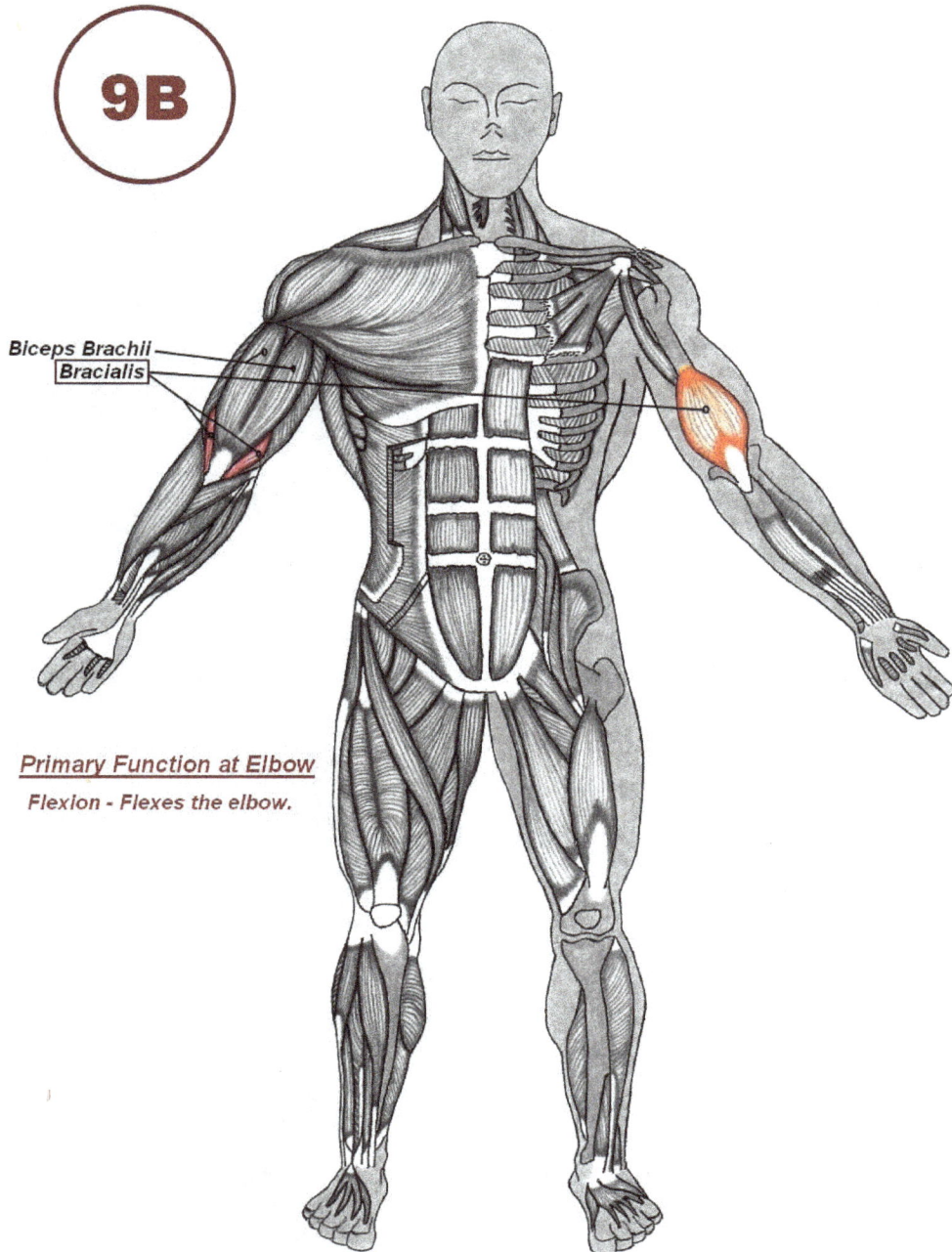

Primary Function at Elbow

Flexion - Flexes the elbow.

9A and B - Exercises

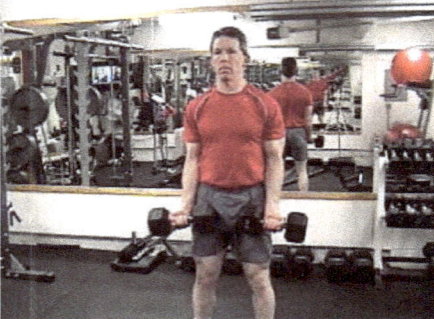

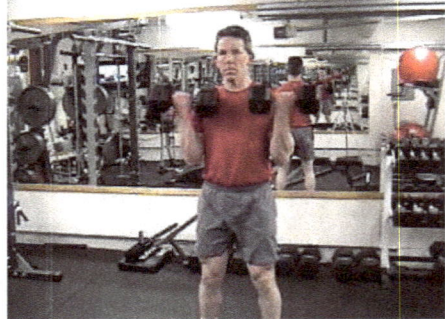

Biceps Standing Double Dumbbell Curl (1-3 Sets 7-15 Reps)

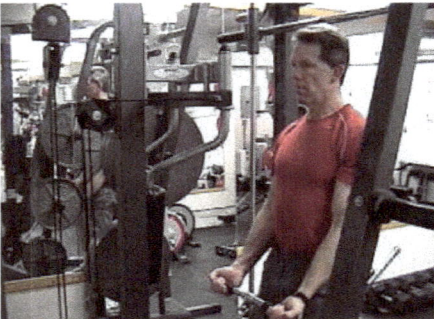

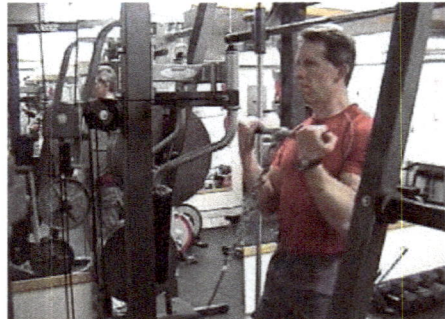

Biceps Standing Cable Curl (1-3 Sets 7-15 Reps)

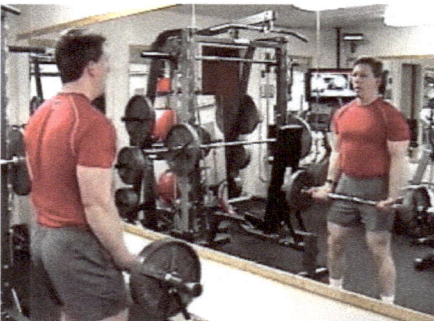

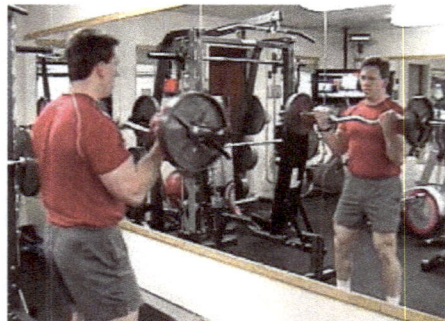

Biceps Standing EZ-Bar Curl (1-3 Sets 7-15 Reps)

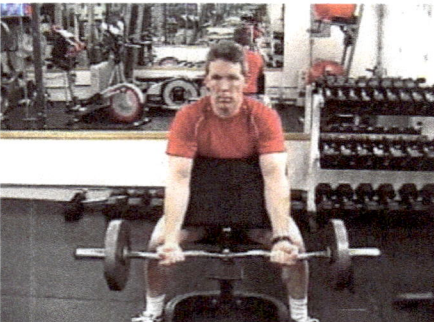

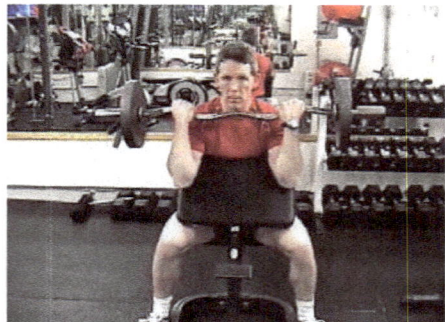

Biceps Seated EZ-Bar Preacher Curl (1-3 Sets 7-15 Reps)

9A and B - Exercises

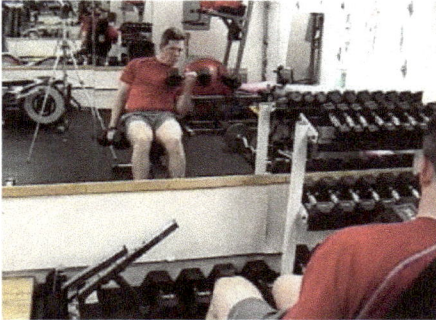

Biceps Seated Incline Dumbbell Curl (1-3 Sets 7-10 Reps)

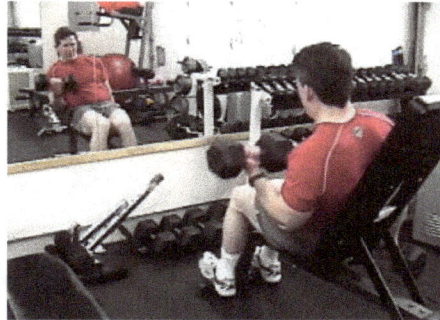

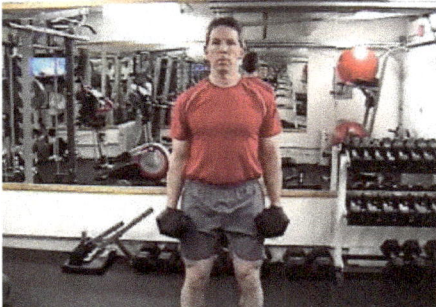

Biceps Standing Dumbbell Hammer Curl (1-3 Sets 7-10 Reps)

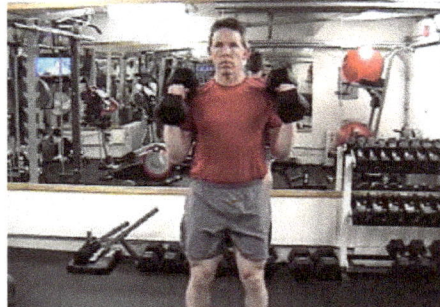

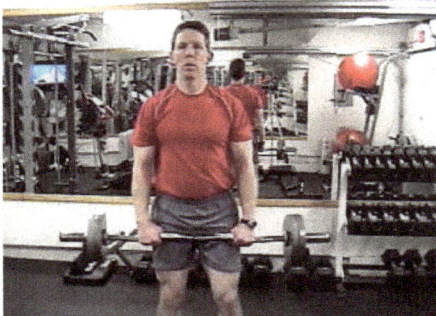

Biceps Standing Reverse EZ-Bar Curl (1-3 Sets 7-10 Reps)

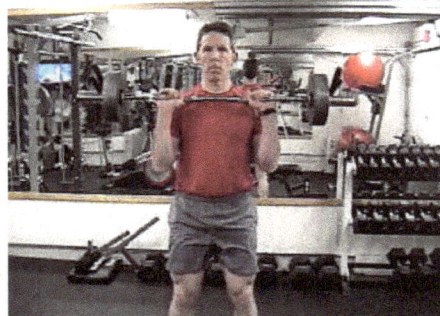

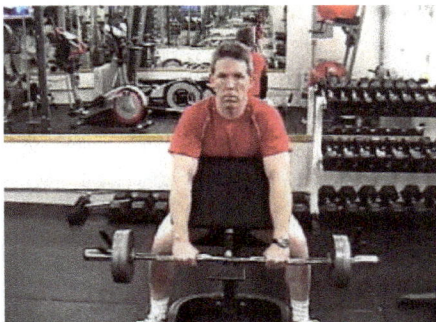

Biceps Seated Reverse EZ-Bar Preacher Curl (1-3 Sets 7-10 Reps)

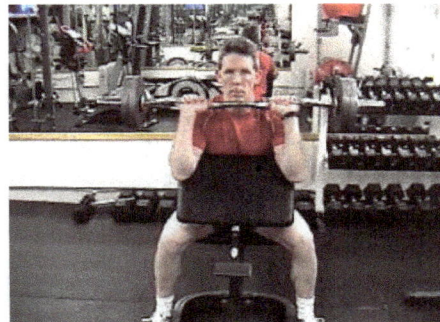

9A and B - Exercises

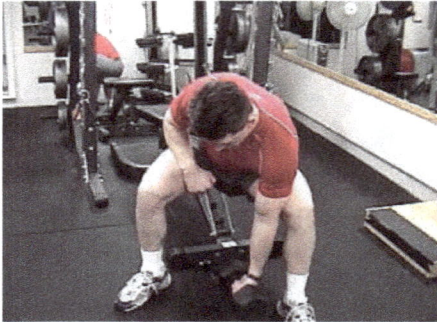

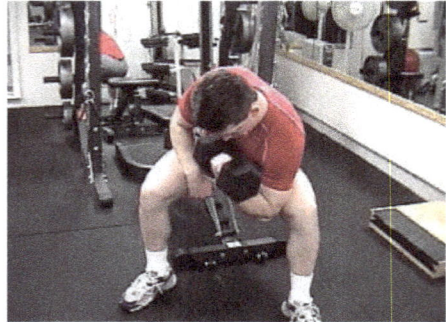

Biceps Seated Concentration Curl (1-3 Sets 7-15 Reps)

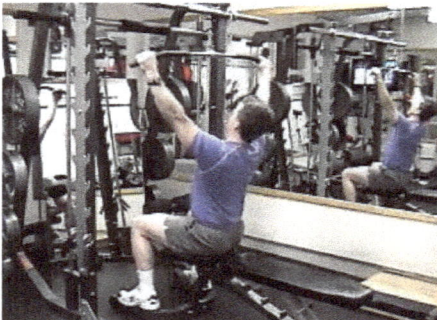

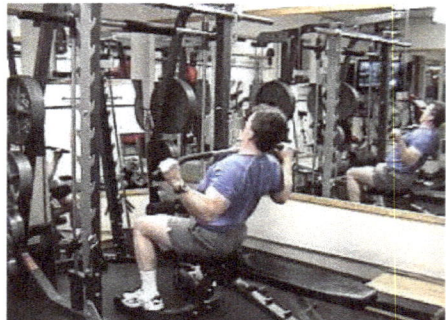

Lat Wide Grip Front Pull Down (1-3 Sets 7-15 Reps)

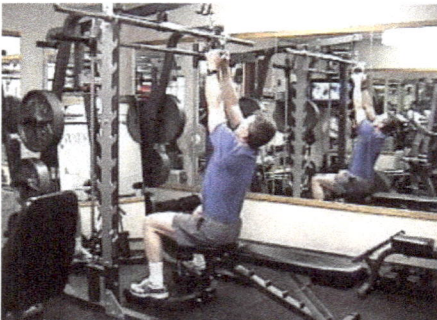

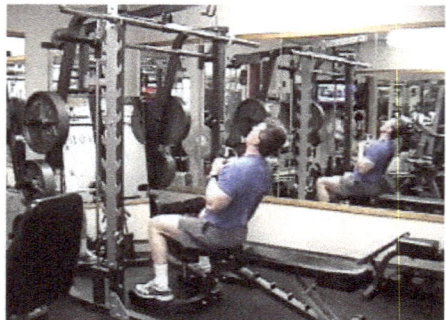

Lat Close Grip Front Pull Down (1-3 Sets 7-15 Reps)

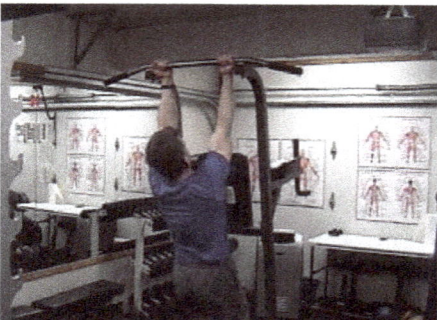

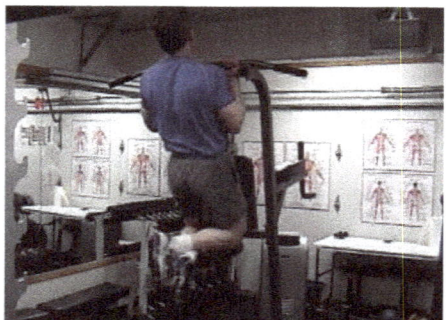

Reverse Chin Ups (1-3 Sets 7-15 Reps)

Forearm - Brachioradialis

10

Brachioradialis

Primary Function at Elbow

Flexion - Flexes the elbow

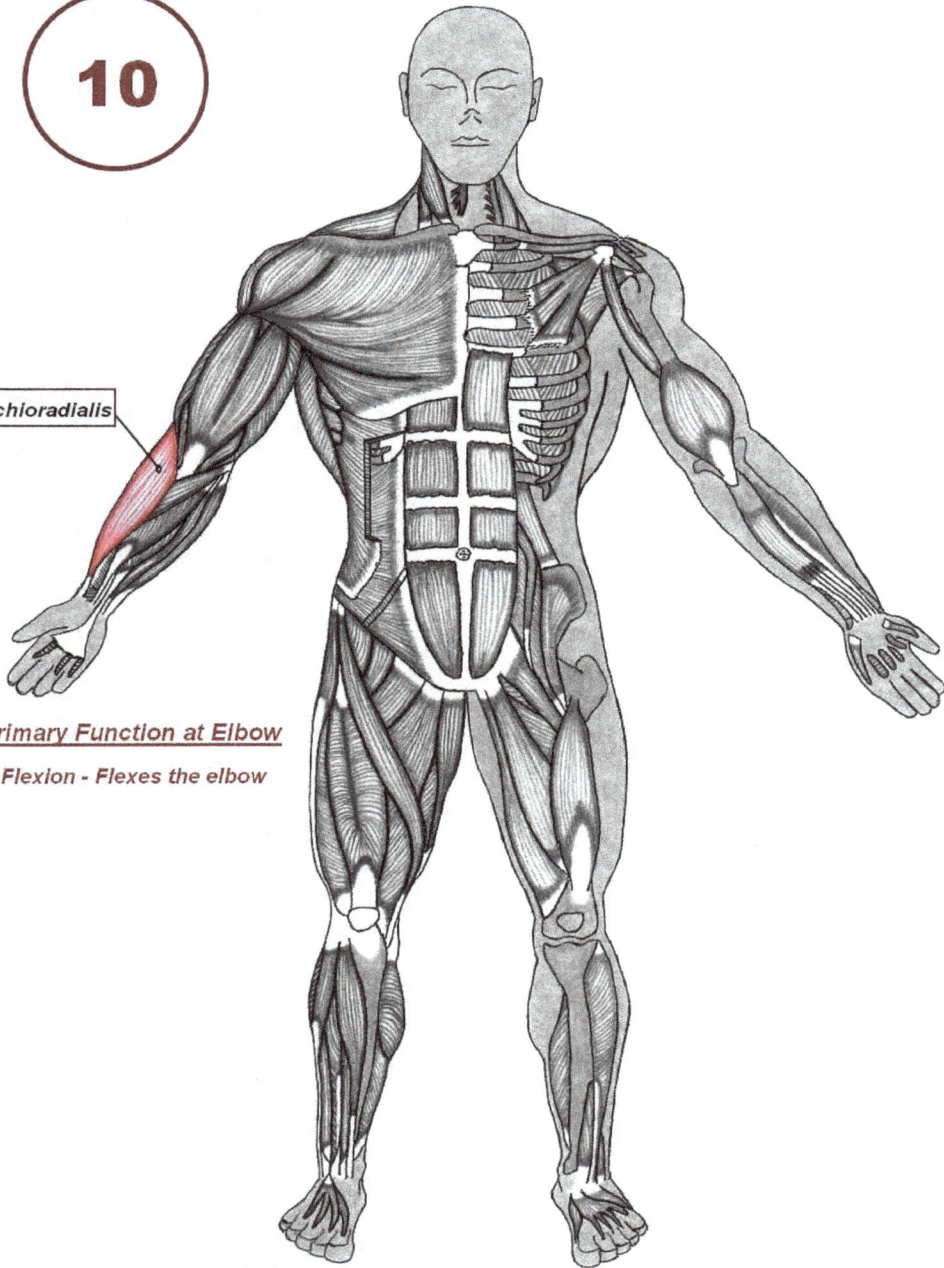

33

10 - Exercises

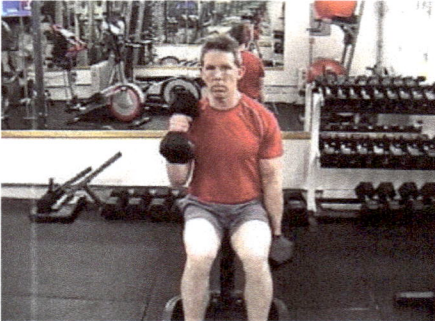

Biceps Seated Alternating Hammer Curl (1-3 Sets 7-10 Reps)

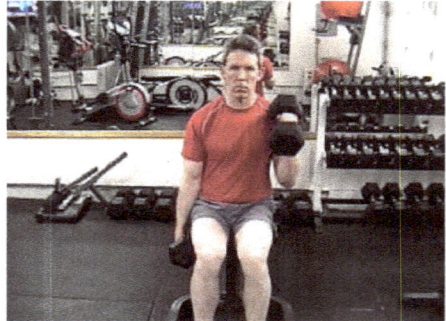

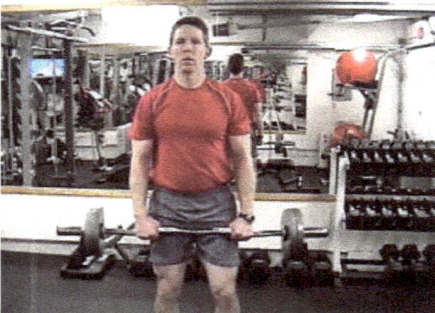

Biceps Standing Reverse EZ-Bar Curl (1-3 Sets 7-10 Reps)

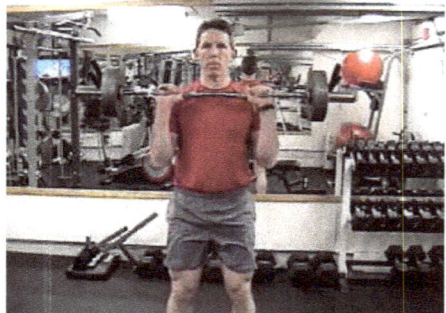

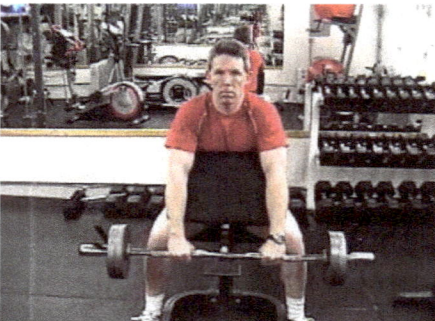

Biceps Seated Reverse EZ-Bar Preacher Curl (1-3 Sets 7-10 Reps)

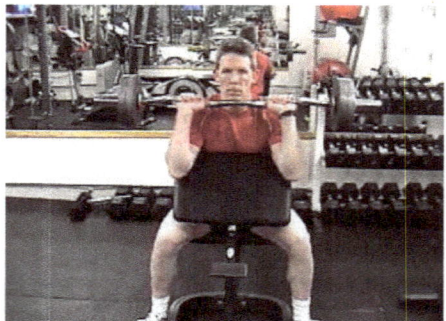

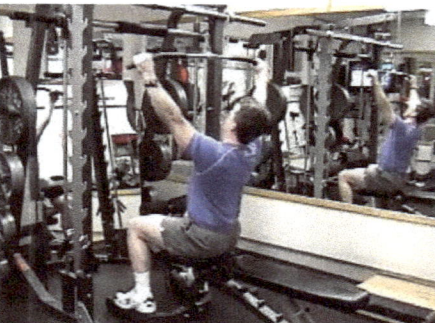

Lat Wide Grip Front Pull Down (1-3 Sets 7-15 Reps)

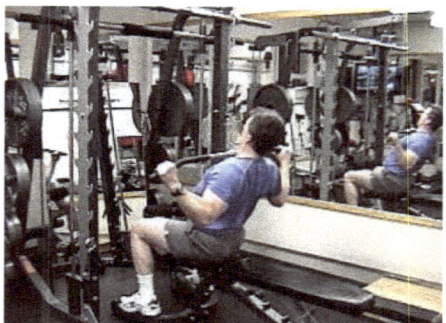

Pronator Teres

11A

Pronator Teres

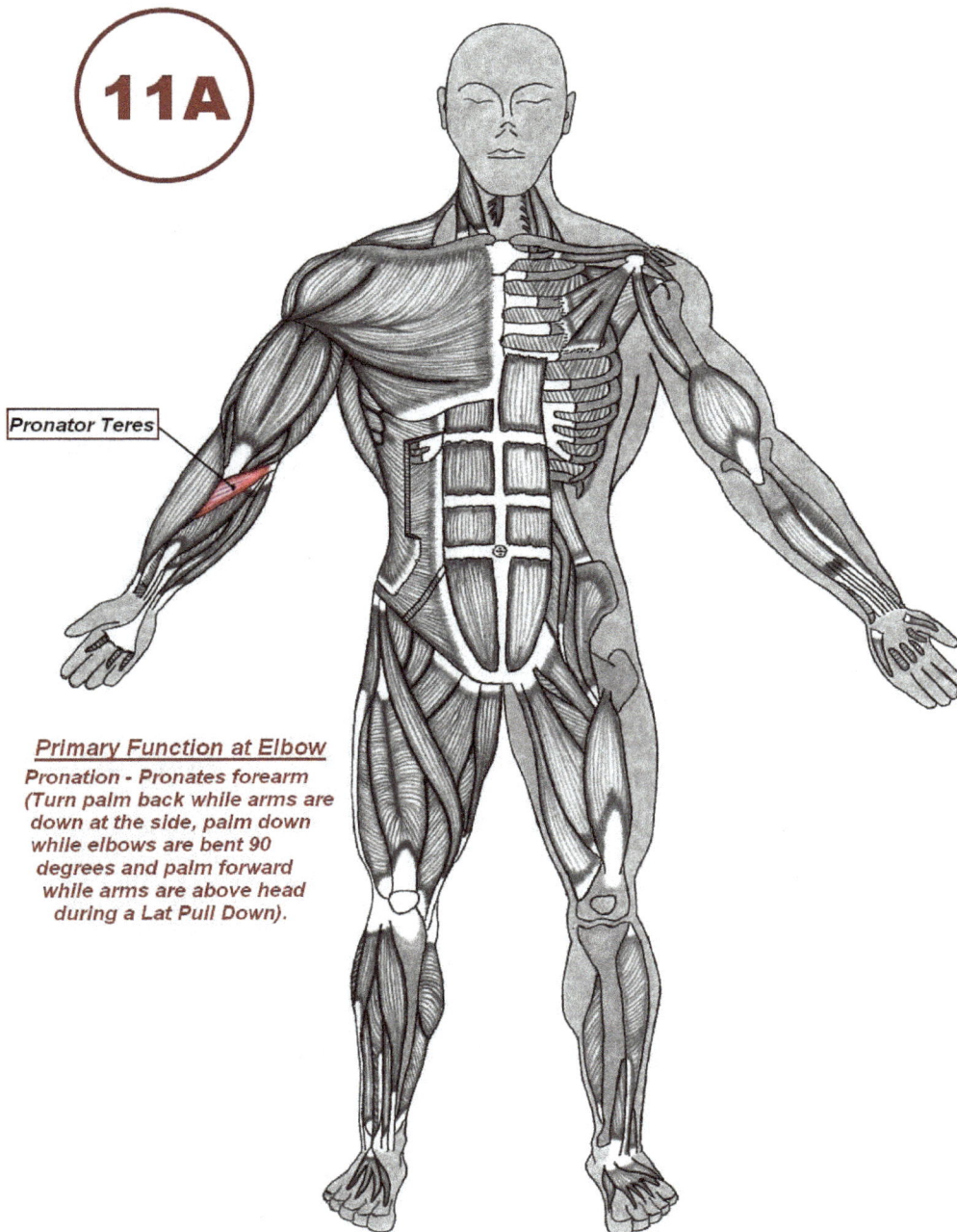

Primary Function at Elbow
*Pronation - Pronates forearm
(Turn palm back while arms are
down at the side, palm down
while elbows are bent 90
degrees and palm forward
while arms are above head
during a Lat Pull Down).*

Forearm - Pronator Quadratus

11B

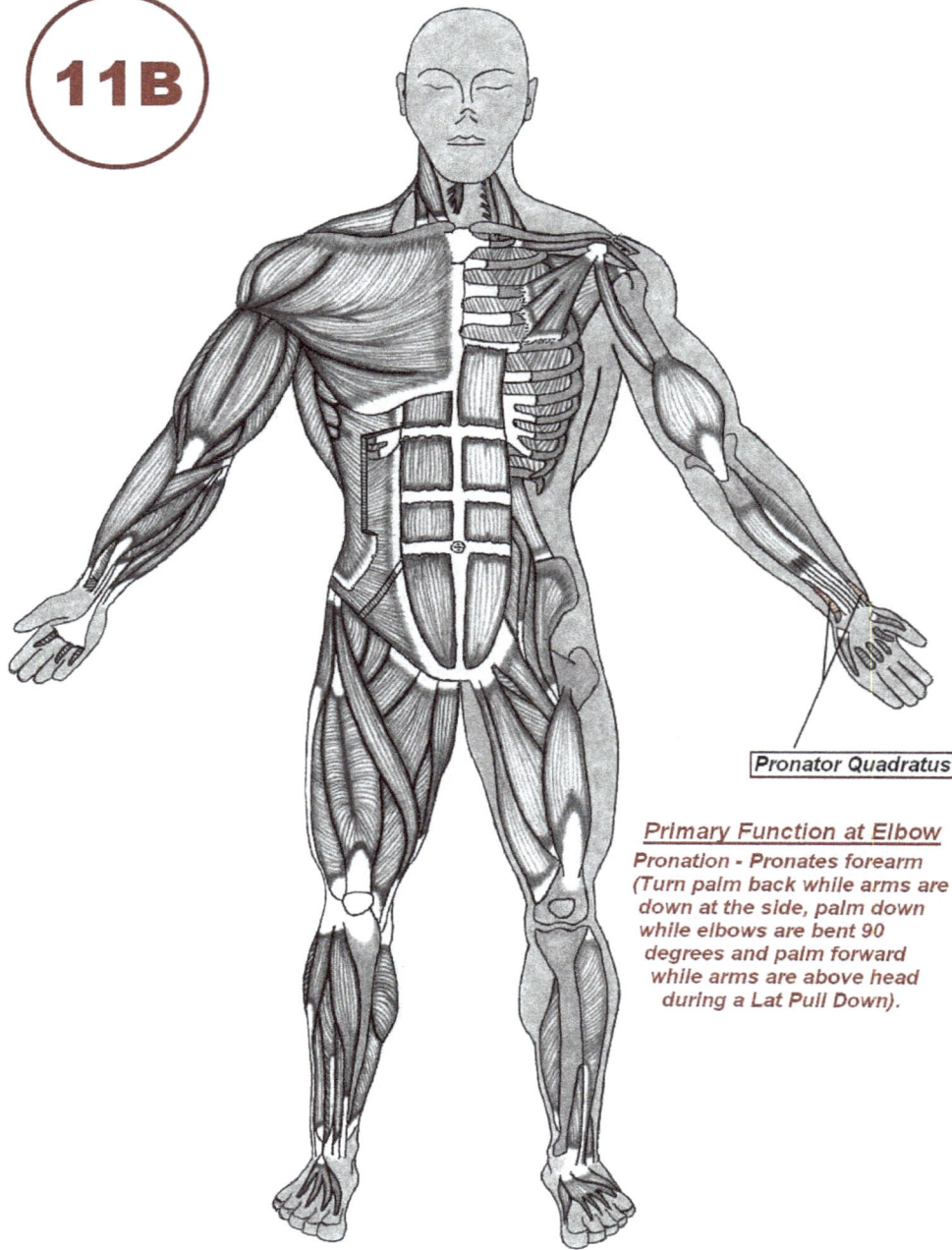

Pronator Quadratus

Primary Function at Elbow

Pronation - Pronates forearm (Turn palm back while arms are down at the side, palm down while elbows are bent 90 degrees and palm forward while arms are above head during a Lat Pull Down).

11A and B - Exercises

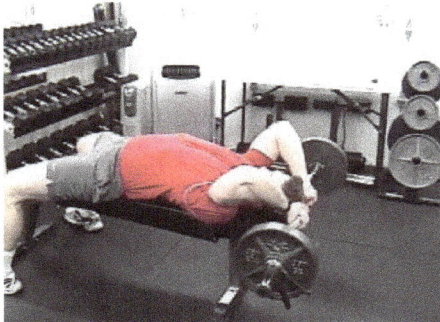

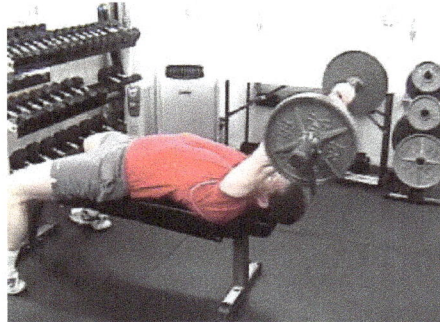

Triceps Lying 45 Deg Bar Extension (Turns Hands Palms Away: 1-3 Sets 7-15 Reps)

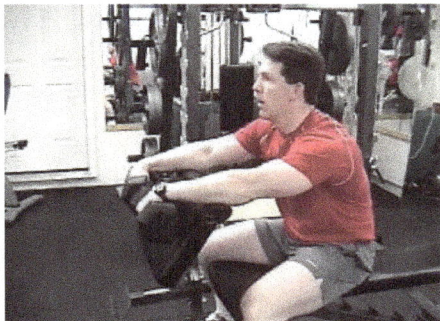

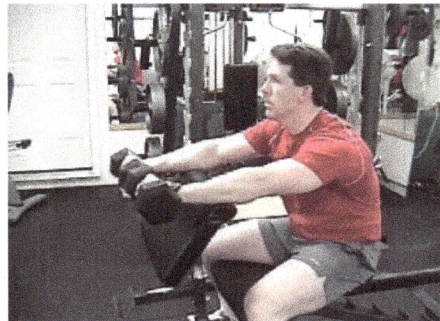

Forearm Extension (Turns Hands Palms Down: 1-3 Sets 7-10 Reps)

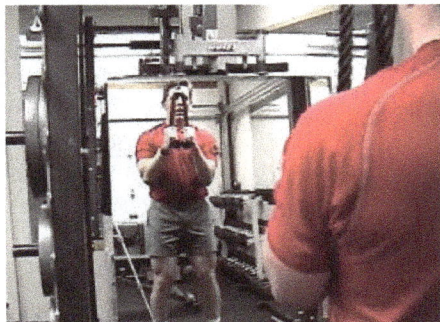

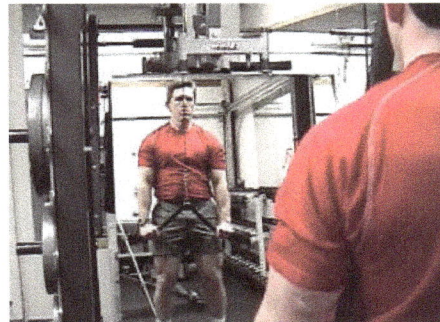

Triceps "Rope" Cable Press (Turns Hands Palms Down: 1-3 Sets 7-15 Reps)

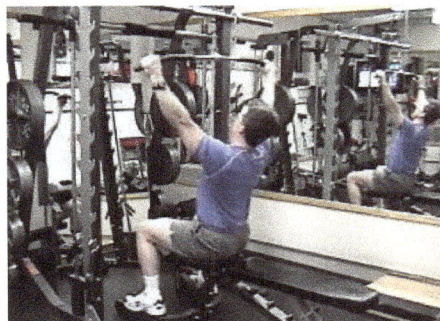

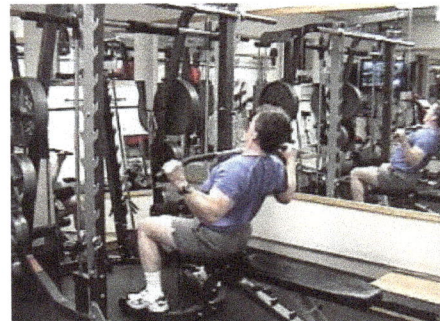

Lat Wide Grip Front Pull Down (Turns Hands Palms Away: 1-3 Sets 7-15 Reps)

Wrist Flexors

12

Flexor Carpi Ulnaris
Primary Function at Wrist

Flexion - Flexes the wrist and the 2 proximal (closest) joints of each of the 4 fingers.

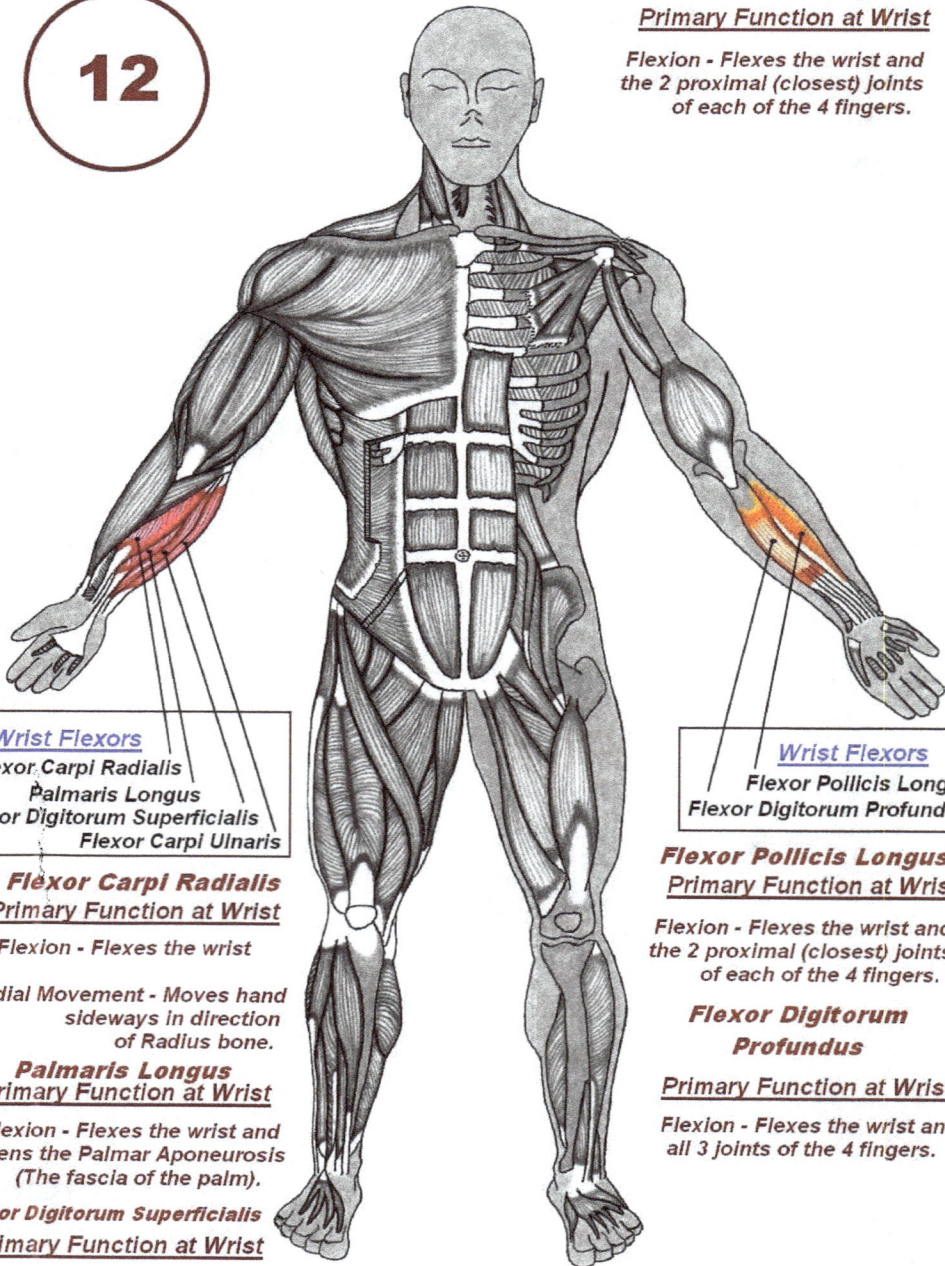

Wrist Flexors
Flexor Carpi Radialis
Palmaris Longus
Flexor Digitorum Superficialis
Flexor Carpi Ulnaris

Wrist Flexors
Flexor Pollicis Longus
Flexor Digitorum Profundus

Flexor Carpi Radialis
Primary Function at Wrist

Flexion - Flexes the wrist

Radial Movement - Moves hand sideways in direction of Radius bone.

Palmaris Longus
Primary Function at Wrist

Flexion - Flexes the wrist and tightens the Palmar Aponeurosis (The fascia of the palm).

Flexor Digitorum Superficialis
Primary Function at Wrist

Flexion - Flexes the wrist and the 2 proximal (closest) joints of each of the 4 fingers.

Flexor Pollicis Longus
Primary Function at Wrist

Flexion - Flexes the wrist and the 2 proximal (closest) joints of each of the 4 fingers.

Flexor Digitorum Profundus
Primary Function at Wrist

Flexion - Flexes the wrist and all 3 joints of the 4 fingers.

12 - Exercises

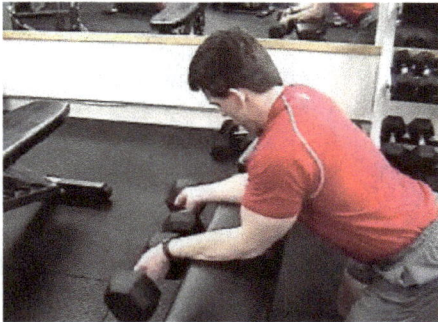

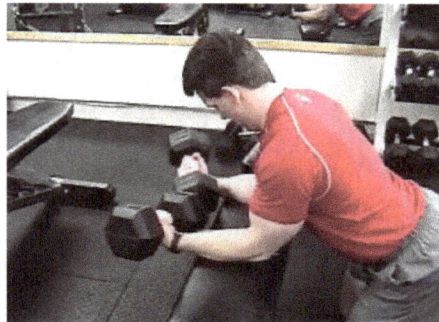

Wrist Curl on Bench (1-3 Sets 7-10 Reps)

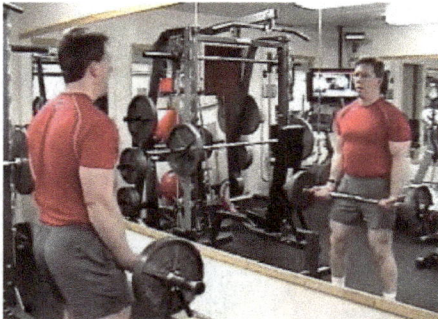

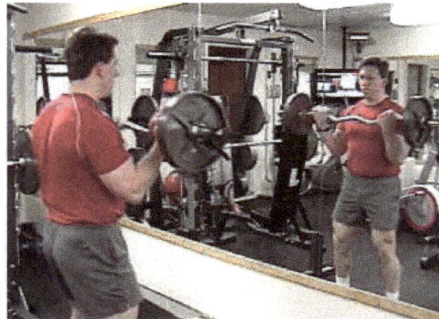

Biceps Standing EZ-Bar Curl (1-3 Sets 7-15 Reps)

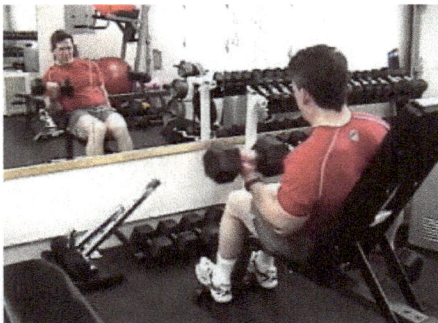

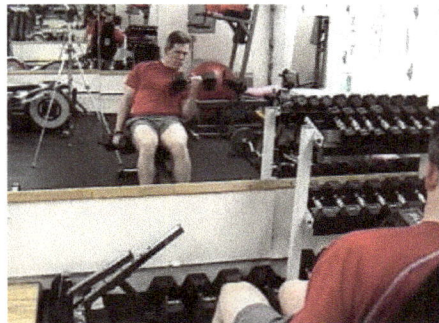

Biceps Seated Incline Dumbbell Curl (1-3 Sets 7-10 Reps)

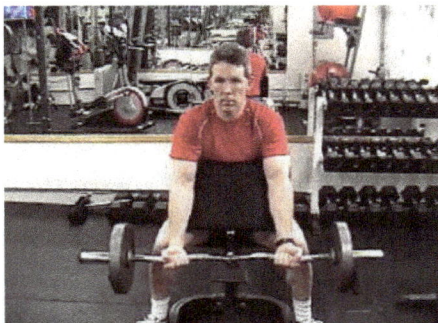

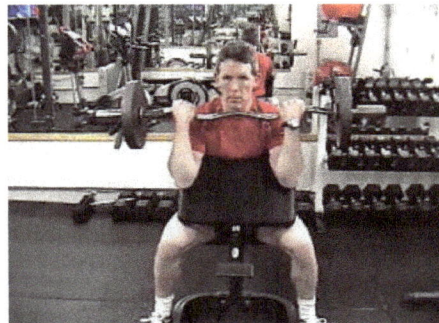

Biceps Seated EZ-Bar Preacher Curl (1-3 Sets 7-15 Reps)

12 - Exercises

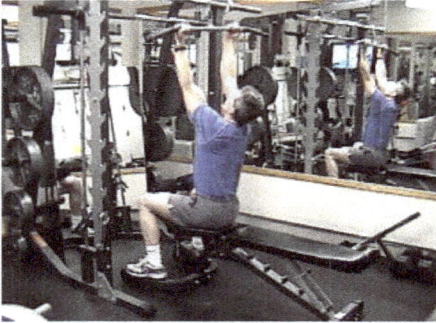

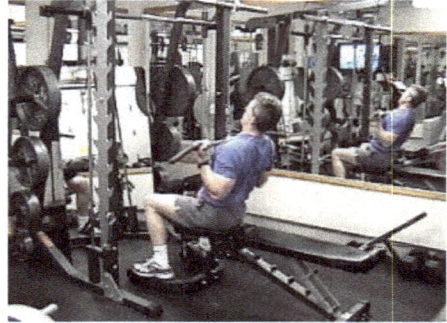

Lat Reverse Grip Pull Down (1-3 Sets 7-15 Reps)

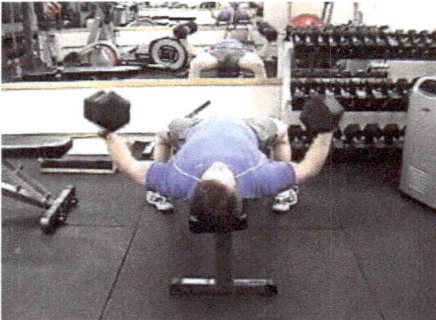

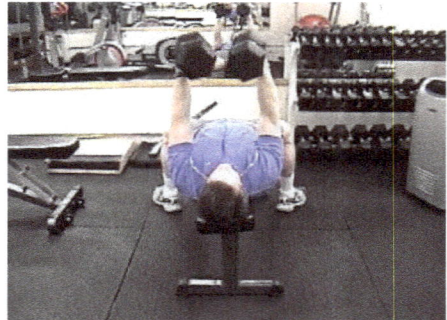

Chest Flat Flye (1-3 Sets 7-15 Reps)

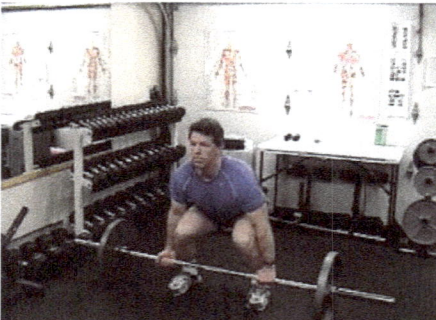

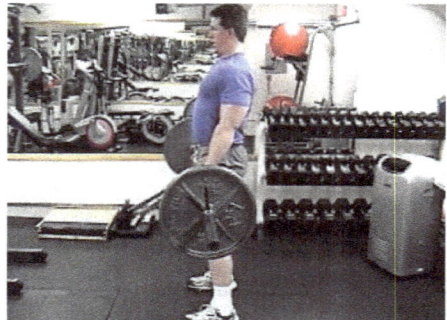

Dead-Lift (1-3 Sets 7-10 Reps)

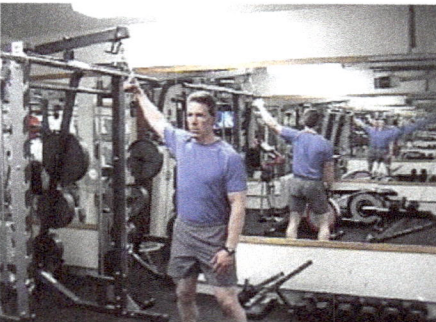

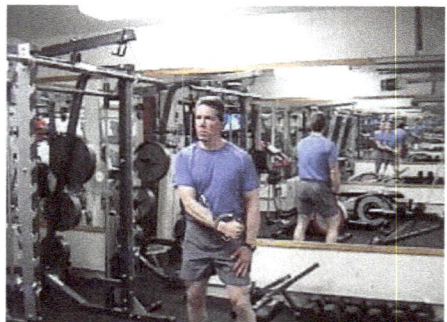

Cable Cross-Over (1-3 Sets 7-15 Reps)

AB's - Rectus Abdominis

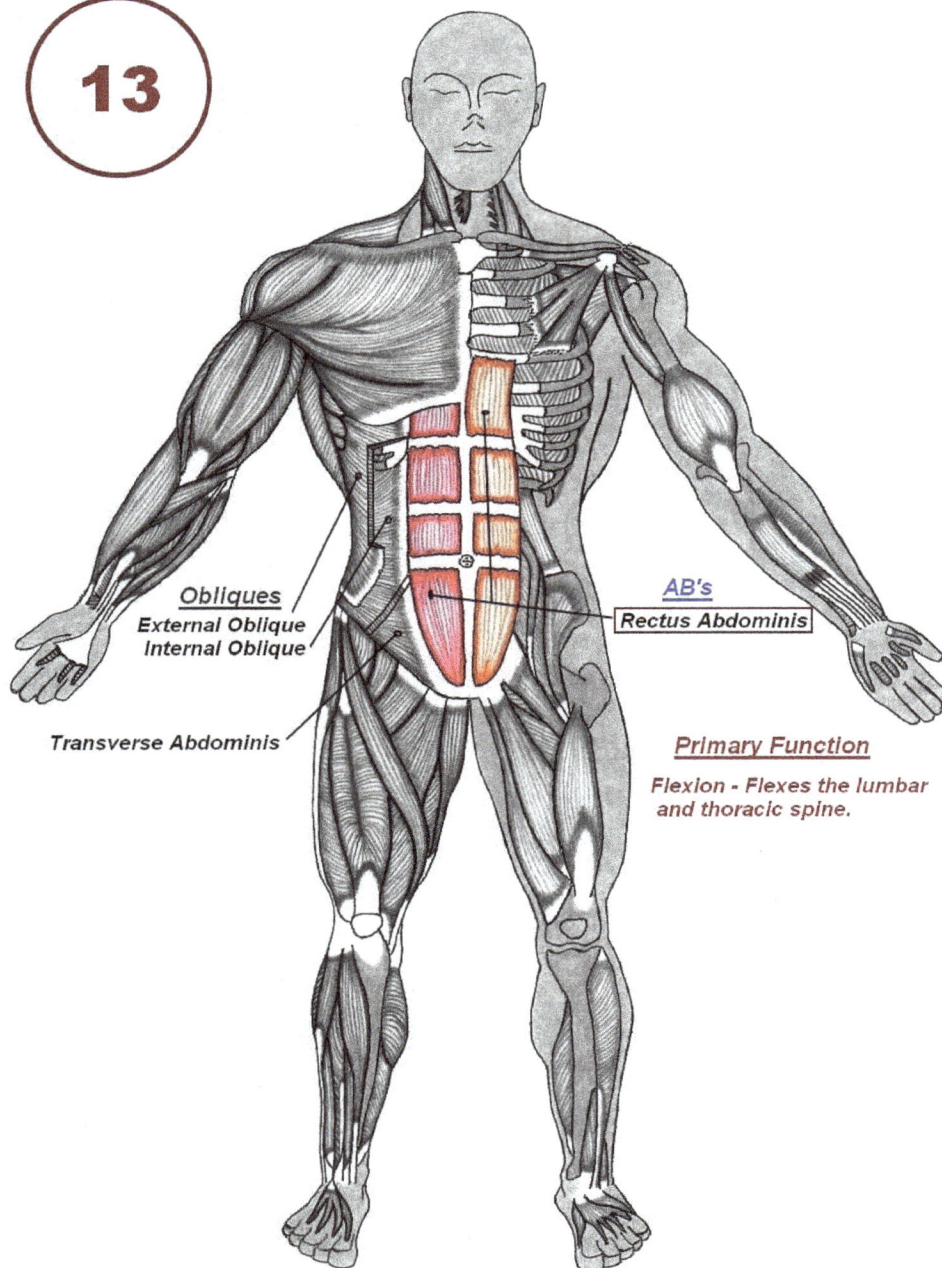

13

Obliques
External Oblique
Internal Oblique

Transverse Abdominis

<u>AB's</u>
Rectus Abdominis

Primary Function

Flexion - Flexes the lumbar
and thoracic spine.

13 - Exercises

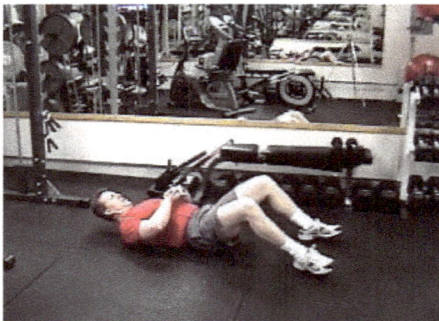

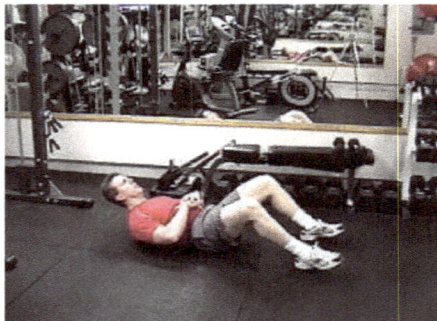

Ab Crunch on Floor (1-3 Sets 10-30 Reps)

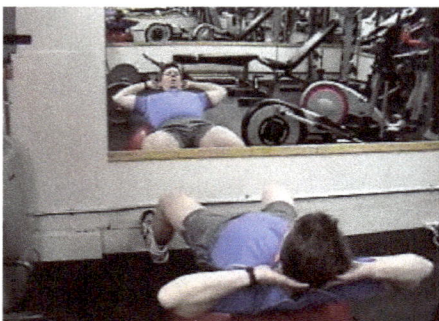

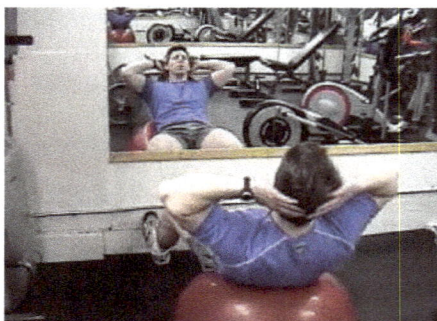

Ab Crunch on Stability Ball (1-3 Sets 10-30 Reps)

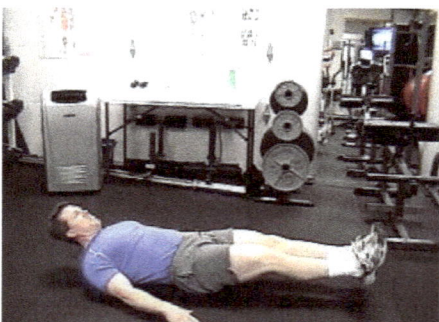

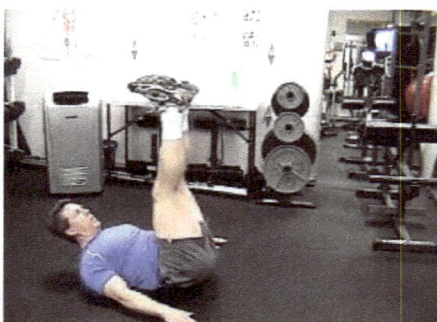

Straight Leg Lift on Floor (Lower Ab Focus: 1-3 Sets 10-15 Reps)

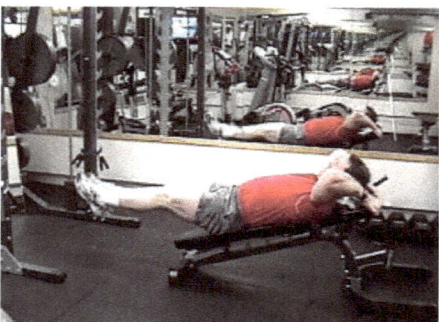

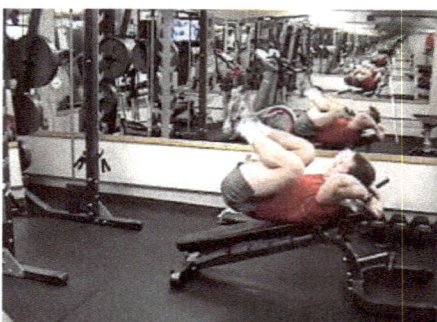

Reverse Crunch on Incline Bench (Lower Ab Focus: 1-3 Sets 10-15 Reps)

13 - Exercises

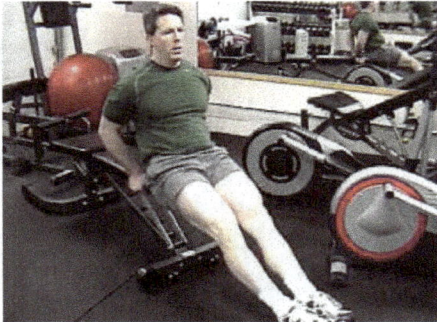

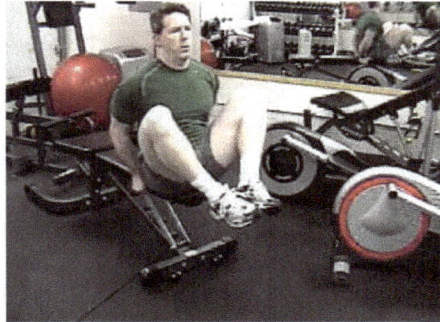

Seated Leg Tuck (Lower Ab Focus: 1-3 Sets 10-15 Reps)

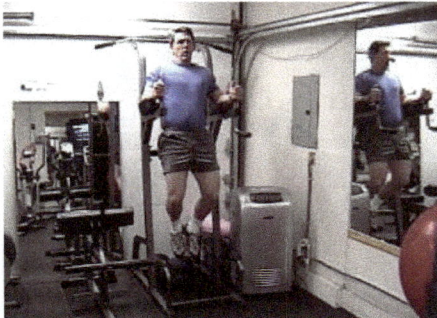

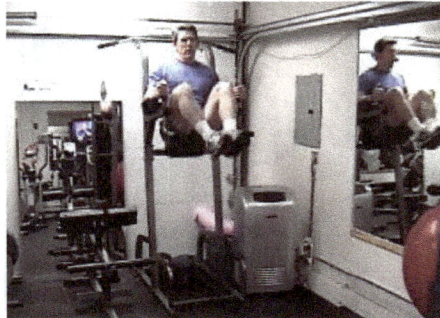

Upright Reverse Crunch (Lower Ab Focus: 1-3 Sets 10-15 Reps)

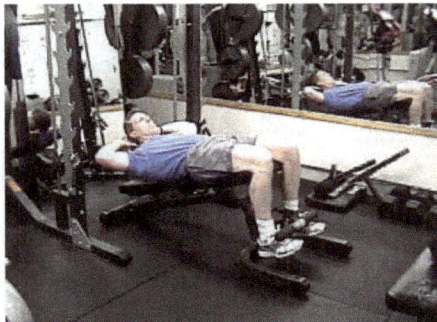

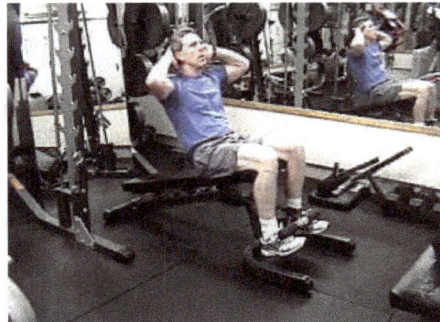

Decline Sit Ups (Hands support, but don't pull head: 1-3 Sets 10-30 Reps)

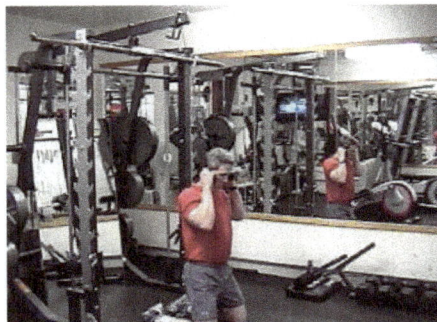

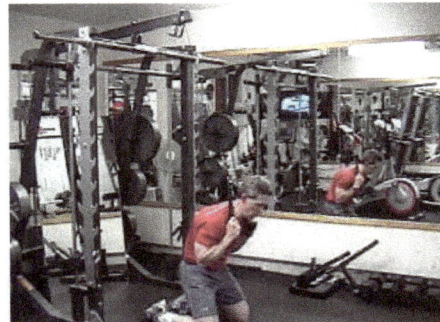

Kneeling Cable Crunch (1-3 Sets 10-30 Reps)

13 - Exercises

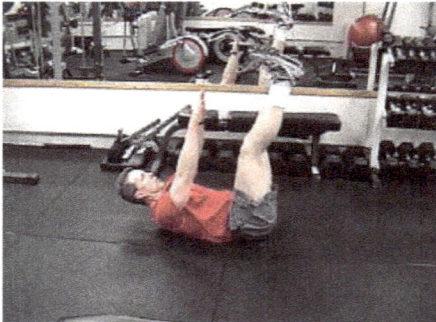

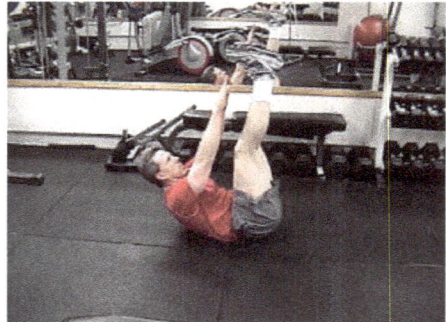

Partial V-Ups (1-3 Sets 10-15 Reps)

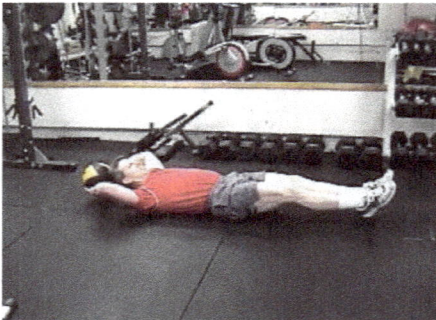

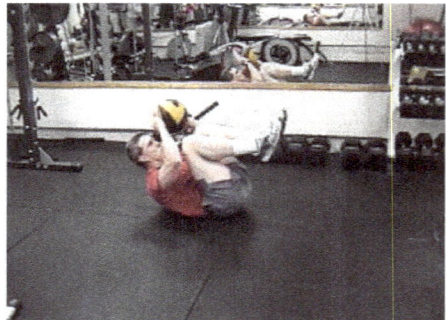

Medicine Ball Full Crunch (1-3 Sets 10-30 Reps)

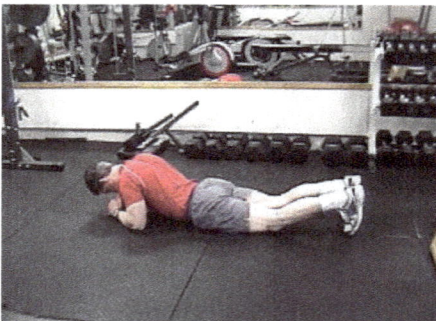

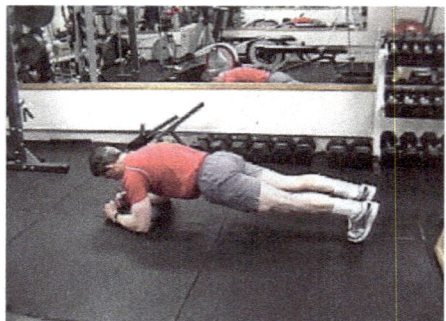

Prone Planks (1-3 Sets, Hold 30-60 Seconds/Set)

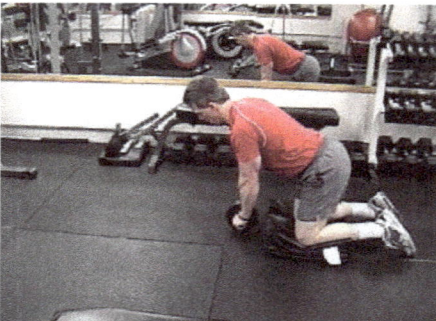

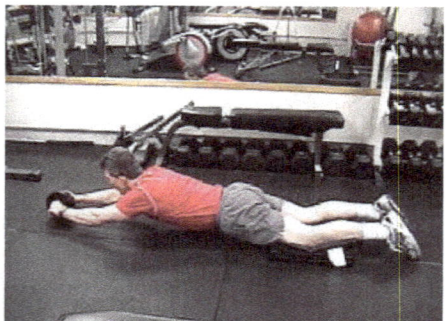

Ab Roller (1-3 Sets 7-10 Reps)

Obliques - External and Internal

14

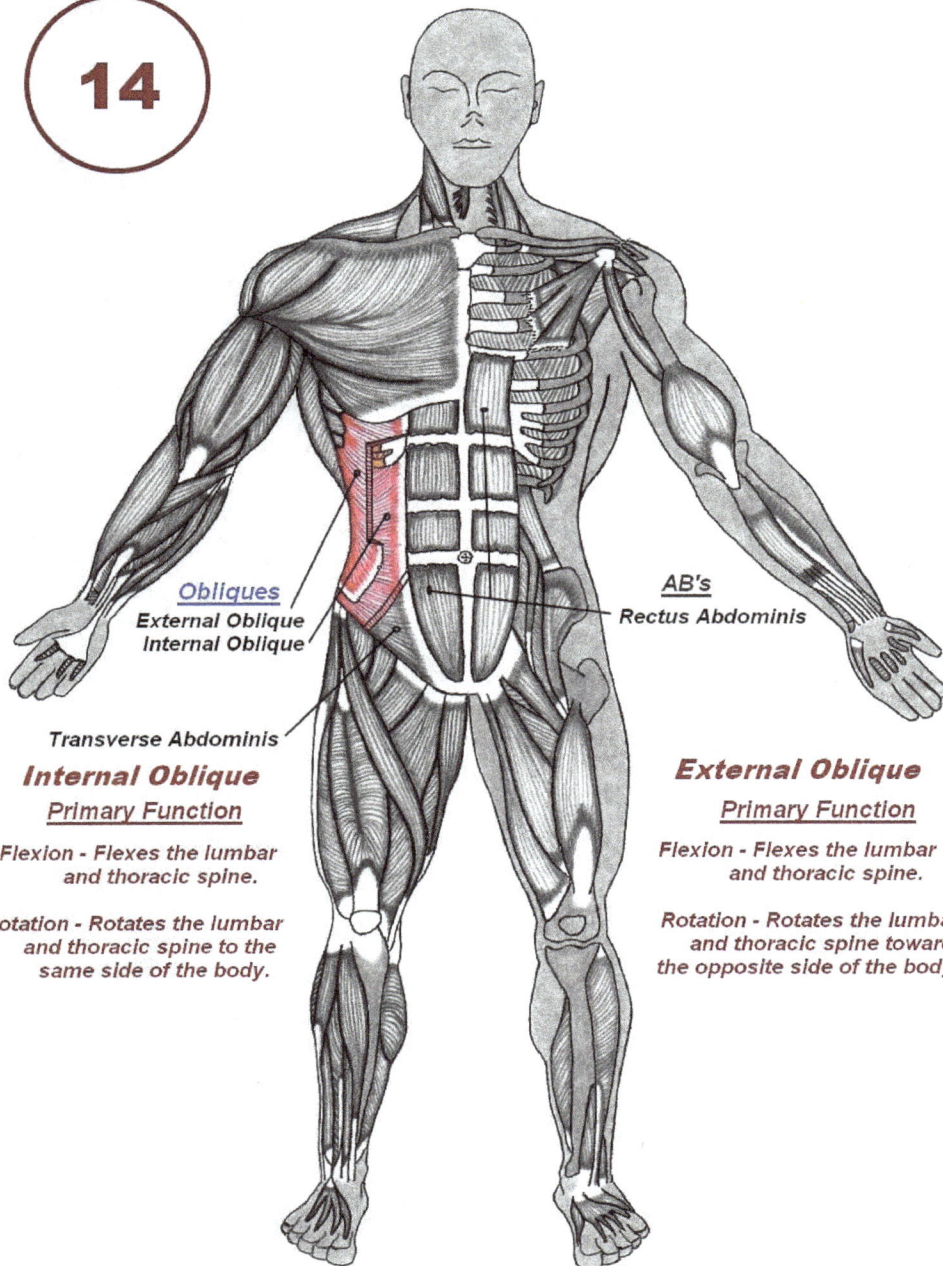

Obliques
External Oblique
Internal Oblique

Transverse Abdominis

AB's
Rectus Abdominis

Internal Oblique

Primary Function

Flexion - Flexes the lumbar
and thoracic spine.

Rotation - Rotates the lumbar
and thoracic spine to the
same side of the body.

External Oblique

Primary Function

Flexion - Flexes the lumbar
and thoracic spine.

Rotation - Rotates the lumbar
and thoracic spine toward
the opposite side of the body.

14 - Exercises

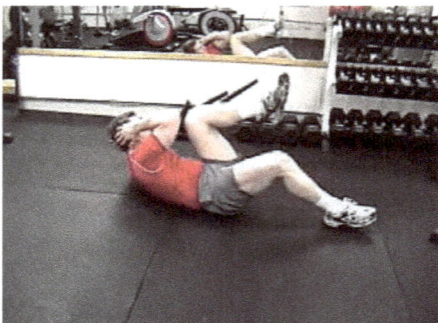

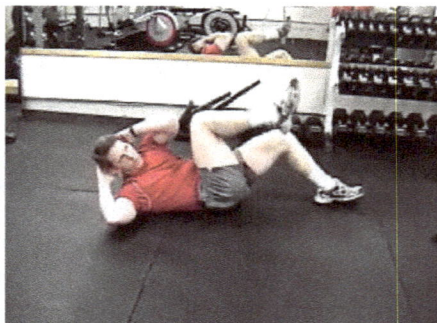

Lying Floor Twist "Bicycles" (1-3 Sets 10-15 Reps Each Side)

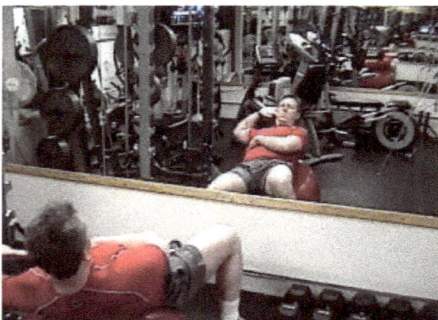

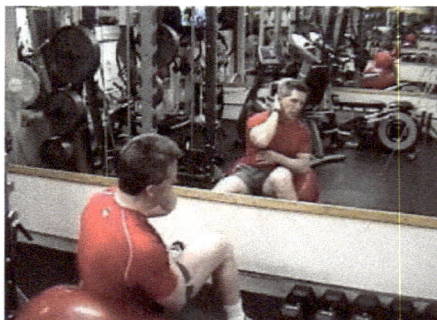

Stability Ball Twist (1-3 Sets 10-15 Reps Each Side)

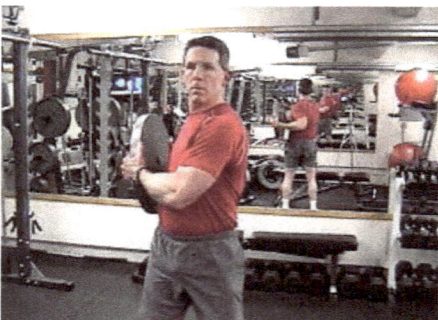

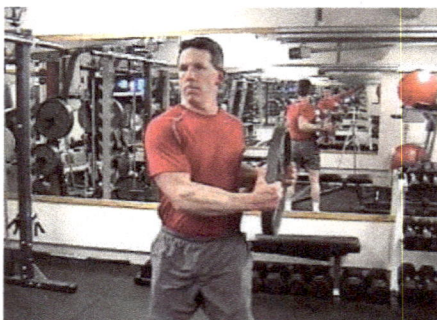

Standing Plate Twist (1-3 Sets 10-15 Reps Each Side)

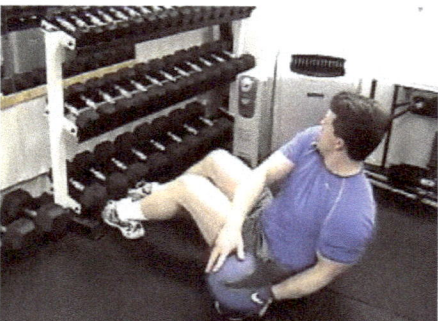

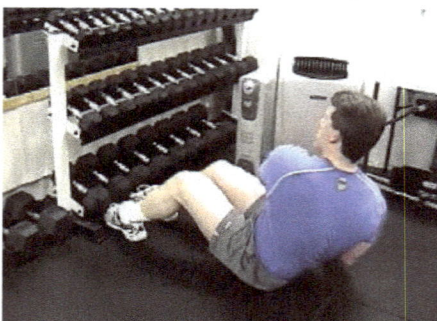

Seated Floor Twist With Medicine Ball (1-3 Sets 10-15 Reps Each Side)

14 - Exercises

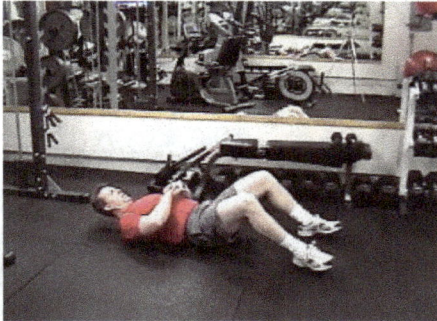

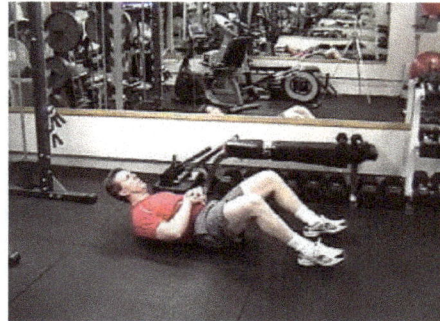

Ab Crunch on Floor (1-3 Sets 10-30 Reps)

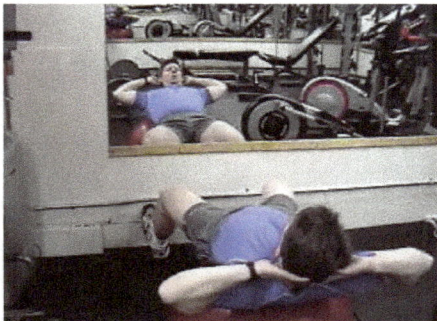

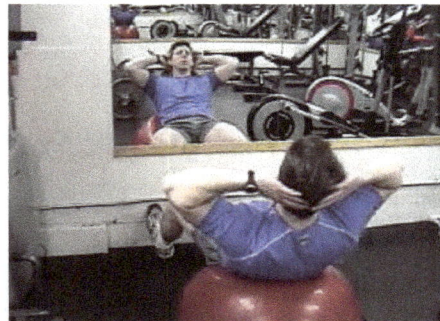

Ab Crunch on Stability Ball (1-3 Sets 10-30 Reps)

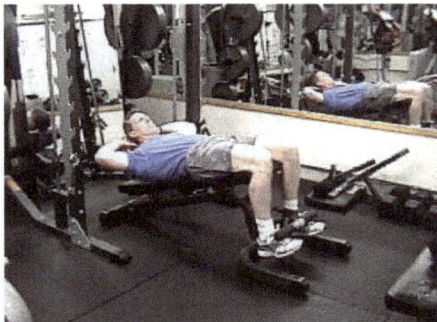

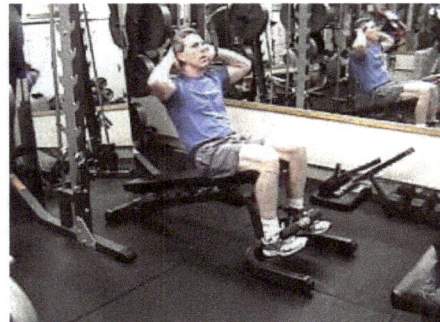

Decline Sit Ups (Hands support, but don't pull head: 1-3 Sets 10-30 Reps)

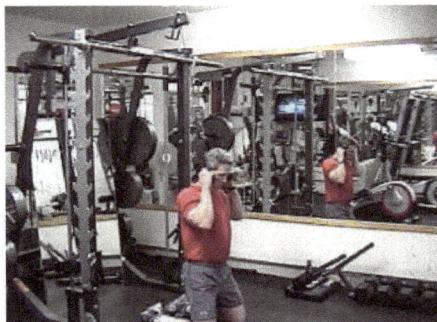

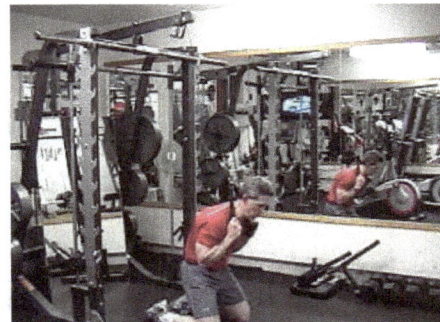

Kneeling Cable Crunch (1-3 Sets 10-30 Reps)

14 - Exercises

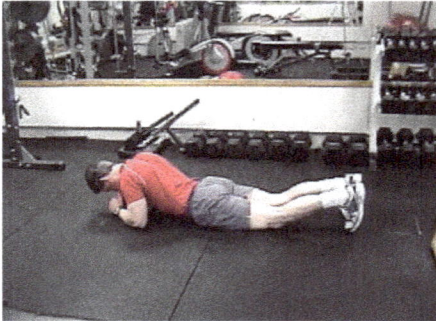

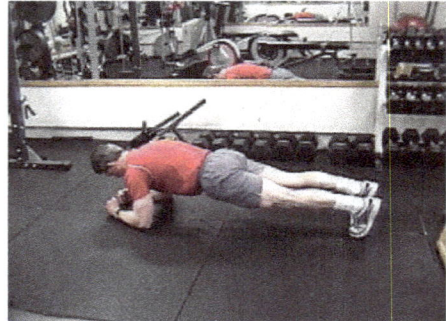

Prone Plank (1-3 Sets, Hold 30-60 Seconds/Set)

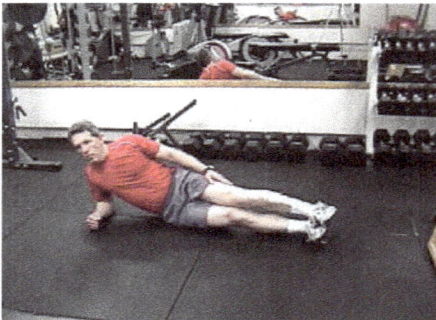

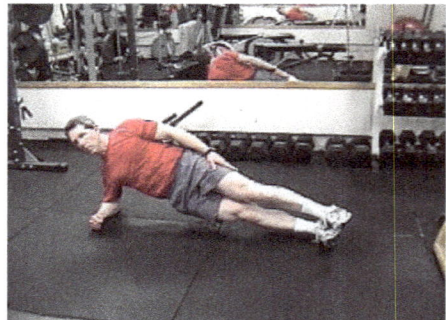

Side-Lying Plank (1-3 Sets, Hold 30-60 Seconds/Set Each Side)

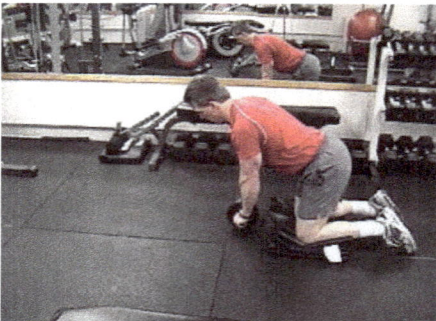

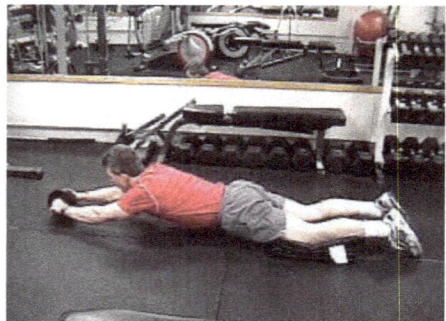

Ab Roller (1-3 Sets 7-10 Reps)

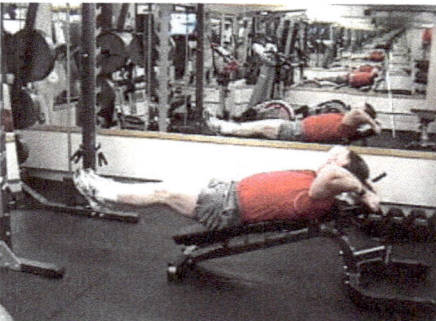

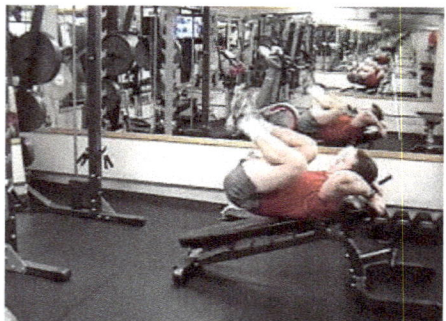

Reverse Crunch on Incline Bench (1-3 Sets 10-15 Reps)

Transverse Abdominis

15

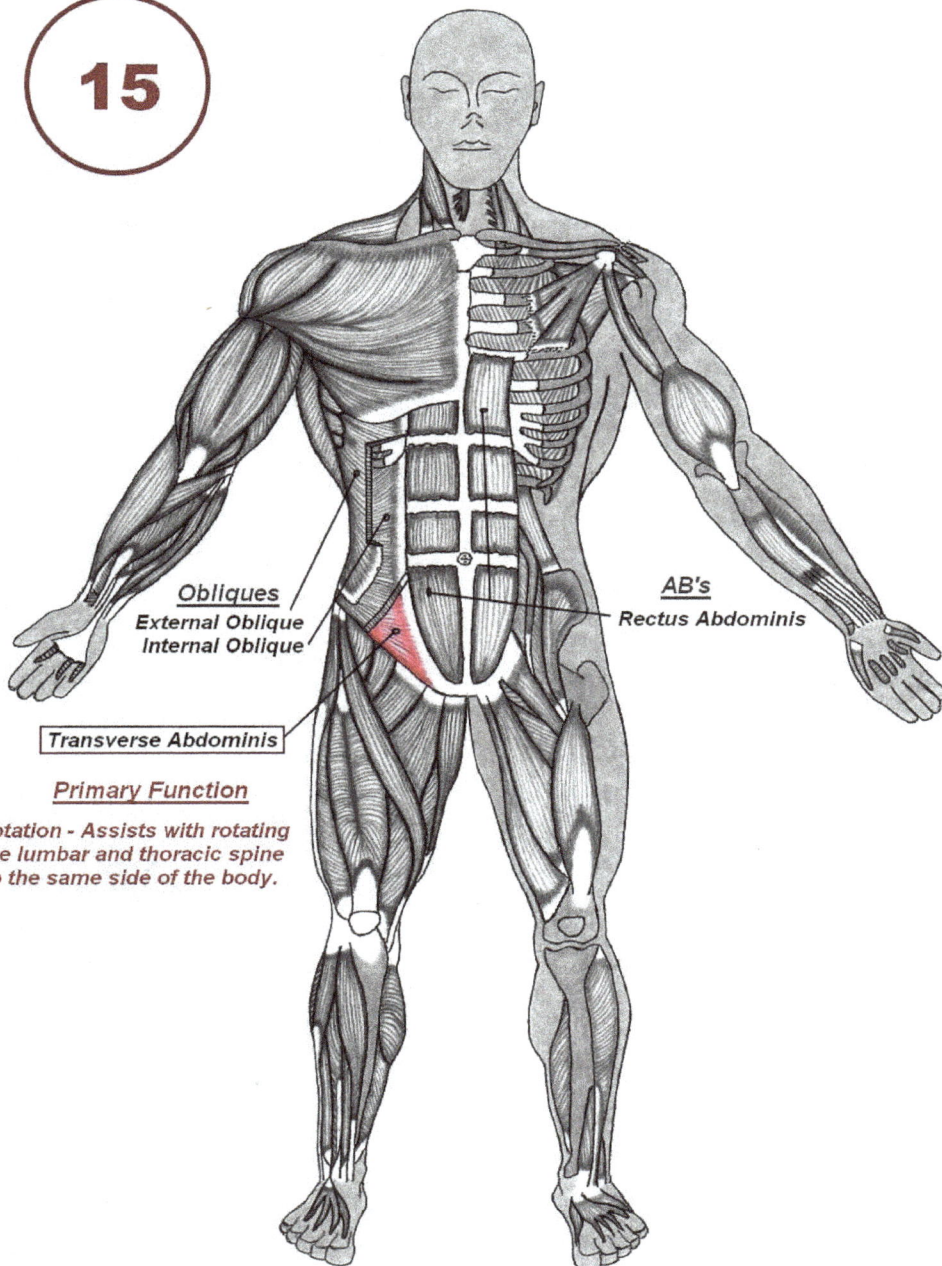

Obliques
External Oblique
Internal Oblique

AB's
Rectus Abdominis

Transverse Abdominis

Primary Function

Rotation - Assists with rotating the lumbar and thoracic spine to the same side of the body.

15 - Exercises

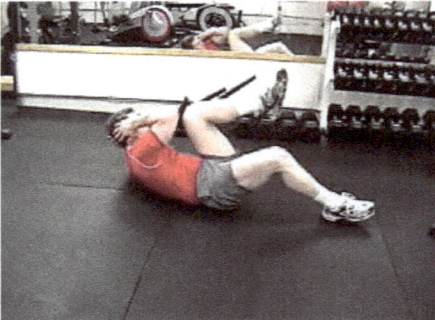

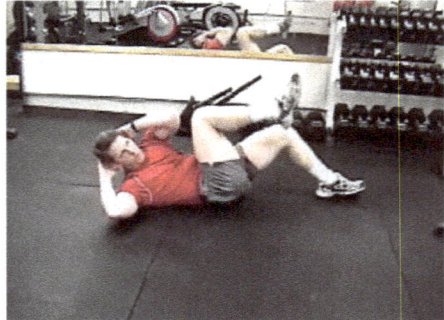

Lying Floor Twist "Bicycles" (1-3 Sets 10-15 Reps Each Side)

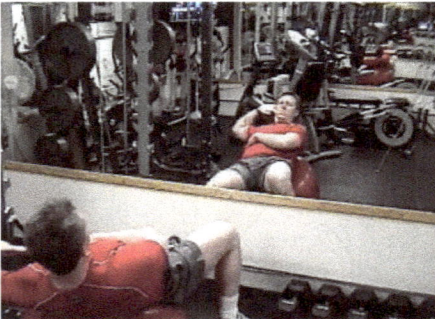

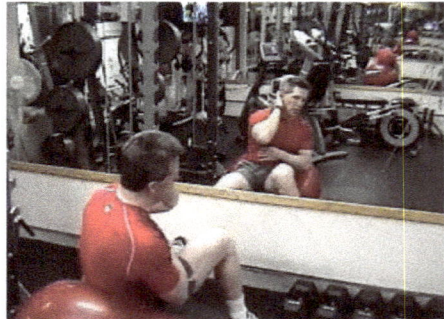

Stability Ball Twist (1-3 Sets 10-15 Reps Each Side)

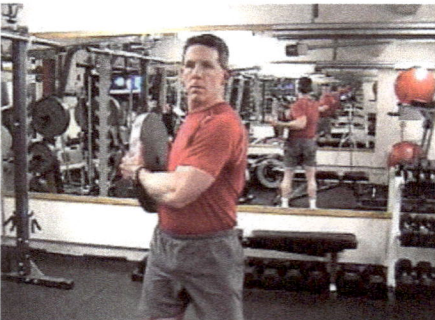

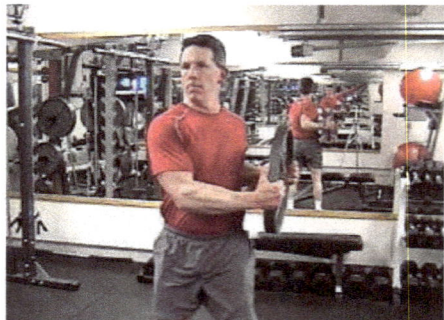

Standing Plate Twist (1-3 Sets 10-15 Reps Each Side)

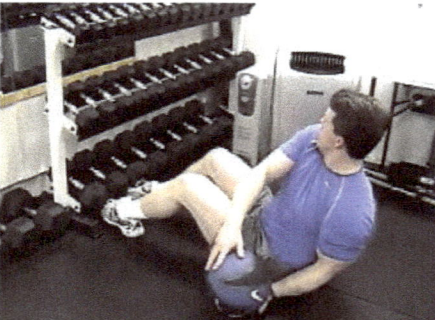

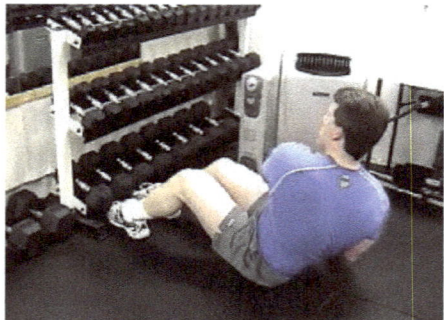

Seated Floor Twist With Medicine Ball (1-3 Sets 10-15 Reps Each Side)

15 - Exercises

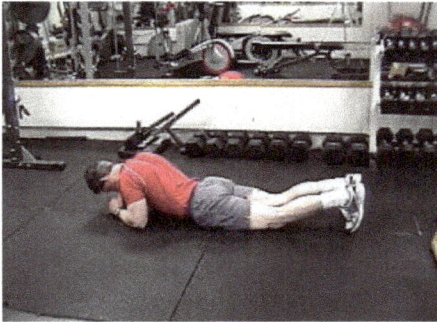

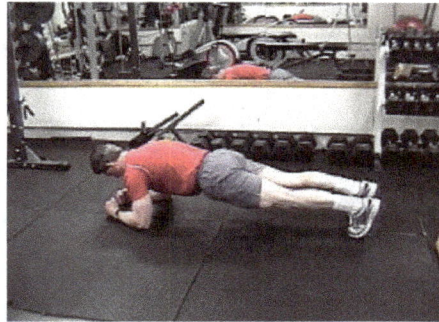

Prone Plank (1-3 Sets, Hold 30-60 Seconds/Set)

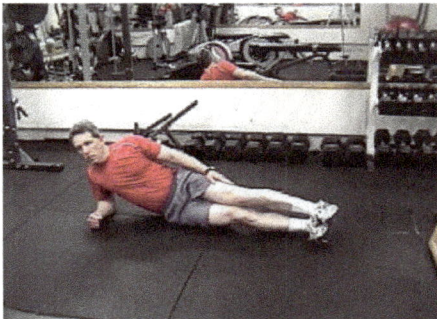

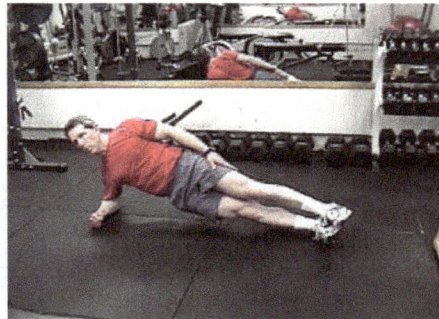

Side-Lying Plank (1-3 Sets, Hold 30-60 Seconds/Set Each Side)

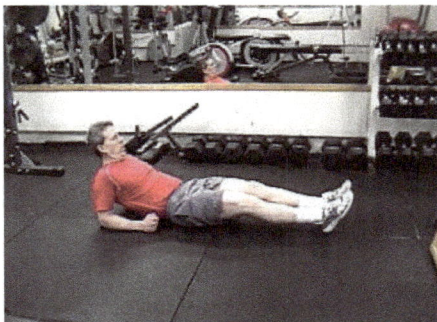

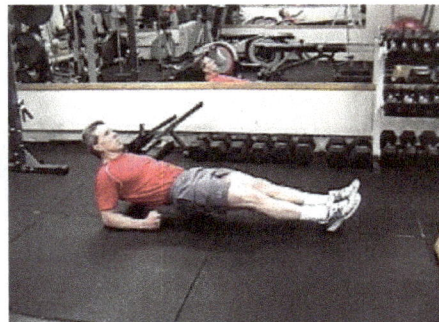

Supine Plank (1-3 Sets, Hold 30-60 Seconds/Set)

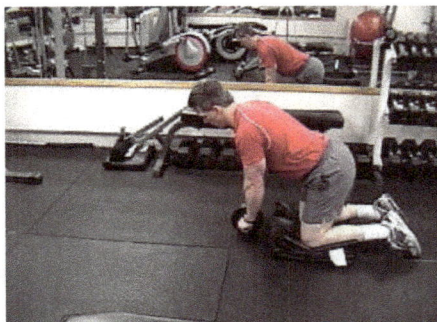

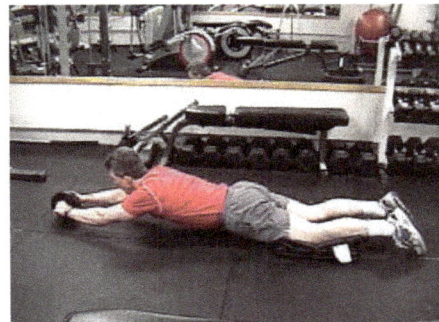

Ab Roller (1-3 Sets 7-10 Reps)

Hip Flexors

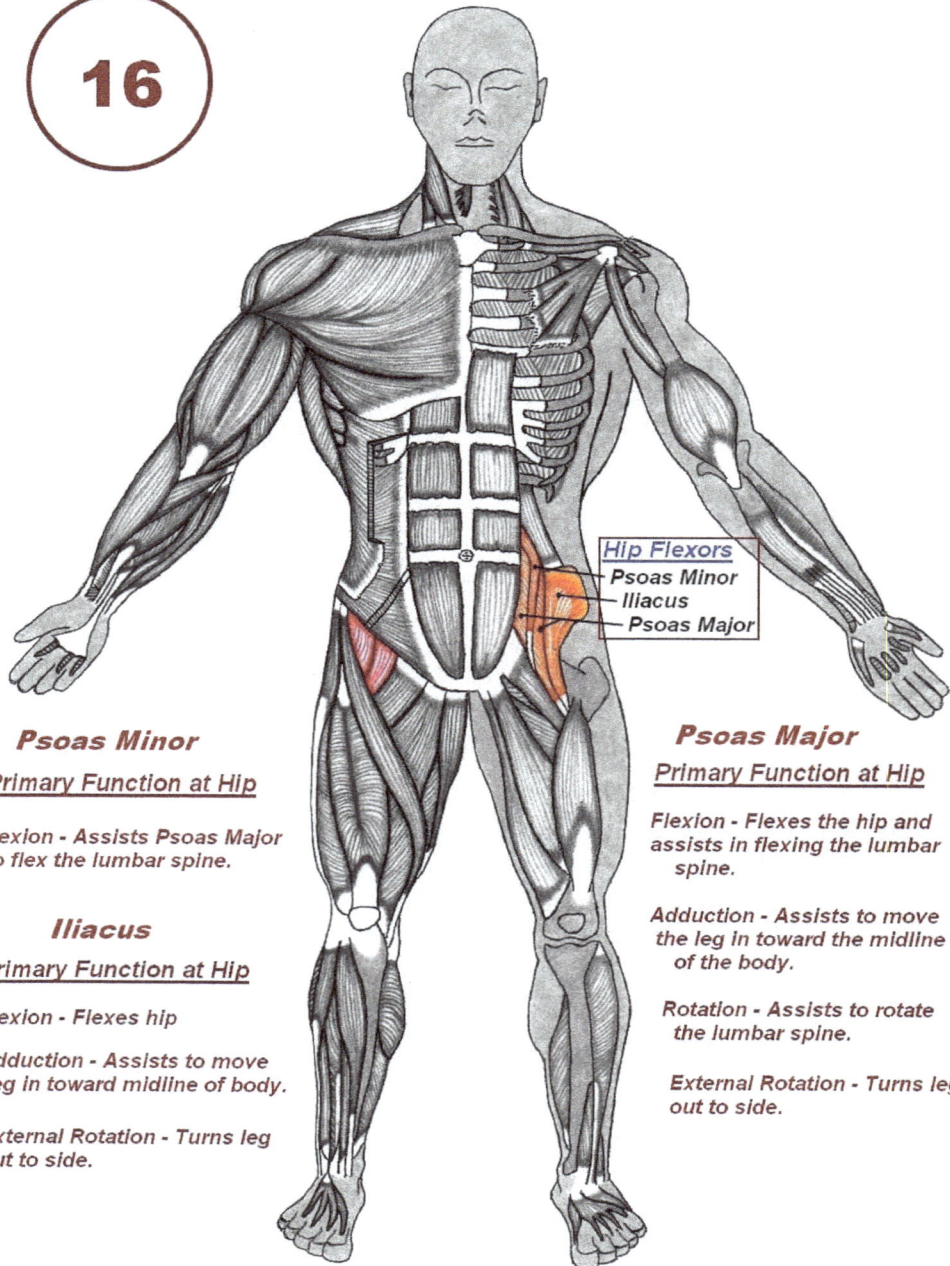

16

Hip Flexors
- Psoas Minor
- Iliacus
- Psoas Major

Psoas Minor

Primary Function at Hip

Flexion - Assists Psoas Major to flex the lumbar spine.

Iliacus

Primary Function at Hip

Flexion - Flexes hip

Adduction - Assists to move leg in toward midline of body.

External Rotation - Turns leg out to side.

Psoas Major

Primary Function at Hip

Flexion - Flexes the hip and assists in flexing the lumbar spine.

Adduction - Assists to move the leg in toward the midline of the body.

Rotation - Assists to rotate the lumbar spine.

External Rotation - Turns leg out to side.

16 - Exercises

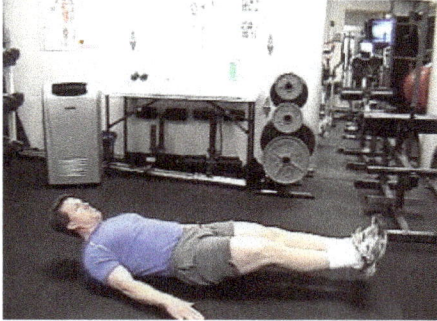

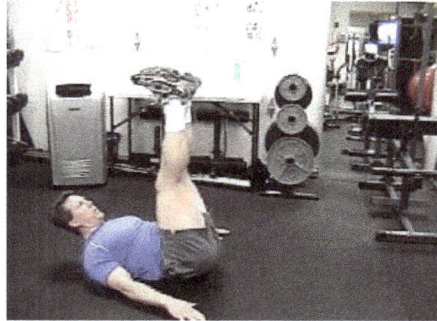

Straight Leg Lift on Floor (1-3 Sets 10-15 Reps)

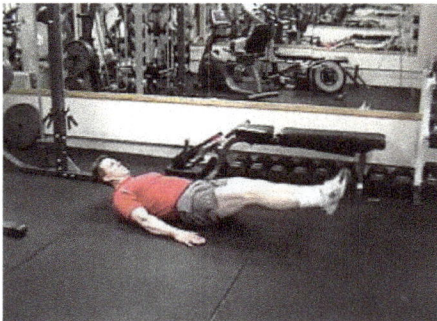

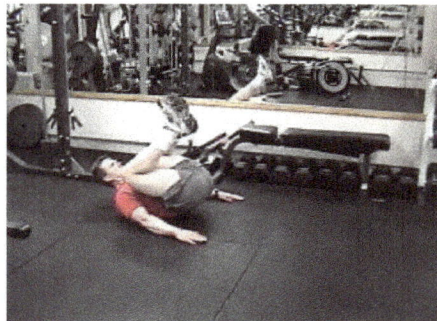

Reverse Crunch on Floor (1-3 Sets 10-15 Reps)

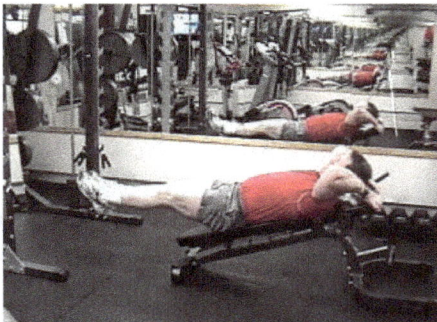

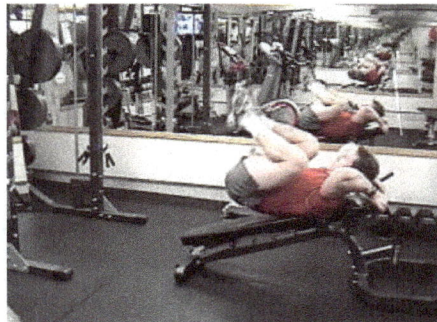

Reverse Crunch on Incline Bench (1-3 Sets 10-15 Reps)

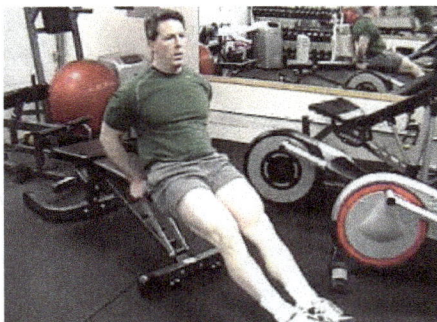

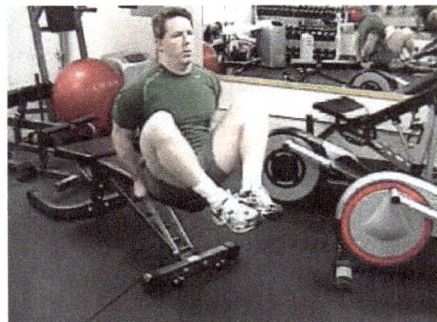

Seated Leg Tuck (1-3 Sets 10-15 Reps)

16 - Exercises

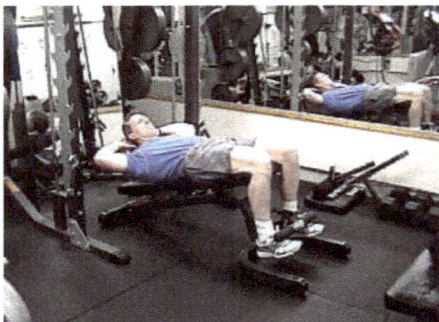

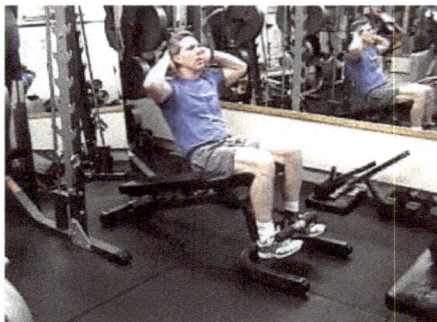

Decline Sit Ups (Hands support, but don't pull head: 1-3 Sets 10-30 Reps)

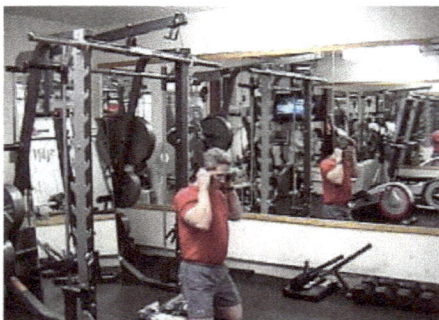

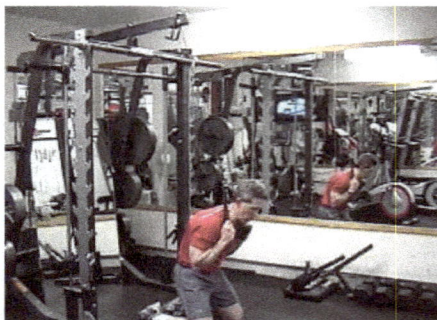

Kneeling Cable Crunch (1-3 Sets 10-30 Reps)

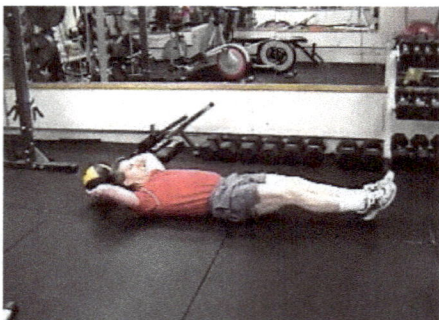

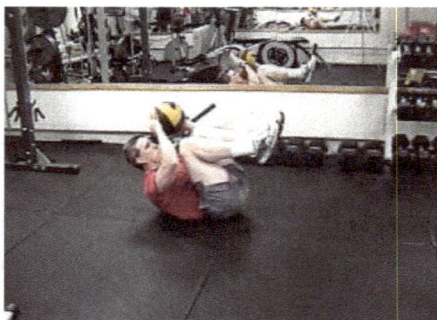

Medicine Ball Full Crunch (1-3 Sets 10-30 Reps)

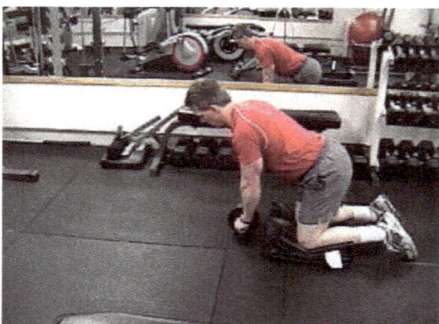

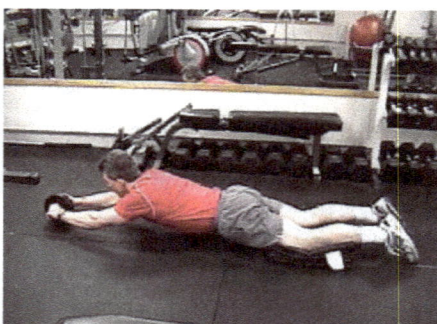

Ab Roller (1-3 Sets 7-10 Reps)

Hip Abductors

17

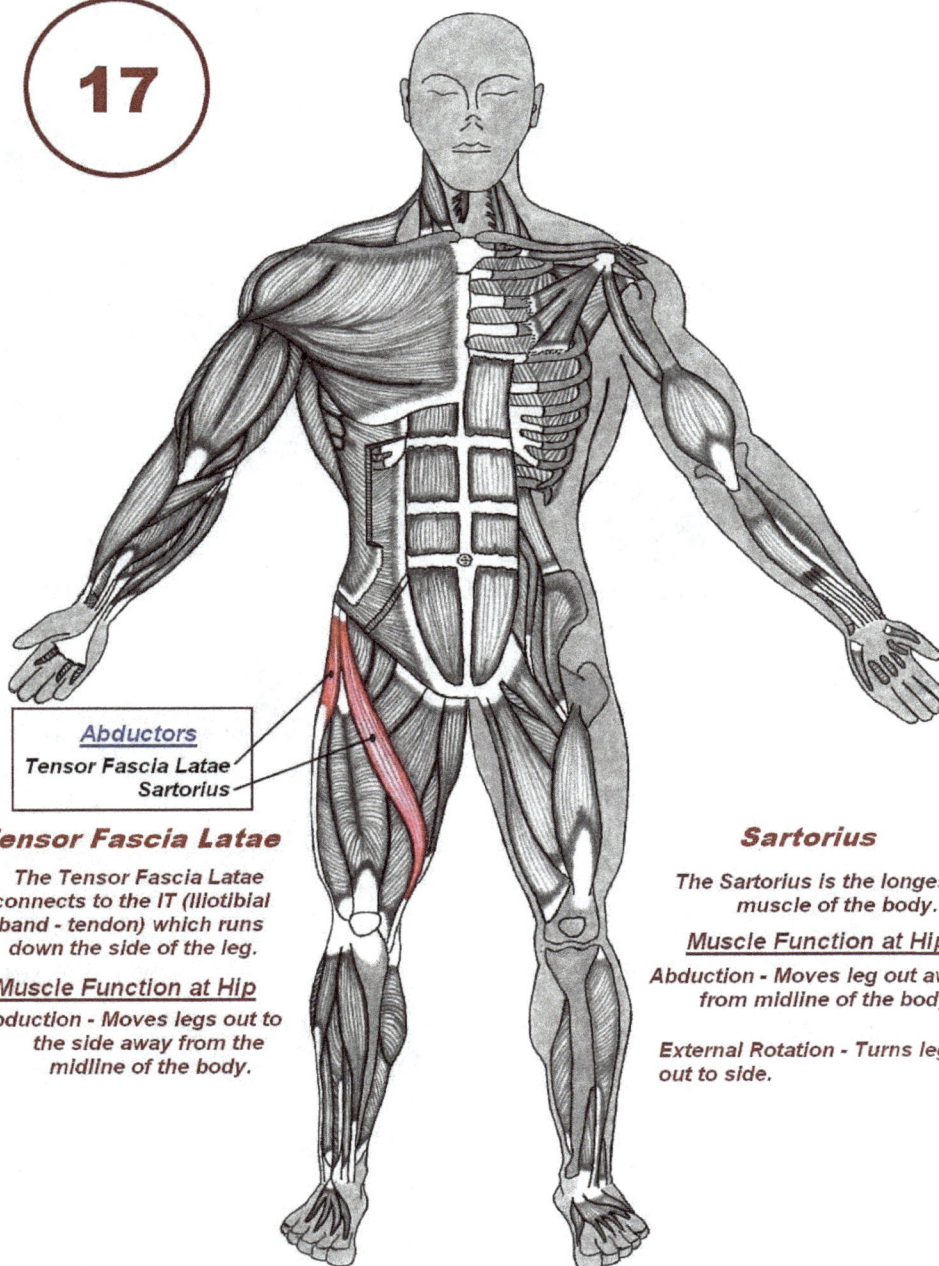

Abductors
Tensor Fascia Latae
Sartorius

Tensor Fascia Latae

The Tensor Fascia Latae connects to the IT (Iliotibial band - tendon) which runs down the side of the leg.

Muscle Function at Hip

Abduction - Moves legs out to the side away from the midline of the body.

Sartorius

The Sartorius is the longest muscle of the body.

Muscle Function at Hip

Abduction - Moves leg out away from midline of the body.

External Rotation - Turns leg out to side.

17 - Exercises

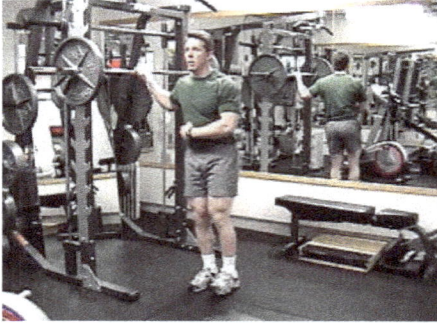
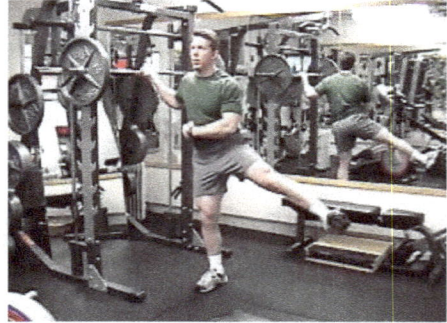

Standing Side Leg Raise (1-3 Sets 10-15 Reps)

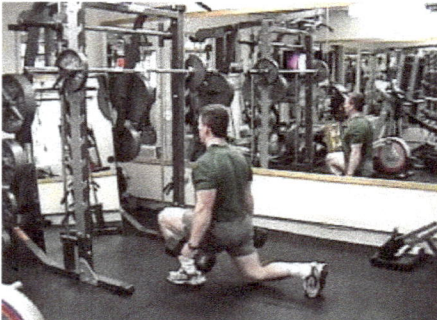
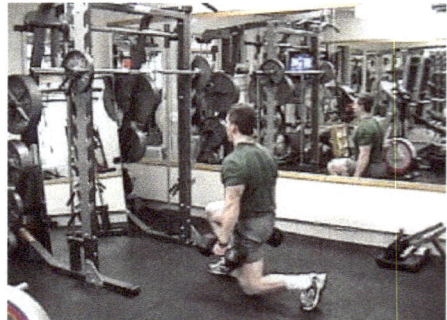

Alternating Dumbbell Lunge (Move Leg Out to Side: 1-3 Sets 7-10 Reps)

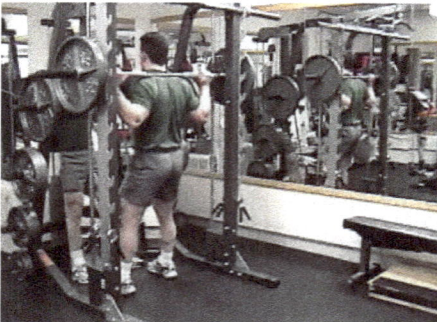
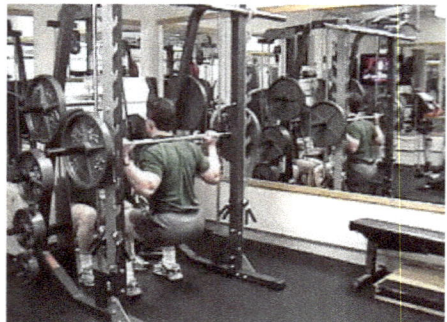

Leg Press With Smith Machine (Move Legs Apart: 1-5 Sets 7-10 Reps)

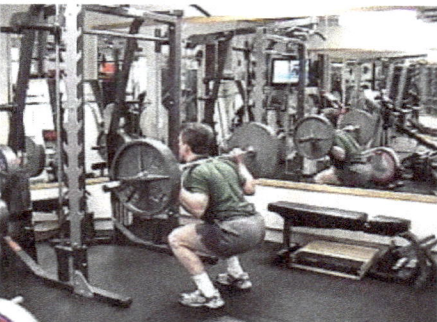
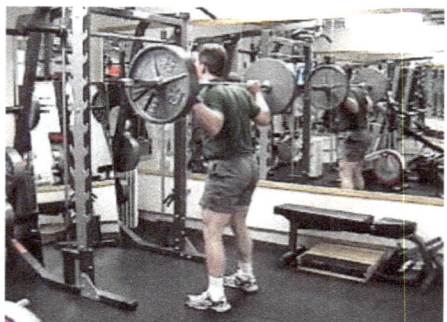

Free Weight Bar Squat (Move Legs Apart: 1-5 Sets 7-10 Reps)

56

17 - Exercises

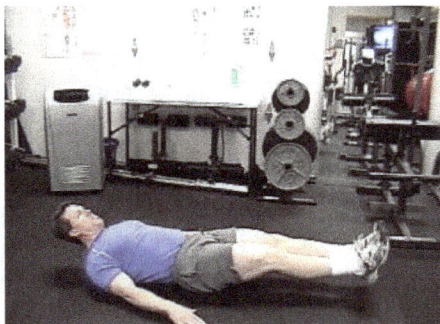

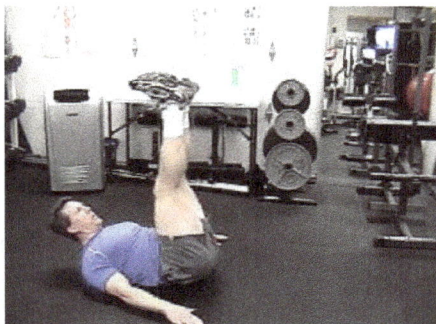

Straight Leg Lift on Floor (1-3 Sets 10-15 Reps)

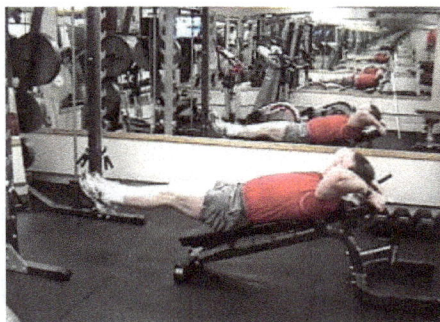

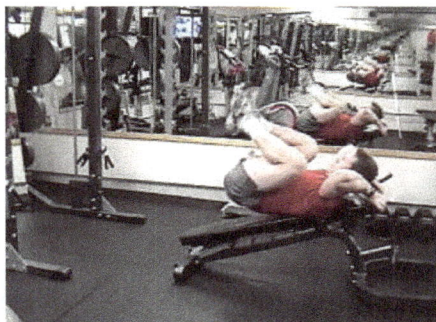

Reverse Crunch Incline Bench (Move Legs Up and Apart: 1-3 Sets 10-15 Reps)

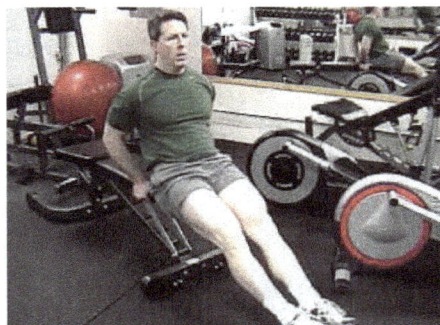

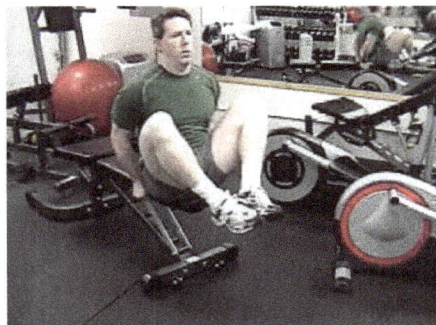

Seated Leg Tuck (Move Legs Up and Apart: 1-3 Sets 10-15 Reps)

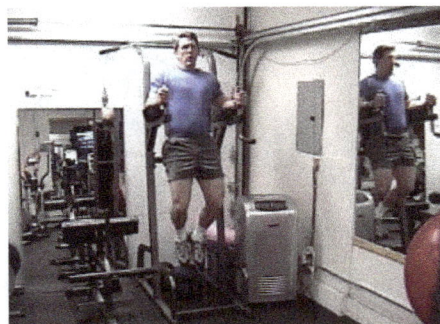

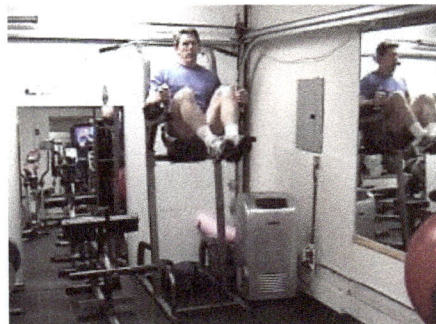

Upright Reverse Crunch (Move Legs Up and Apart: 1-3 Sets 10-15 Reps)

17 - Exercises

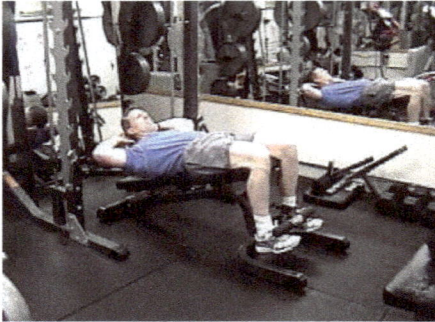

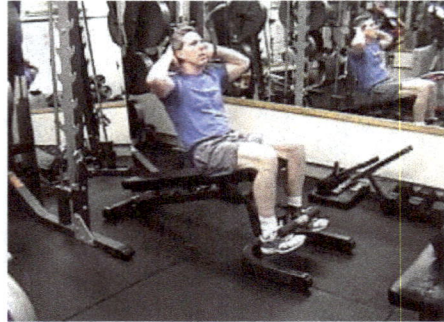

Decline Sit Ups (Hands support, but don't pull head: 1-3 Sets 10-30 Reps)

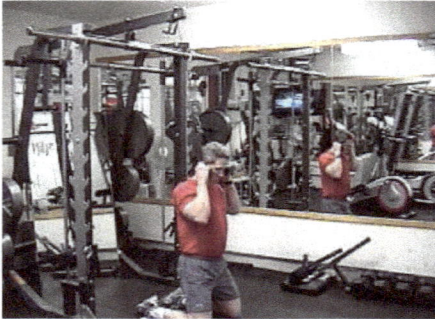

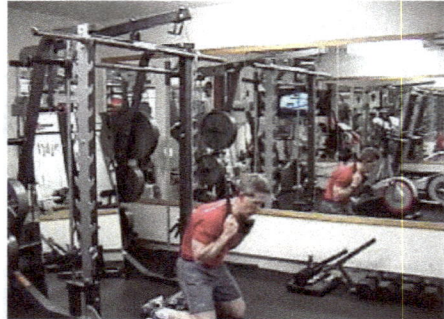

Kneeling Cable Crunch (1-3 Sets 10-30 Reps)

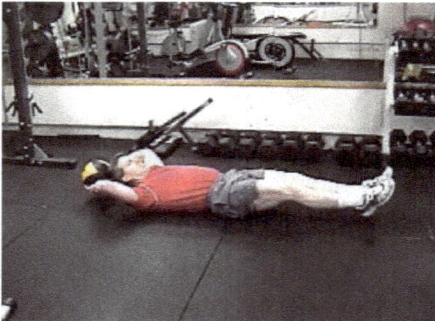

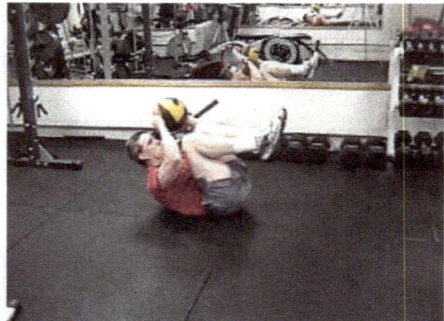

Medicine Ball Full Crunch (1-3 Sets 10-30 Reps)

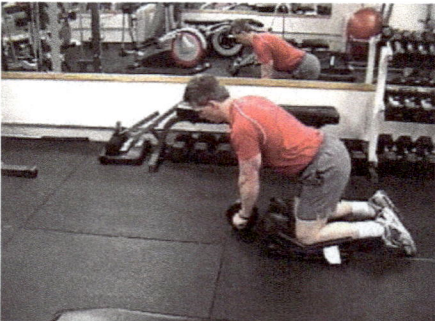

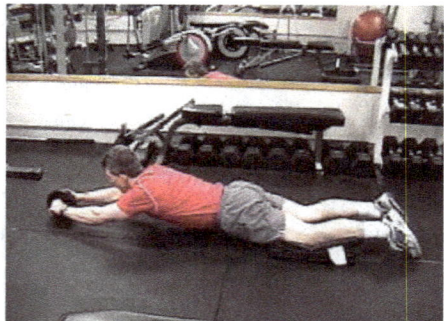

Ab Roller (1-3 Sets 7-10 Reps)

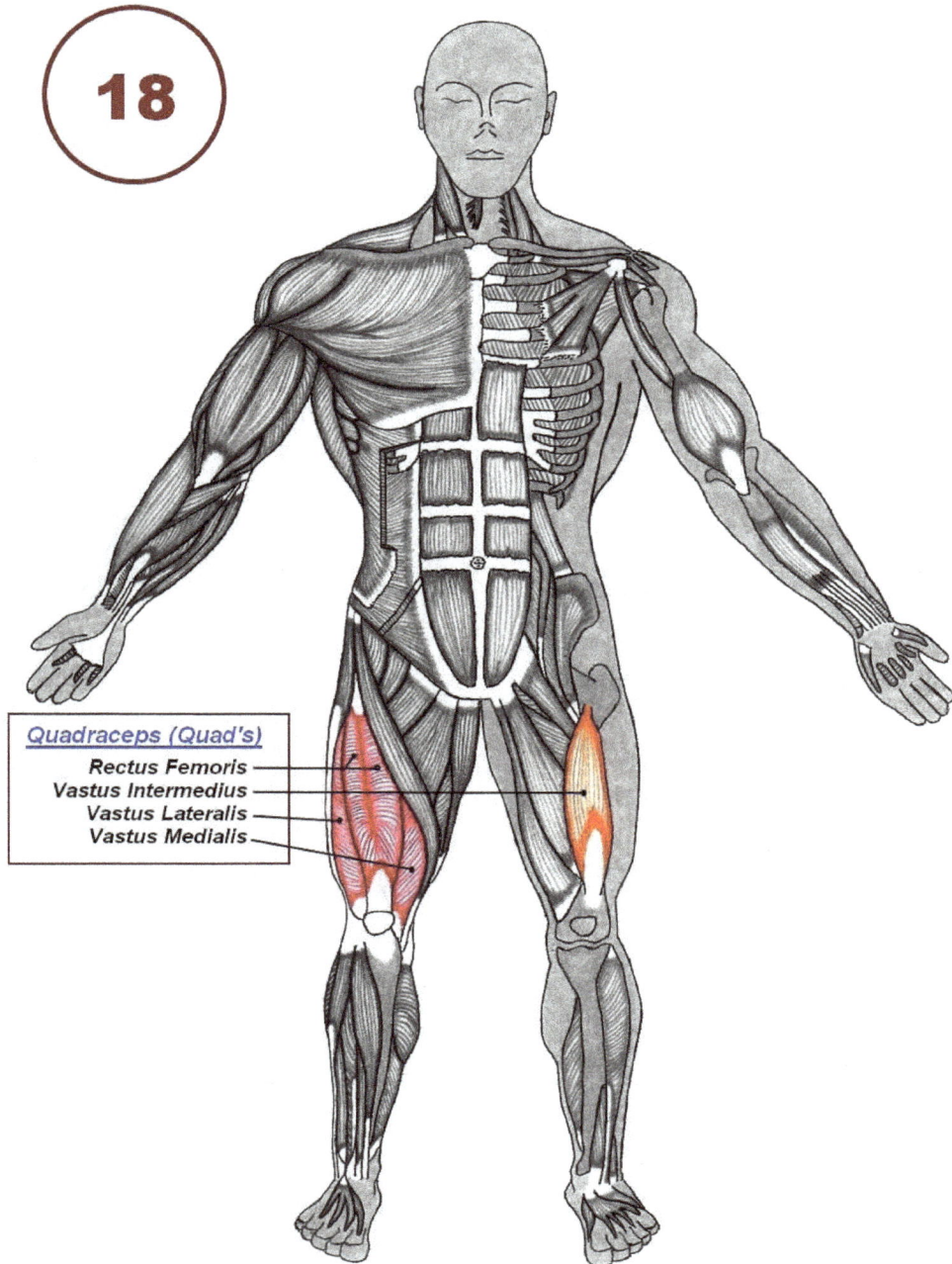

Quadraceps (Quad's)

18

Quadraceps (Quad's)
Rectus Femoris
Vastus Intermedius
Vastus Lateralis
Vastus Medialis

Quadraceps - Rectus Femoris

18A

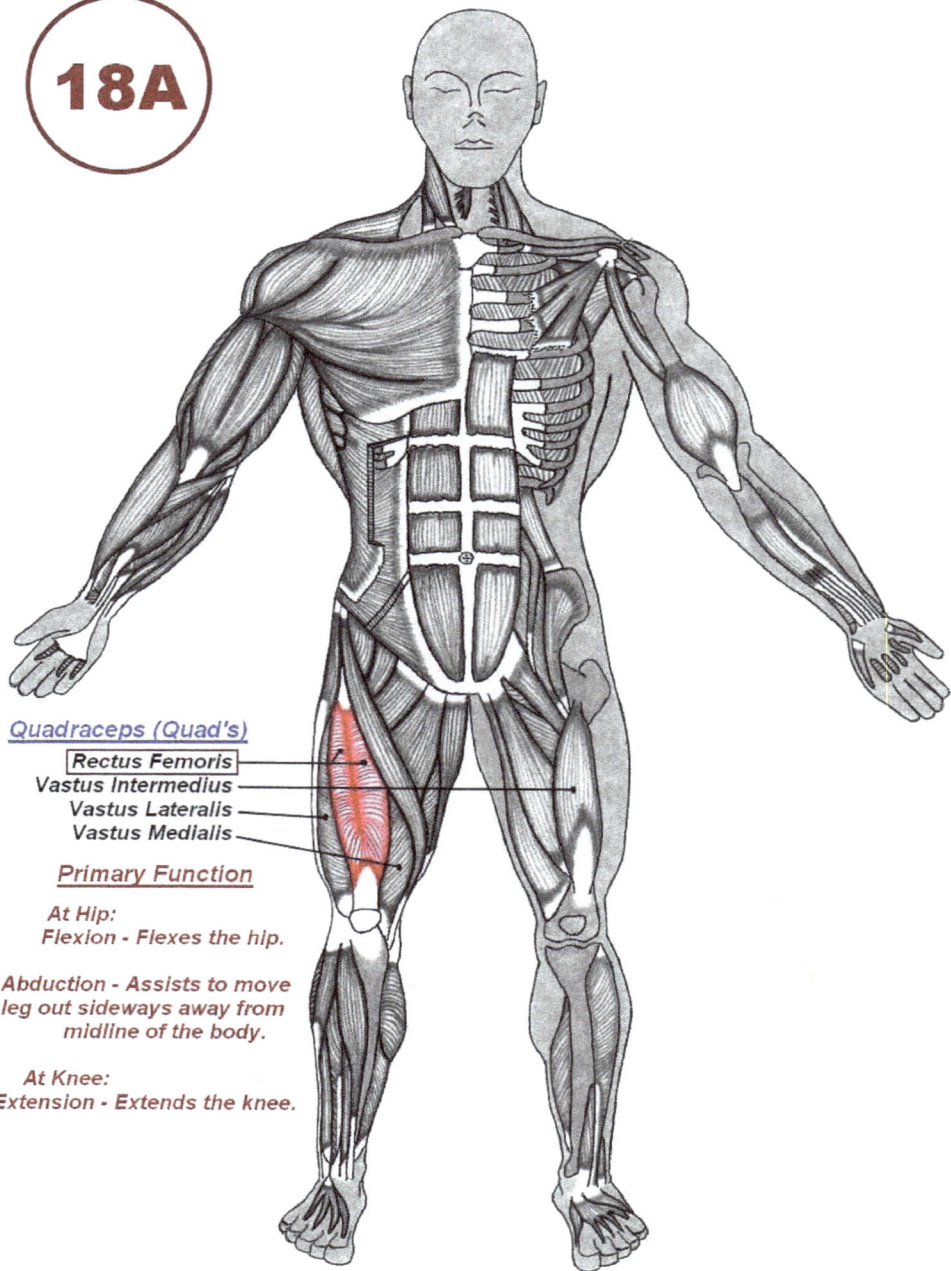

Quadraceps (Quad's)
Rectus Femoris
Vastus Intermedius
Vastus Lateralis
Vastus Medialis

Primary Function

At Hip:
Flexion - Flexes the hip.

Abduction - Assists to move
leg out sideways away from
midline of the body.

At Knee:
Extension - Extends the knee.

18A - Exercises

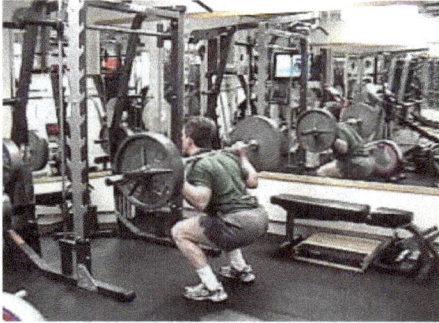

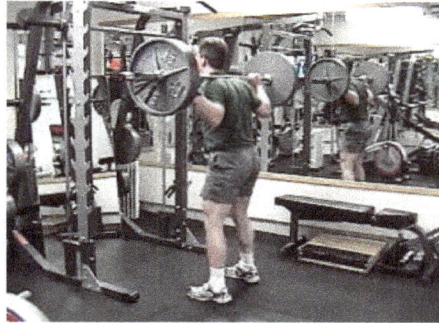

Free Weight Bar Squat (1-5 Sets 7-10 Reps)

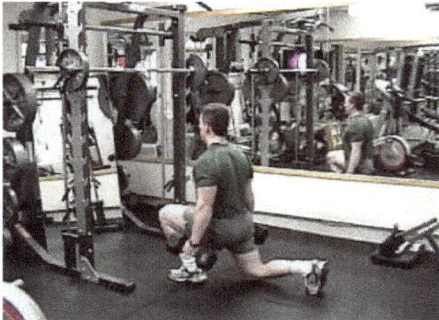

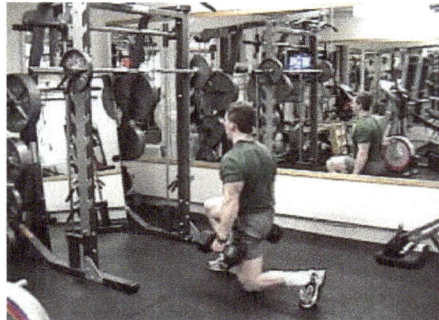

Alternating Dumbbell Lunge (1-3 Sets 7-10 Reps)

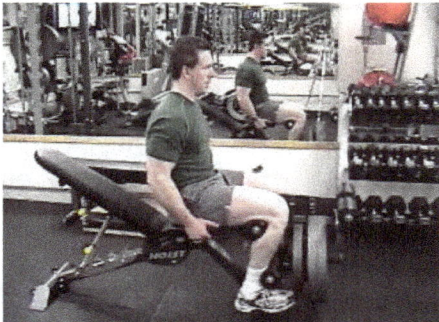

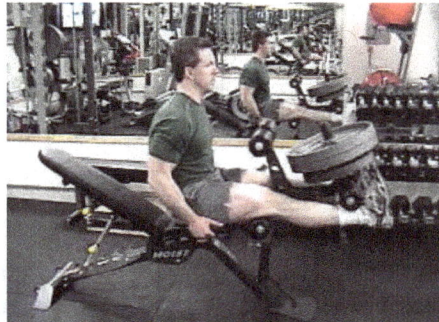

Leg Extension (1-3 Sets 7-10 Reps)

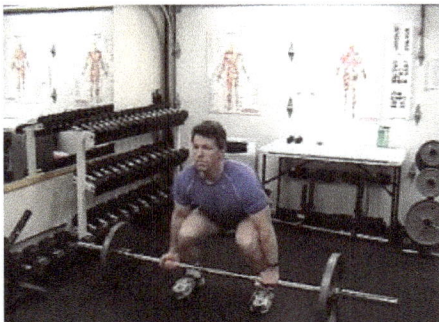

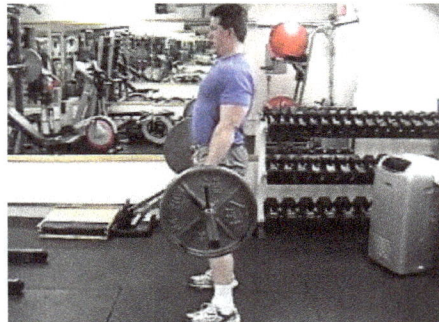

Dead-Lift (1-3 Sets 7-10 Reps)

18A - Exercises

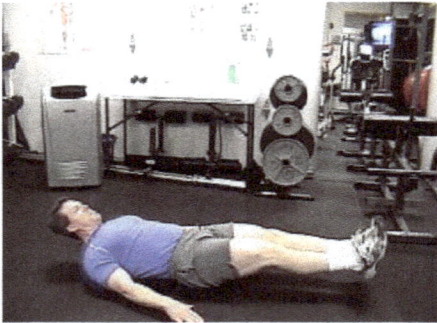

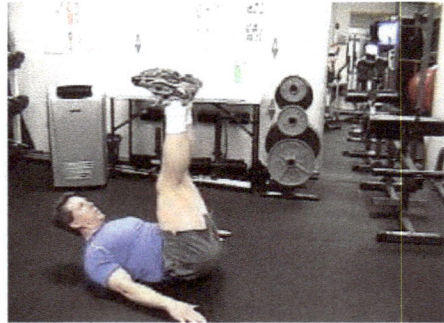

Straight Leg Lift on Floor (Hip Flexor: 1-3 Sets 10-15 Reps)

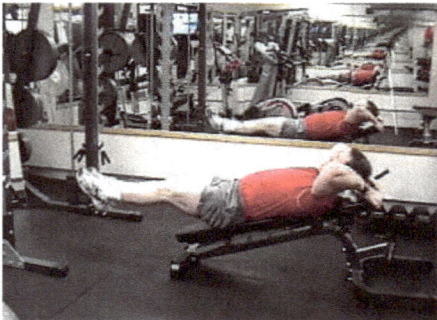

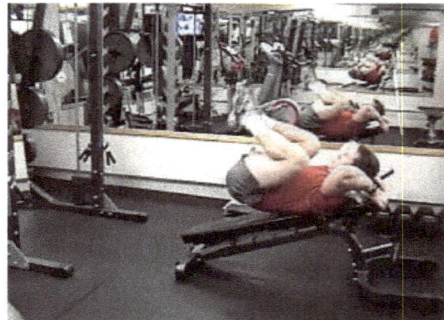

Reverse Crunch on Incline Bench (Hip Flexor: 1-3 Sets 10-15 Reps)

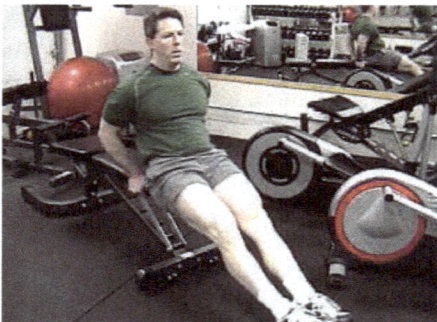

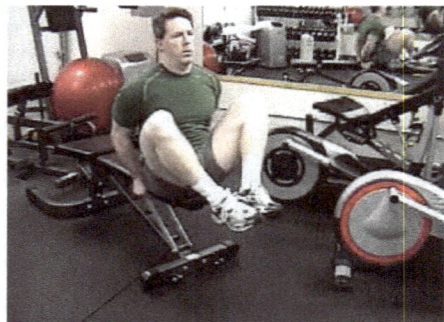

Seated Leg Tuck (Hip Flexor: 1-3 Sets 10-15 Reps)

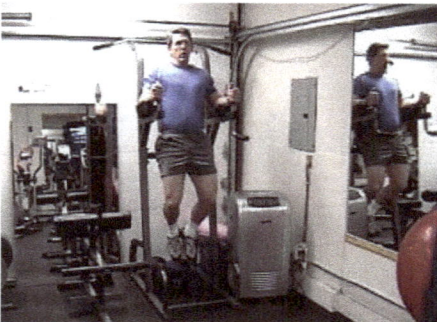

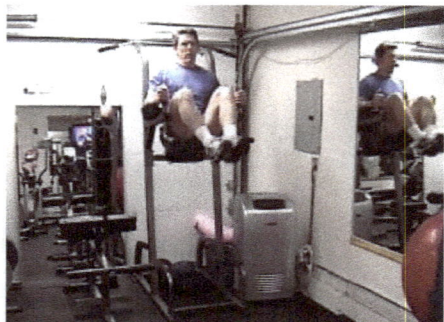

Upright Reverse Crunch (Hip Flexor: 1-3 Sets 10-15 Reps)

18A - Exercises

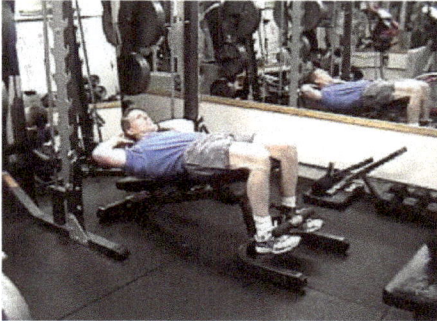

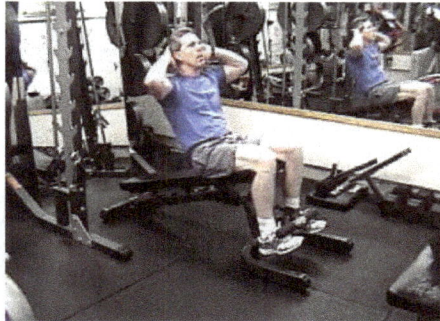

Decline Sit Ups (Hip Flexor: 1-3 Sets 10-30 Reps)

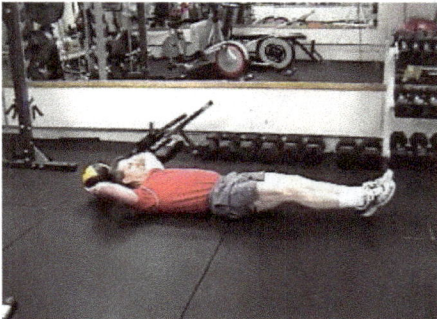

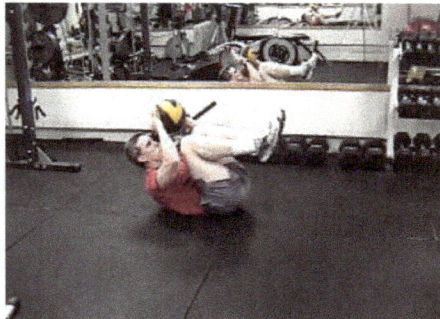

Medicine Ball Full Crunch (Hip Flexor: 1-3 Sets 10-30 Reps)

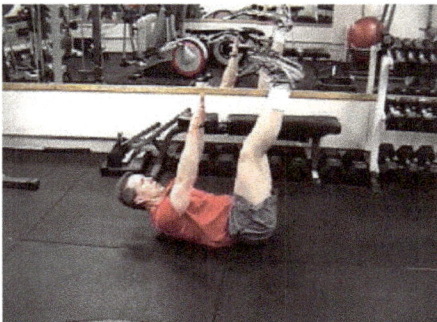

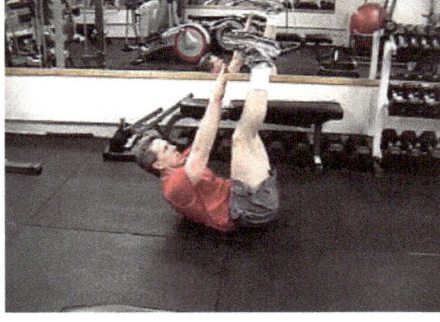

Partial V-Ups (Hip Flexor: 1-3 Sets 10-15 Reps)

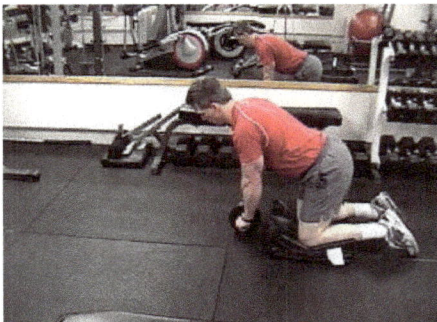

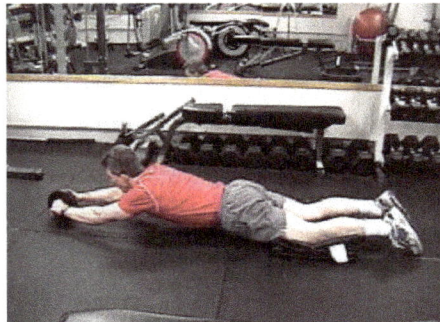

Ab Roller (Hip Flexor: 1-3 Sets 7-10 Reps)

Quadraceps - Vastus Lateralis

18B

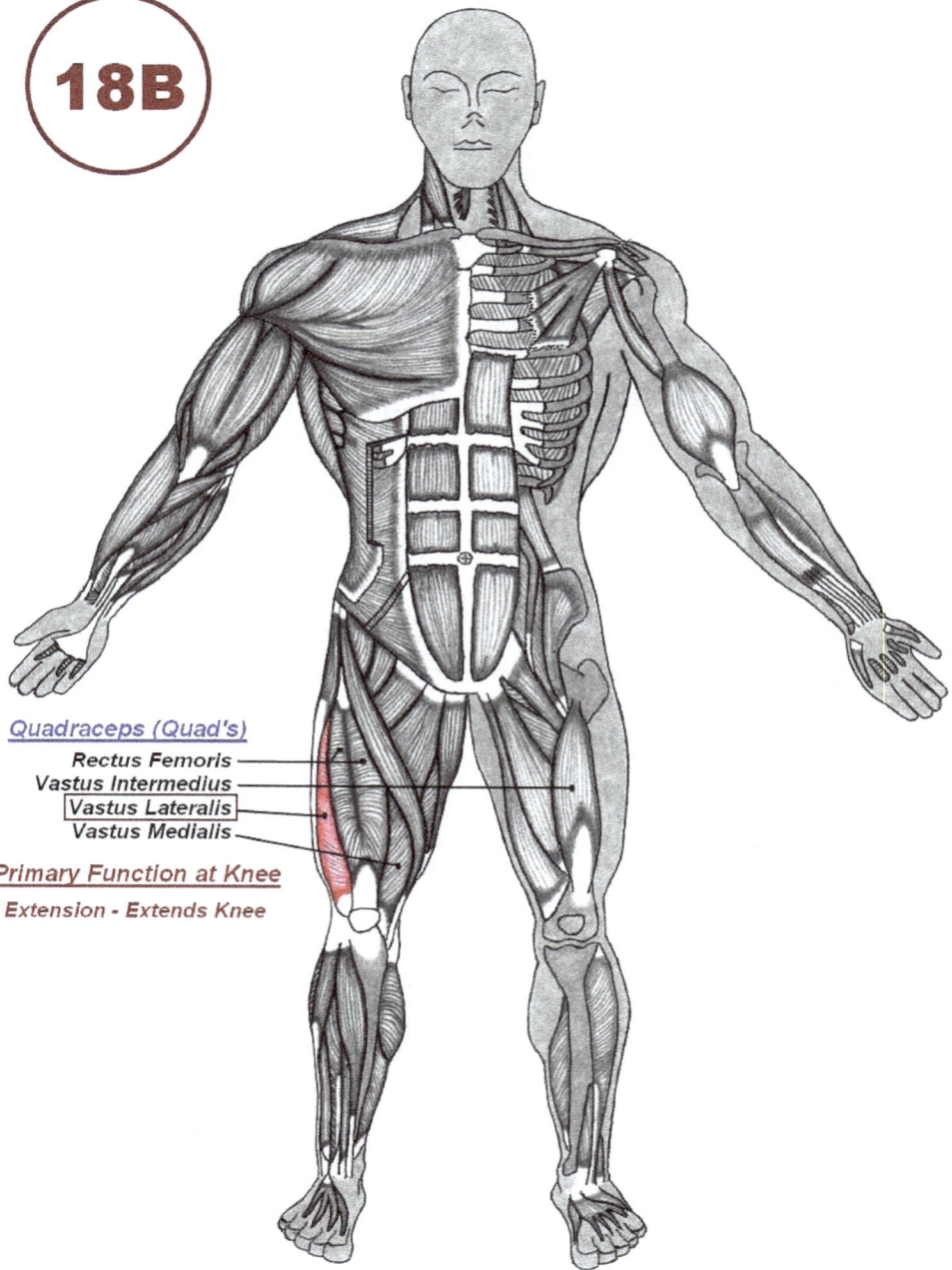

Quadraceps (Quad's)

Rectus Femoris
Vastus Intermedius
Vastus Lateralis
Vastus Medialis

Primary Function at Knee

Extension - Extends Knee

Quadraceps - Vastus Medialis

18C

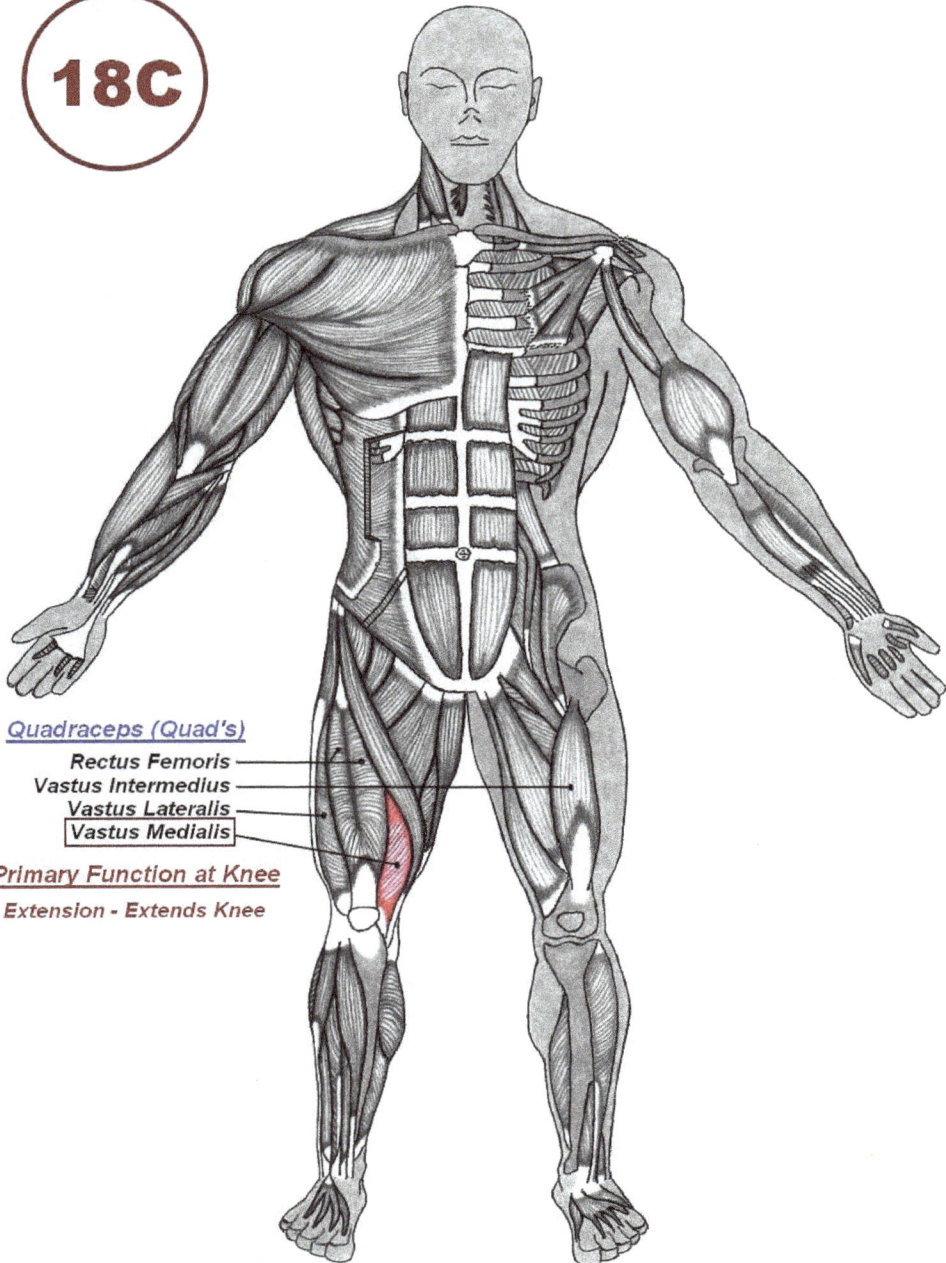

Quadraceps (Quad's)
Rectus Femoris
Vastus Intermedius
Vastus Lateralis
Vastus Medialis

Primary Function at Knee
Extension - Extends Knee

65

Quadraceps - Vastus Intermedius

18D

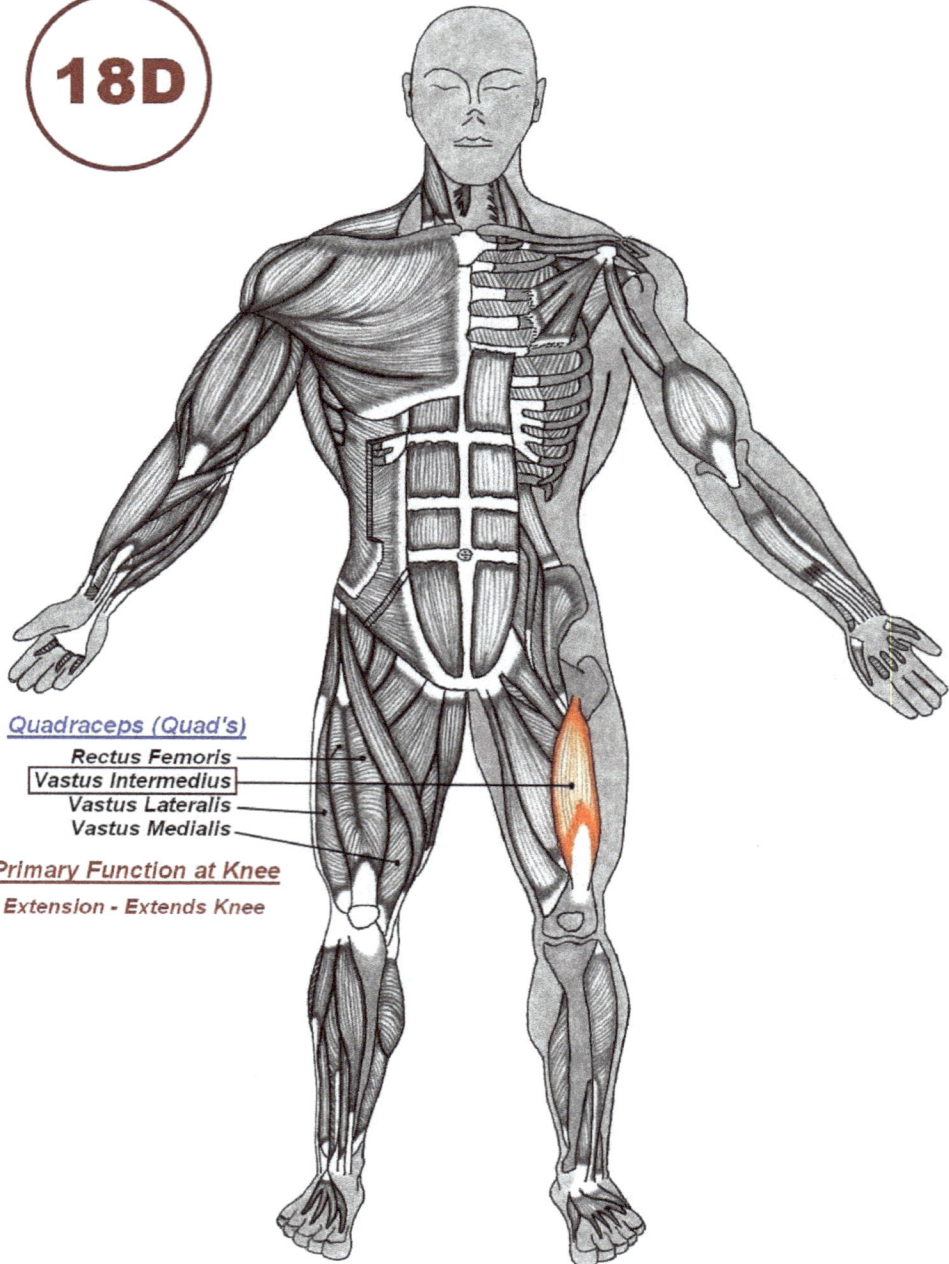

Quadraceps (Quad's)

Rectus Femoris
| Vastus Intermedius |
Vastus Lateralis
Vastus Medialis

Primary Function at Knee

Extension - Extends Knee

18B, C and D - Exercises

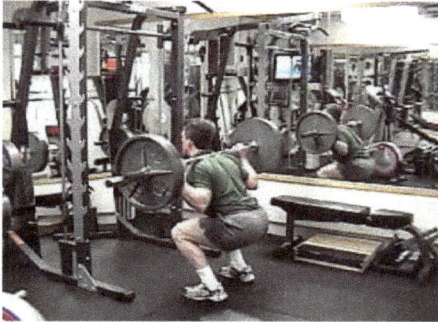

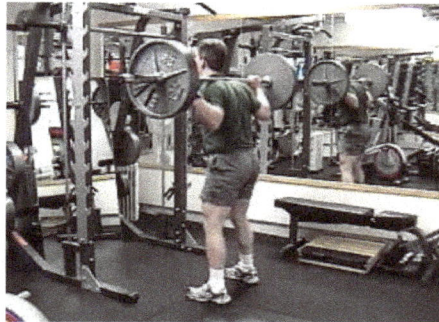

Free Weight Bar Squat (1-5 Sets 7-10 Reps)

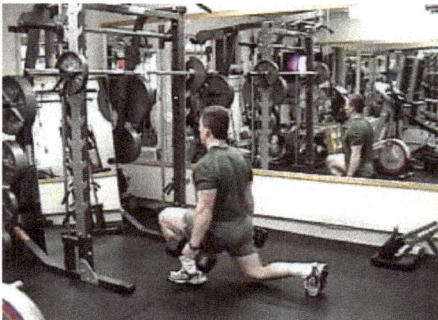

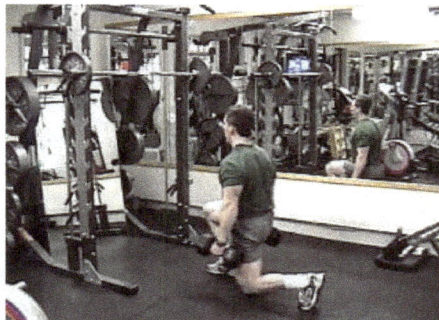

Alternating Dumbbell Lunge (1-3 Sets 7-10 Reps)

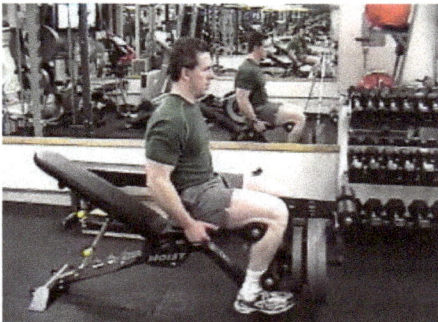

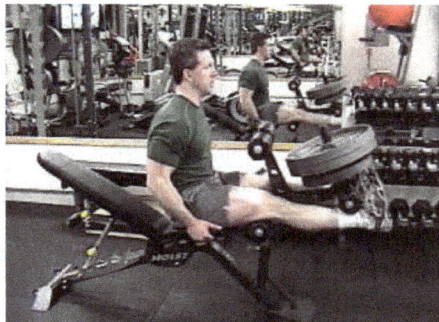

Leg Extension (1-3 Sets 7-10 Reps)

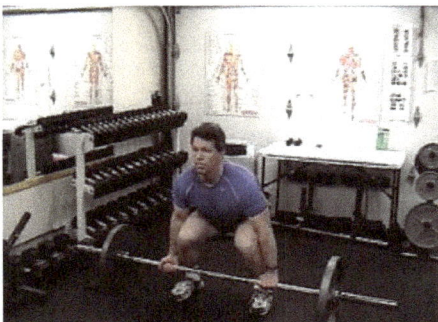

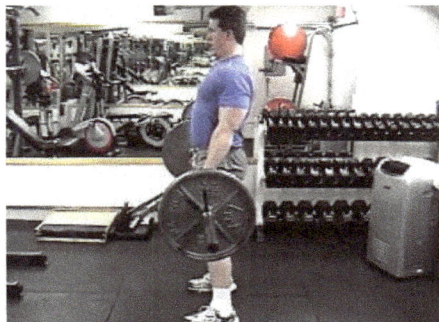

Dead-Lift (1-3 Sets 7-10 Reps)

Hip Adductors

19

The Adductors are the muscles usually felt during a groin strain.

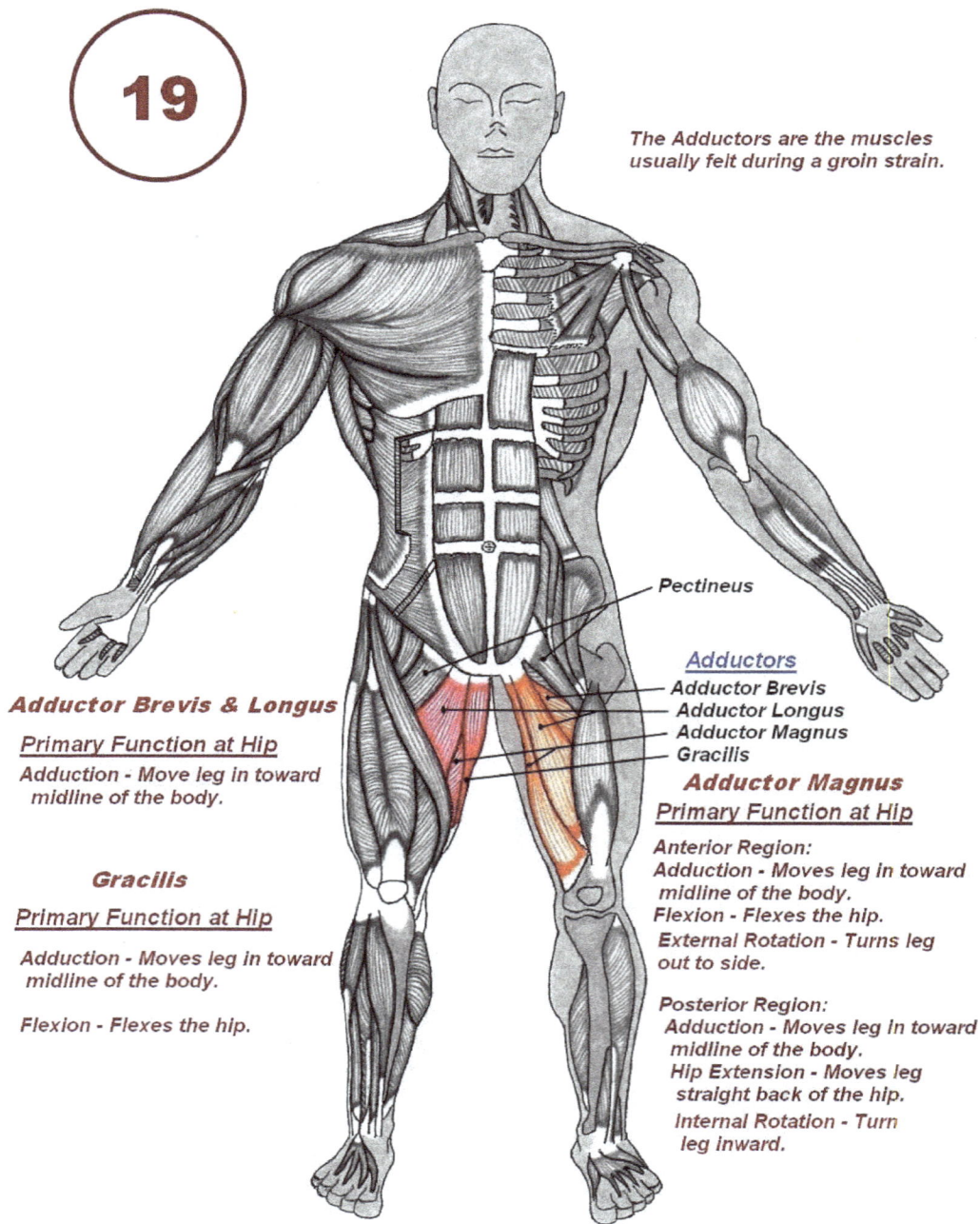

Pectineus

Adductors
Adductor Brevis
Adductor Longus
Adductor Magnus
Gracilis

Adductor Brevis & Longus

Primary Function at Hip

Adduction - Move leg in toward midline of the body.

Gracilis

Primary Function at Hip

Adduction - Moves leg in toward midline of the body.

Flexion - Flexes the hip.

Adductor Magnus

Primary Function at Hip

Anterior Region:
Adduction - Moves leg in toward midline of the body.
Flexion - Flexes the hip.
External Rotation - Turns leg out to side.

Posterior Region:
Adduction - Moves leg in toward midline of the body.
Hip Extension - Moves leg straight back of the hip.
Internal Rotation - Turn leg inward.

19 - Exercises

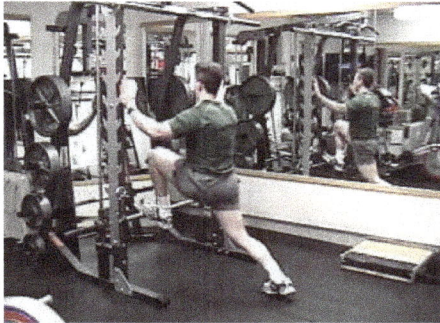

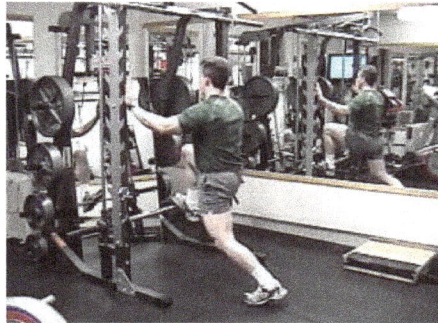

Step Against Locked Smith Bar (1-3 Sets 7-10 Reps)

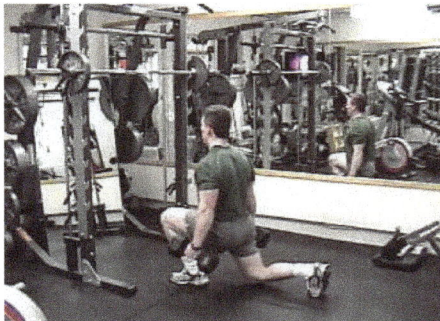

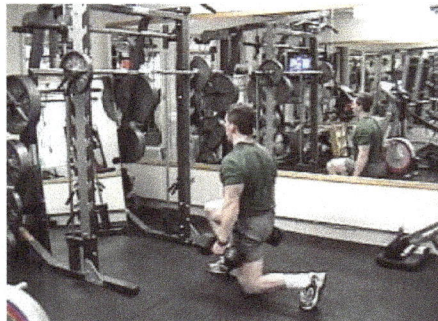

Alternating Dumbbell Lunge (1-3 Sets 7-10 Reps)

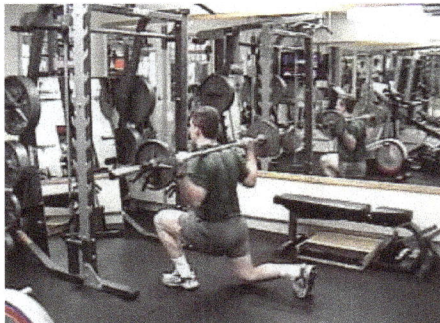

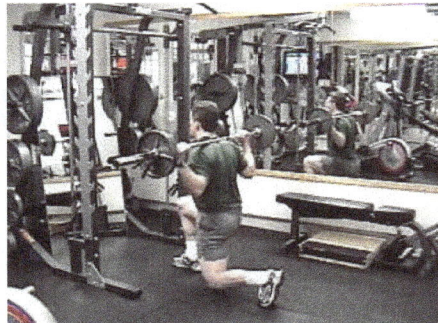

Alternating Bar Lunge (1-3 Sets 7-10 Reps)

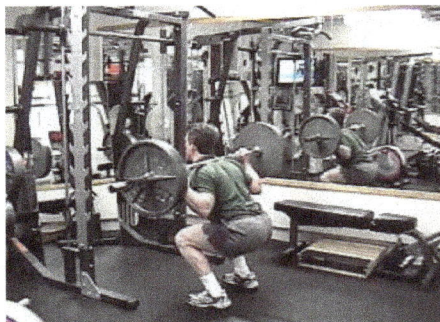

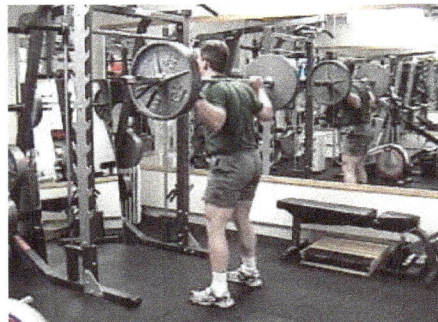

Free Weight Bar "Wide Stance" Power Squat (1-5 Sets 7-10 Reps)

Pectineus

20

Pectineus

Adductors
Adductor Brevis
Adductor Longus
Adductor Magnus
Gracilis

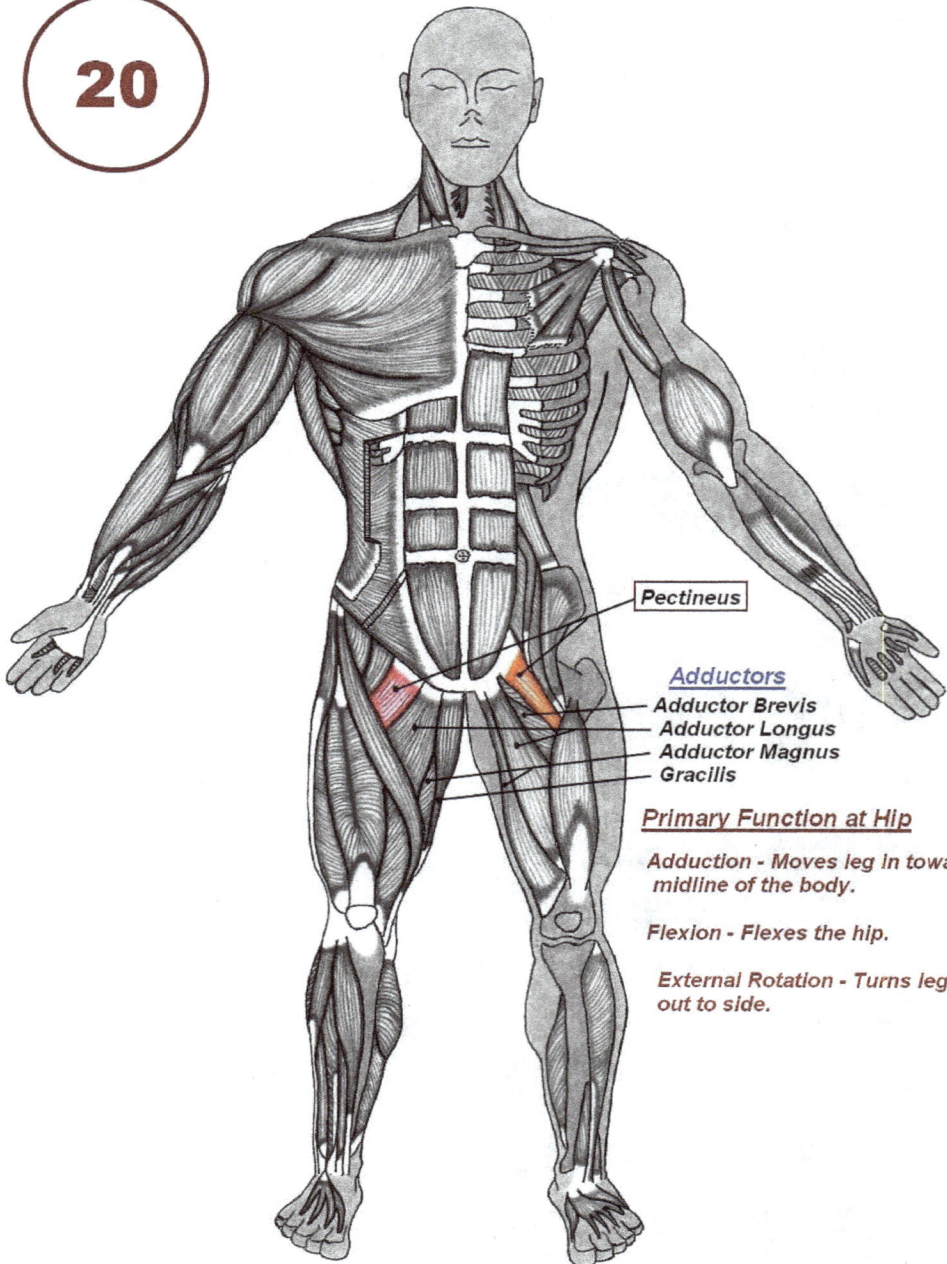

Primary Function at Hip

Adduction - Moves leg in toward midline of the body.

Flexion - Flexes the hip.

External Rotation - Turns leg out to side.

20 - Exercises

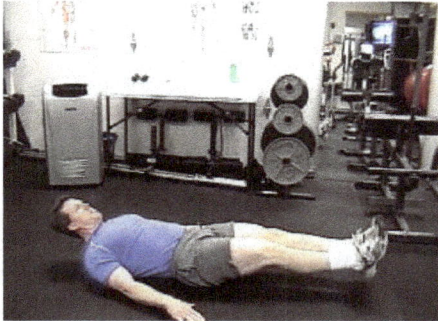

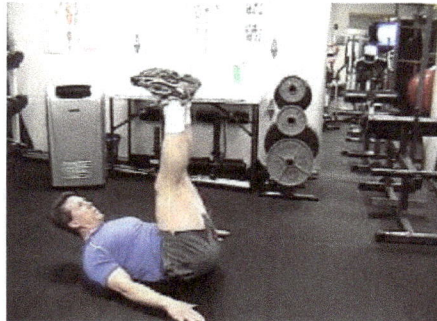

Leg Lift on Floor (Hip Flexor: 1-3 Sets 10-15 Reps)

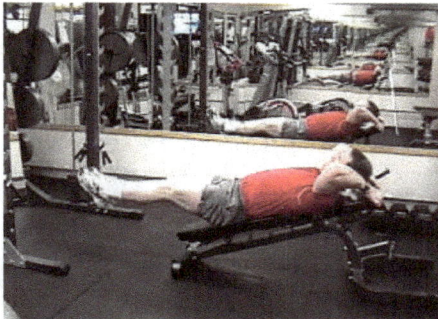

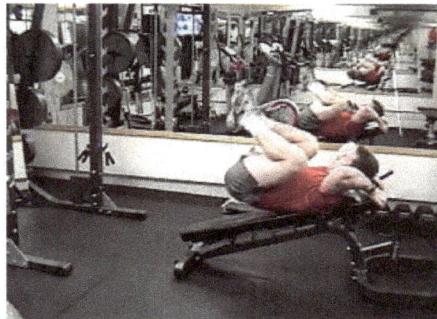

Reverse Crunch on Incline Bench (Hip Flexor: 1-3 Sets 10-15 Reps)

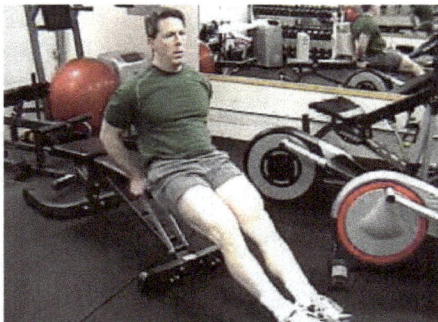

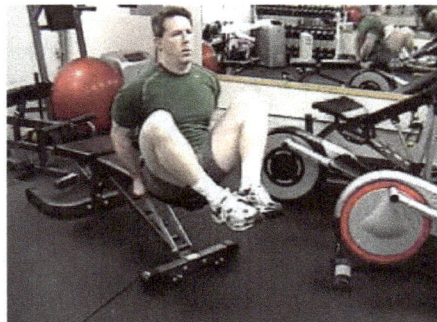

Seated Leg Tuck (Hip Flexor: 1-3 Sets 10-15 Reps)

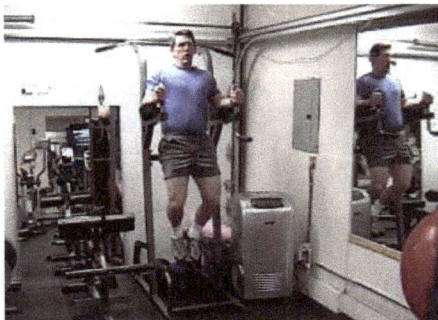

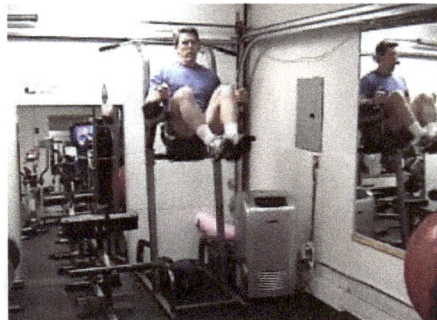

Upright Reverse Crunch (Hip Flexor: 1-3 Sets 10-15 Reps)

20 - Exercises

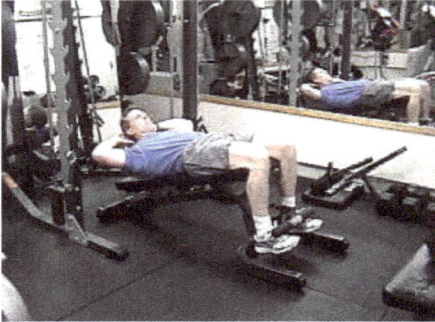

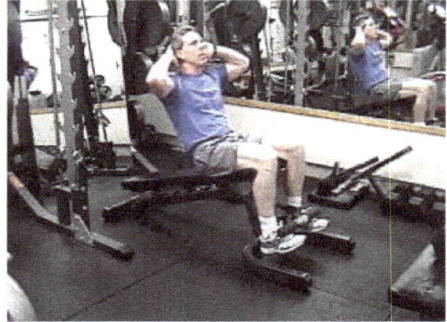

Decline Sit Ups (Hip Flexor: 1-3 Sets 10-30 Reps)

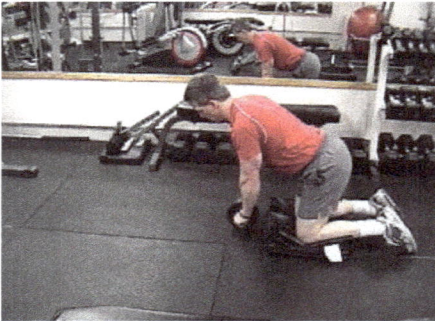

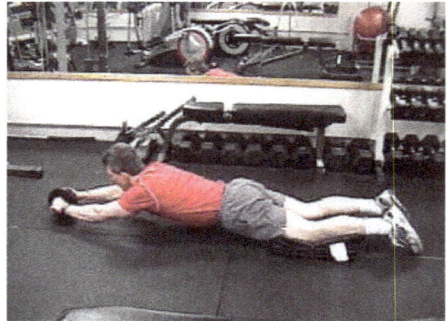

Ab Roller (Hip Flexor: 1-3 Sets 7-10 Reps)

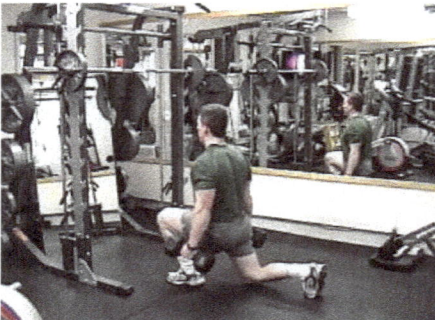

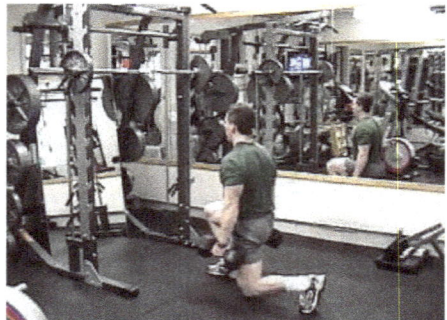

Alternating Dumbbell Lunge (Adductor: 1-3 Sets 7-10 Reps)

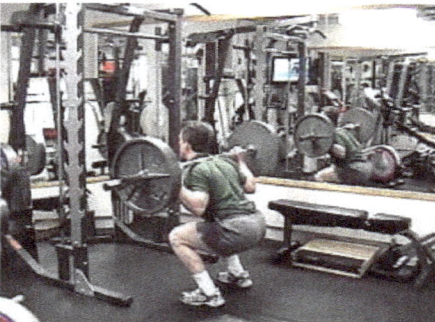

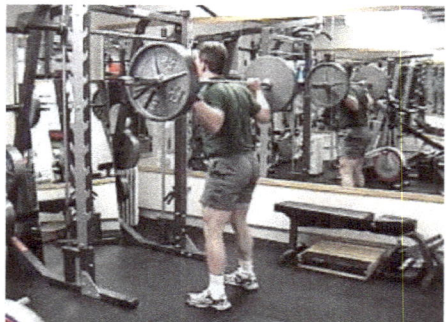

Free Weight Bar "Wide Stance" Power Squat (Adductor: 1-5 Sets 7-10 Reps)

Lower Leg - Tibialis Anterior

21

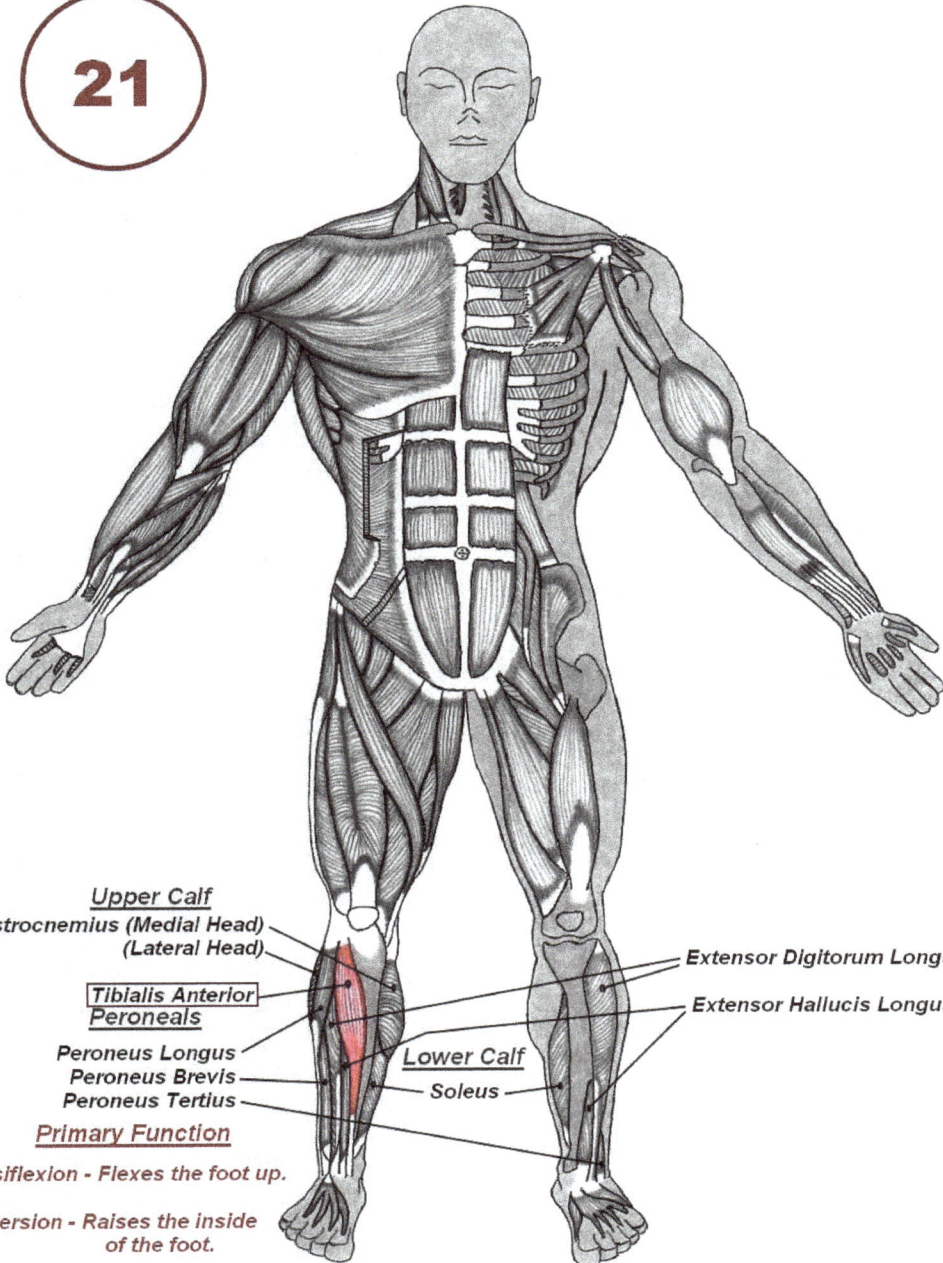

Upper Calf
Gastrocnemius (Medial Head)
(Lateral Head)

Extensor Digitorum Longus

Tibialis Anterior
Peroneals

Extensor Hallucis Longus

Peroneus Longus
Peroneus Brevis
Peroneus Tertius

Lower Calf
Soleus

Primary Function

Dorsiflexion - Flexes the foot up.

Inversion - Raises the inside
of the foot.

73

21 - Exercises

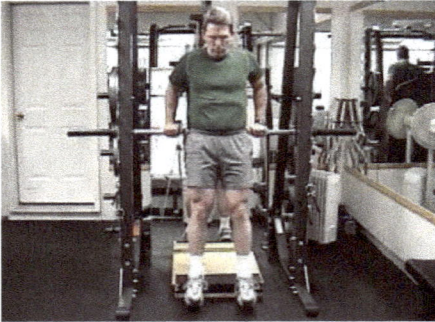

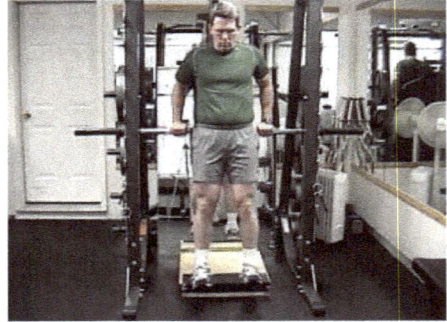

Tibialis Crunch (Flex Foot Up and Invert at Top: 1-3 Sets 10-20 Reps)

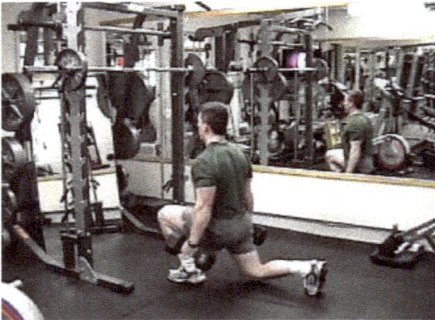

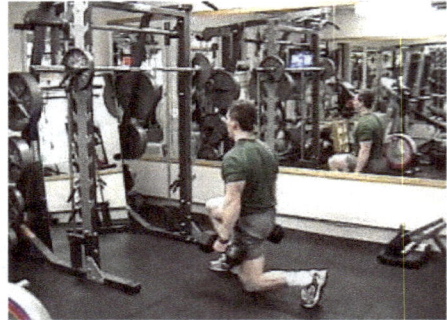

Alternating Dumbbell Lunge (Extend Foot Stepping Out: 1-3 Sets 7-10 Reps)

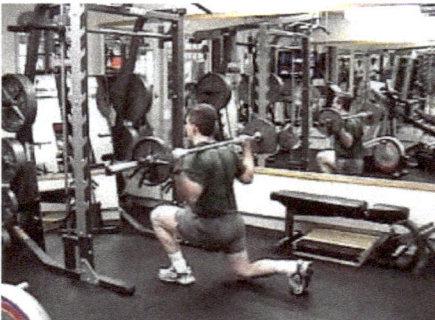

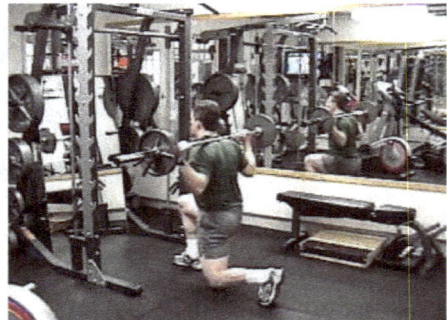

Alternating Bar Lunge (Extend Toes and Foot, Balancing: 1-3 Sets 7-10 Reps)

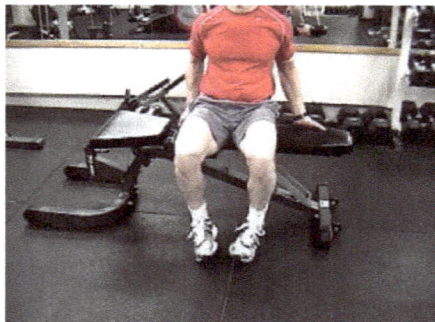

Definition: Inversion "Invert" (Lift Inside of Foot)

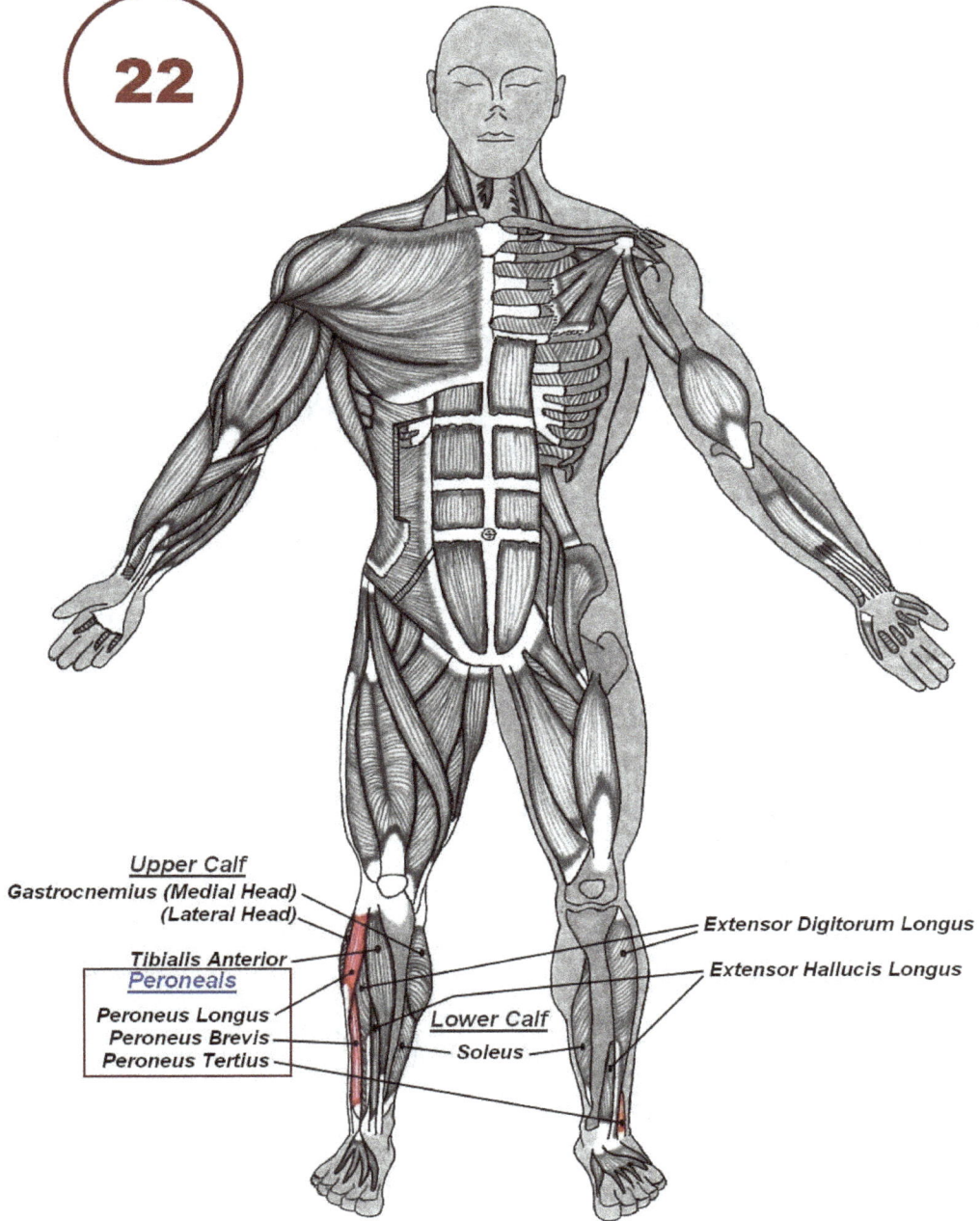

Lower Leg Peroneal Muscles

22

Upper Calf
Gastrocnemius (Medial Head)
(Lateral Head)

Tibialis Anterior
Peroneals

Peroneus Longus
Peroneus Brevis
Peroneus Tertius

Lower Calf
Soleus

Extensor Digitorum Longus
Extensor Hallucis Longus

75

Lower Leg Peroneals - Peroneus Longus

22A

Upper Calf
Gastrocnemius (Medial Head)
(Lateral Head)

Tibialis Anterior
Peroneals

Peroneus Longus
Peroneus Brevis
Peroneus Tertius

Extensor Digitorum Longus

Extensor Hallucis Longus

Lower Calf
Soleus

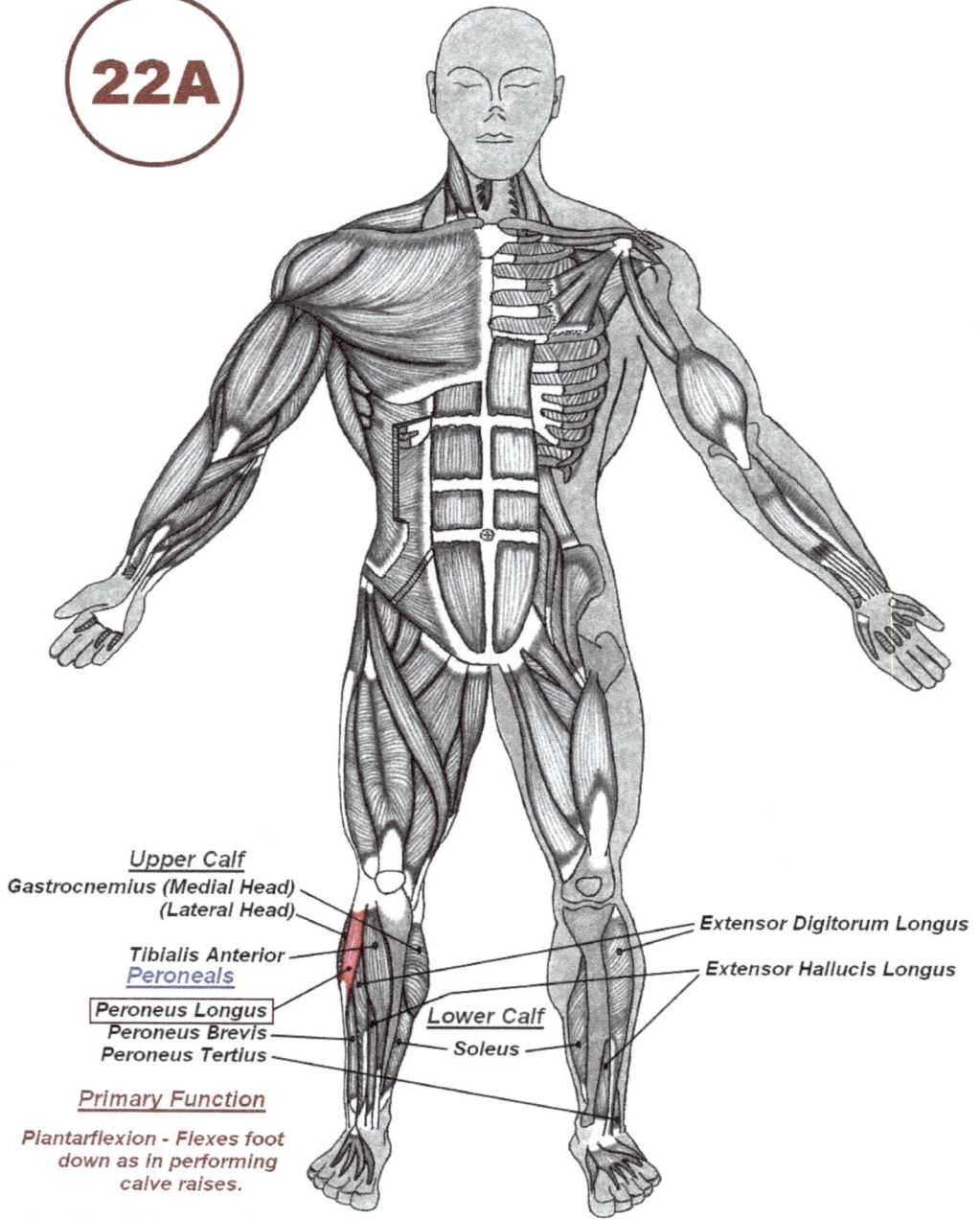

Primary Function

Plantarflexion - Flexes foot
down as in performing
calve raises.

Eversion - Raises outside
of foot.

Lower Leg Peroneals - Peroneus Brevis

22B

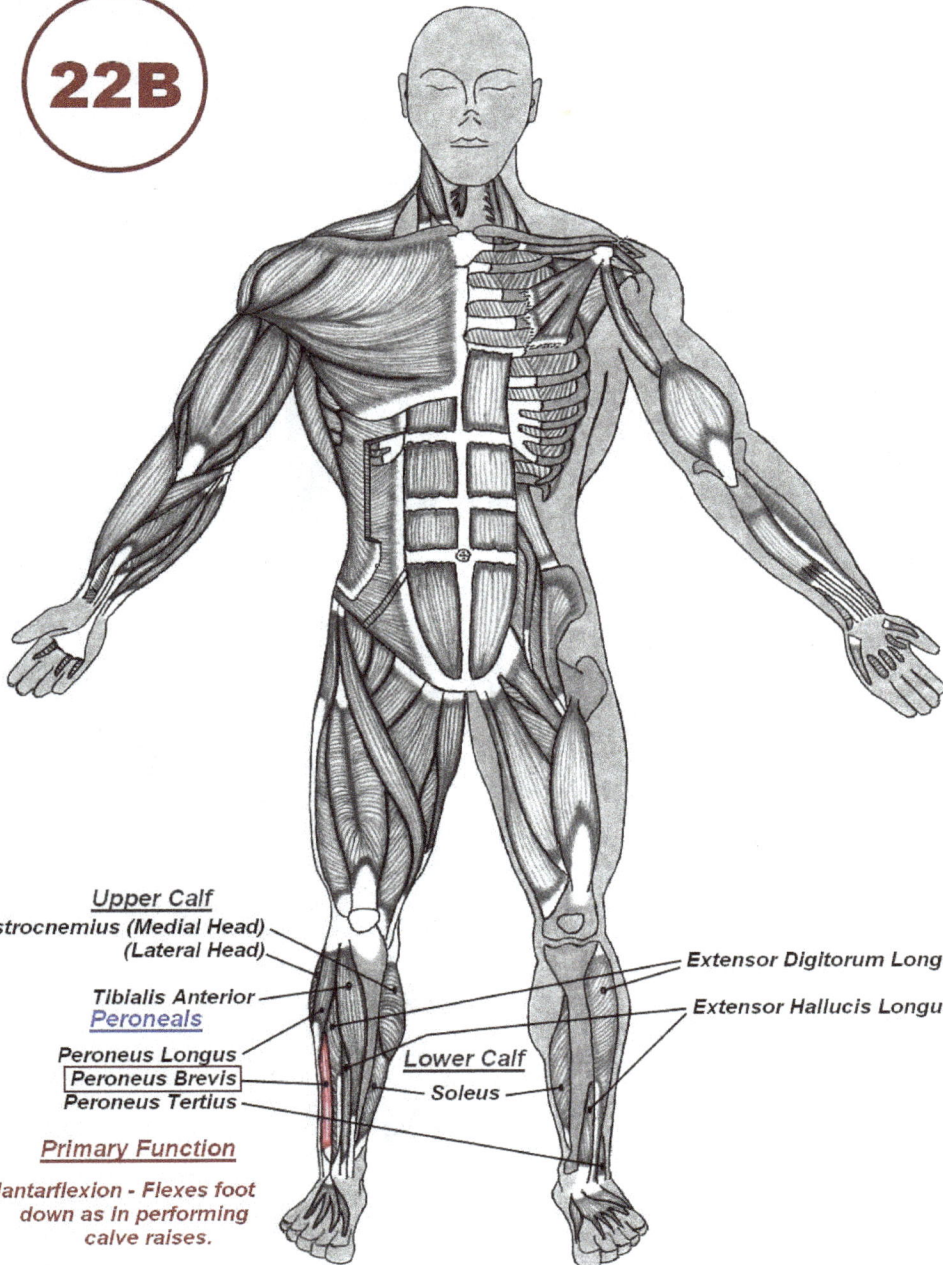

Upper Calf
Gastrocnemius (Medial Head)
(Lateral Head)

Tibialis Anterior
<u>Peroneals</u>

Peroneus Longus
| Peroneus Brevis |
Peroneus Tertius

Extensor Digitorum Longus

Extensor Hallucis Longus

Lower Calf
Soleus

<u>Primary Function</u>

Plantarflexion - Flexes foot
down as in performing
calve raises.

Eversion - Raises outside
of foot.

22A and B - Exercises

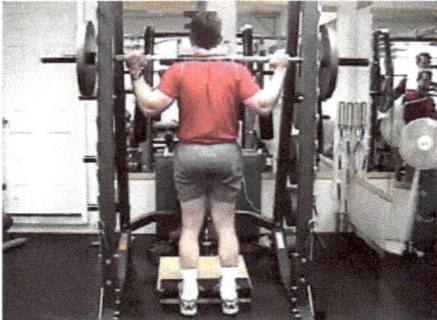
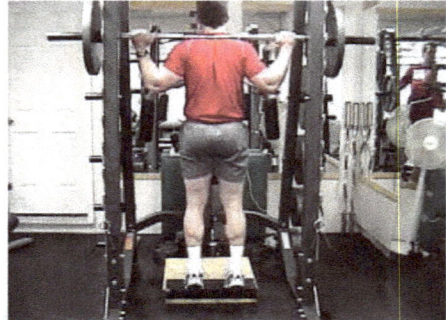

Standing Weighted Calve Raise (Flex Bottom of Foot: 1-3 Sets 10-15 Reps)

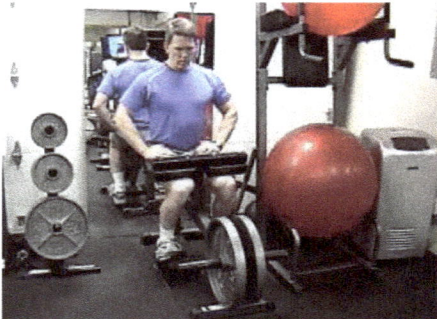
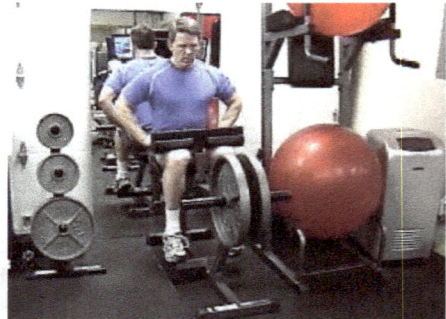

Seated Calve Raise (Flex Bottom of Foot: 1-3 Sets 10-15 Reps)

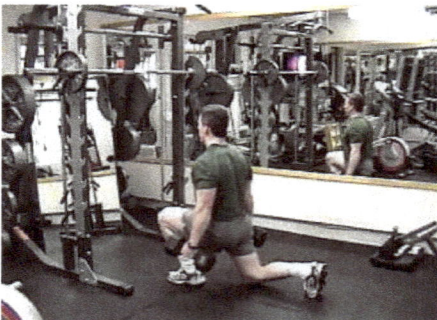
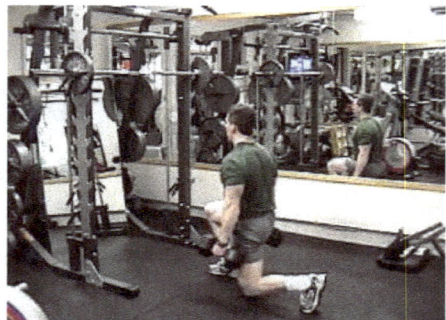

Alternating Dumbbell Lunge (Involved in Balancing: 1-3 Sets 7-10 Reps)

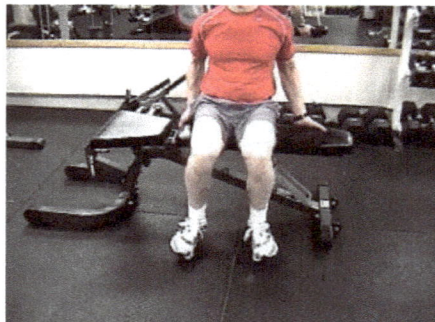

Definition: Eversion "Evert" (Lift Outside of Foot)

Lower Leg Peroneals - Peroneus Tertius

22C

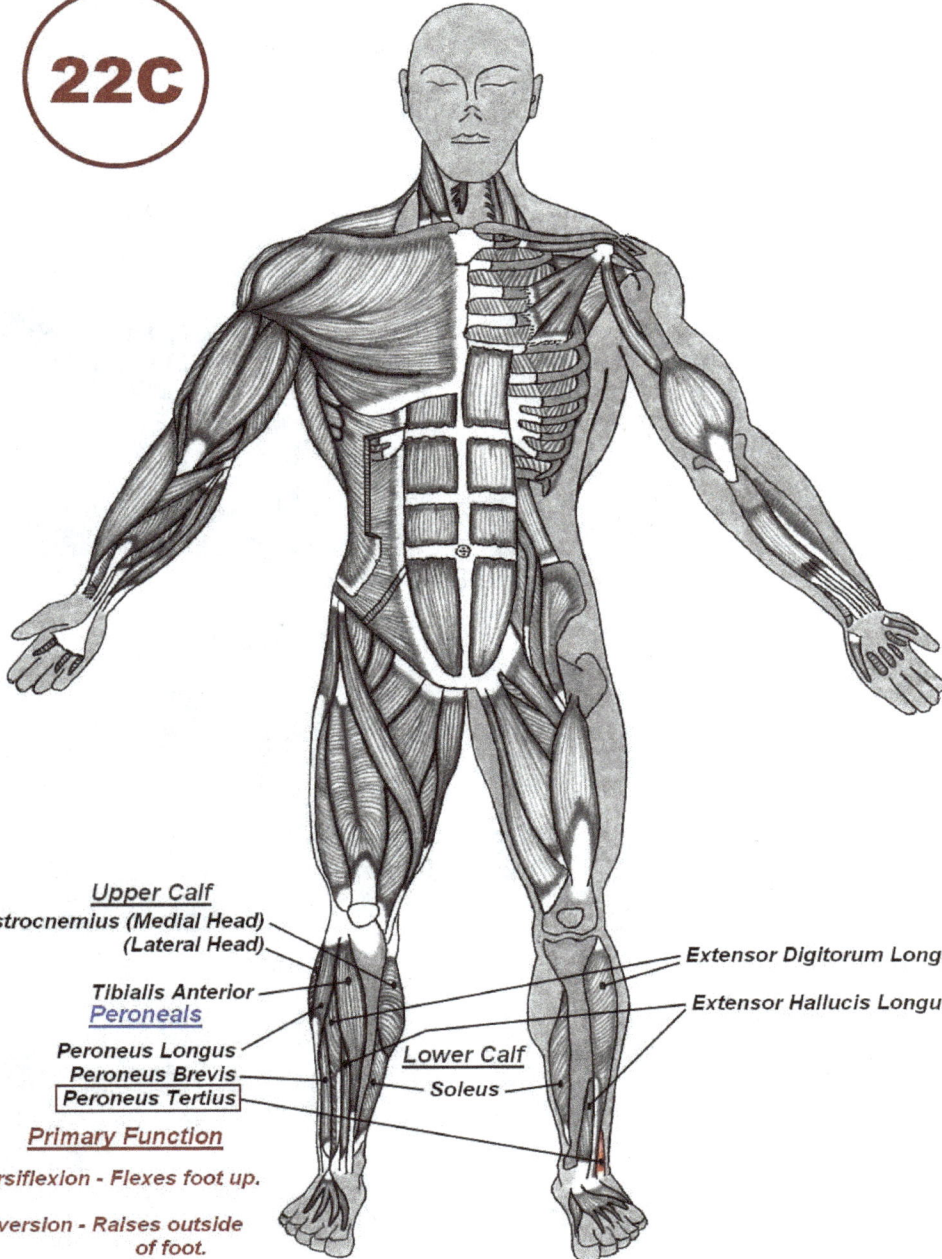

Upper Calf
Gastrocnemius (Medial Head)
(Lateral Head)

Tibialis Anterior
Peroneals

Peroneus Longus
Peroneus Brevis
Peroneus Tertius

Lower Calf
Soleus

Extensor Digitorum Longus

Extensor Hallucis Longus

Primary Function

Dorsiflexion - Flexes foot up.

Eversion - Raises outside of foot.

22C - Exercises

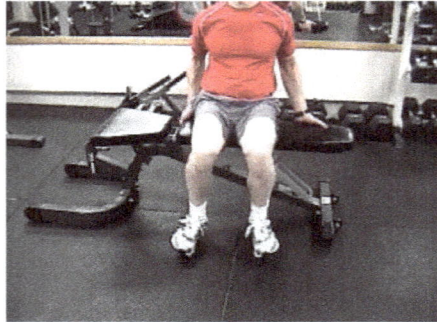

Definition: Eversion "Evert" (Lift Outside of Foot)

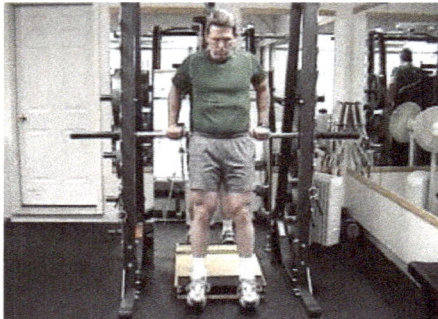

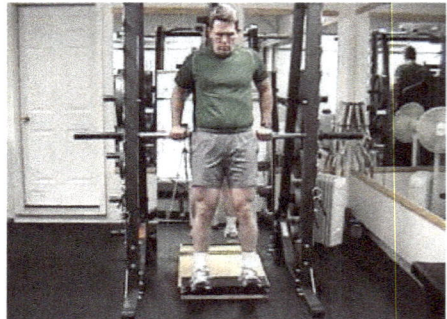

Tibialis Crunch (Flex Foot Up and Evert at Top: 1-3 Sets 10-20 Reps)

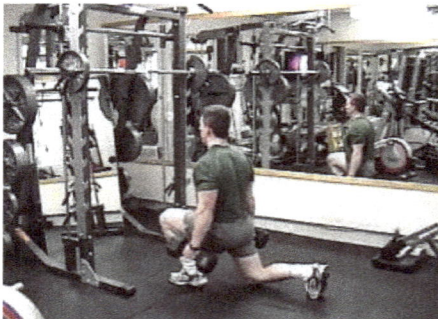

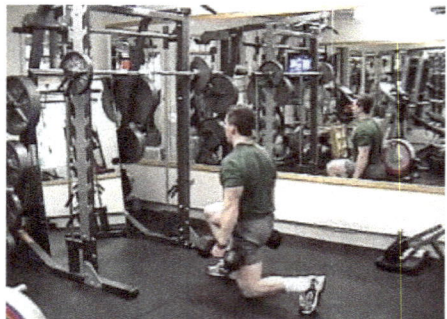

Alternating Dumbbell Lunge (Involved in Balancing: 1-3 Sets 7-10 Reps)

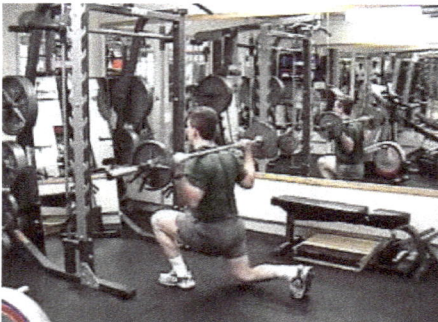

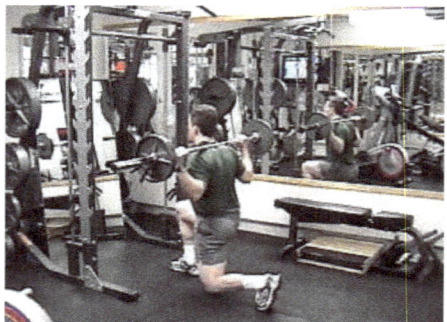

Alternating Bar Lunge (Extend Toes and Foot, Balancing: 1-3 Sets 7-10 Reps)

Lower Leg - Extensor Digitorum Longus

23A

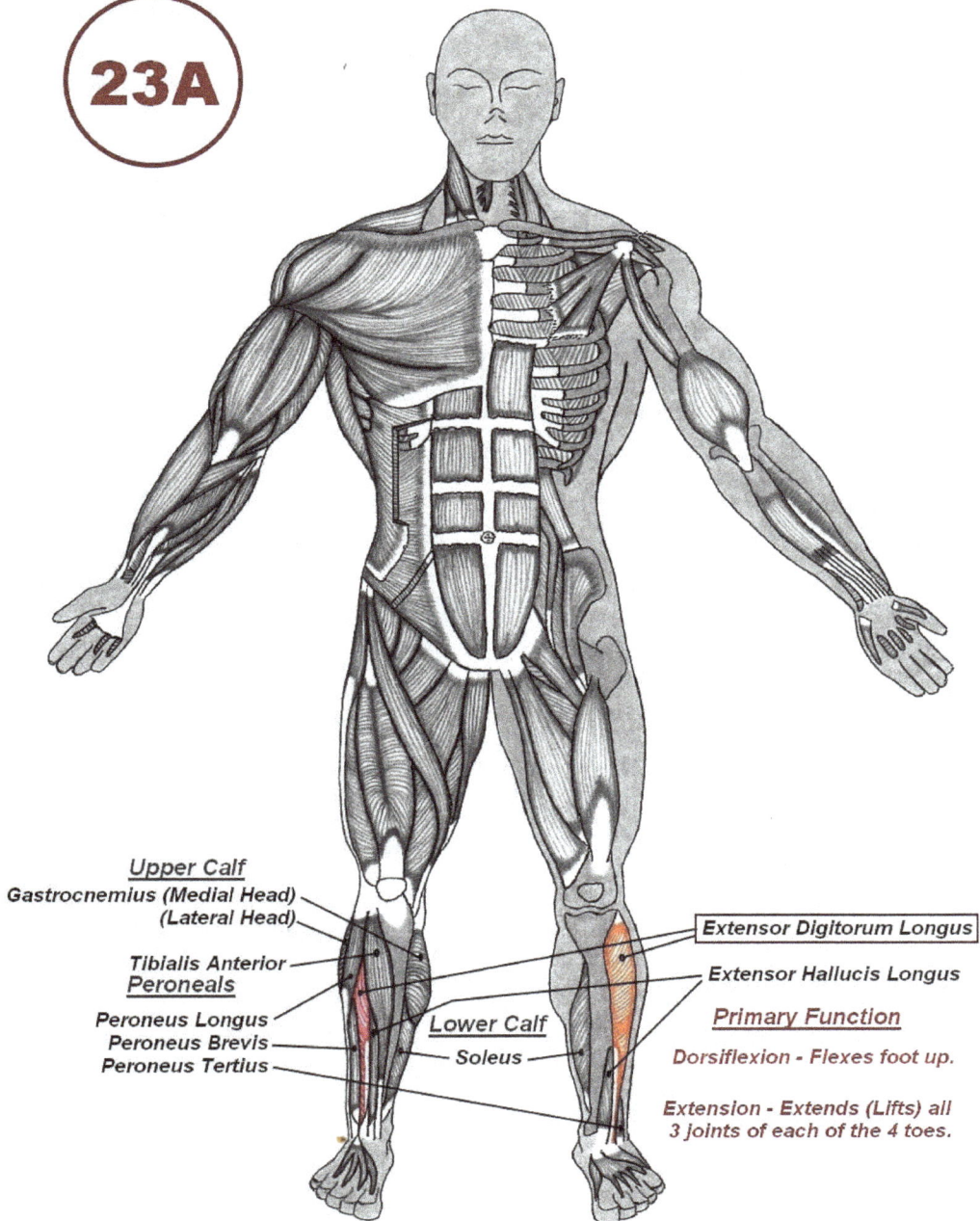

Upper Calf
Gastrocnemius (Medial Head)
(Lateral Head)

Tibialis Anterior
Peroneals

Peroneus Longus
Peroneus Brevis
Peroneus Tertius

Lower Calf
Soleus

Extensor Digitorum Longus

Extensor Hallucis Longus

Primary Function

Dorsiflexion - Flexes foot up.

Extension - Extends (Lifts) all
3 joints of each of the 4 toes.

81

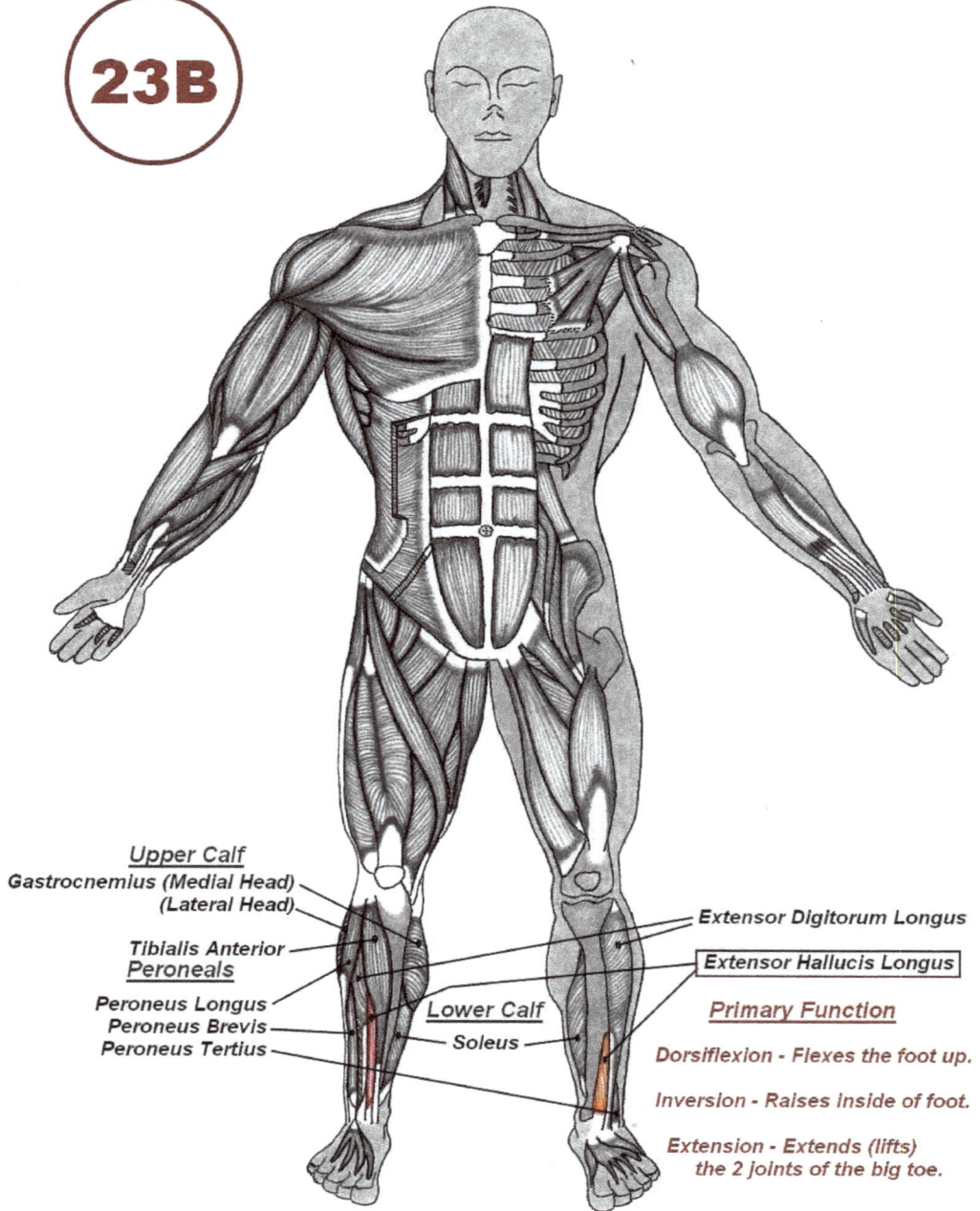

Lower Leg - Extensor Hallucis Longus

23B

Upper Calf
Gastrocnemius (Medial Head)
(Lateral Head)

Tibialis Anterior
Peroneals

Peroneus Longus
Peroneus Brevis
Peroneus Tertius

Lower Calf
Soleus

Extensor Digitorum Longus

Extensor Hallucis Longus

Primary Function

Dorsiflexion - Flexes the foot up.

Inversion - Raises inside of foot.

Extension - Extends (lifts)
the 2 joints of the big toe.

23A and B - Exercises

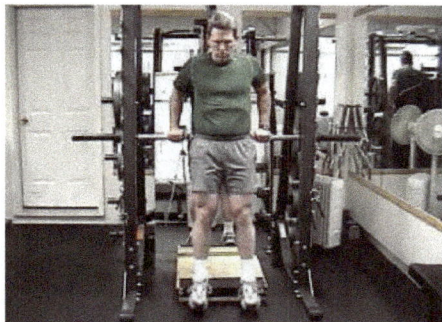
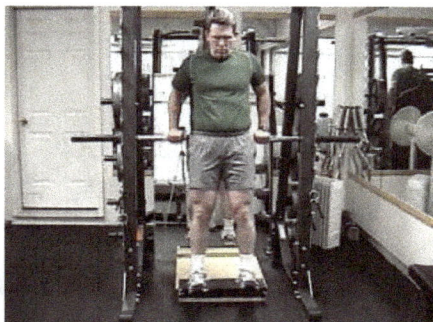

Tibialis Crunch (Flex Foot Up & Invert at Top, Extend Toes: 1-3 Sets 10-20 Reps)

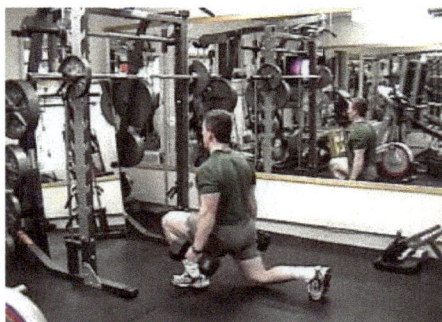
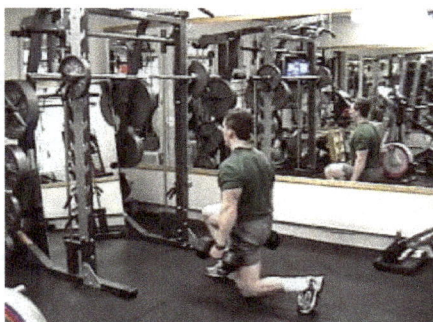

Alternating Dumbbell Lunge (Extend Toes & Foot, Balancing: 1-3 Sets 7-10 Reps)

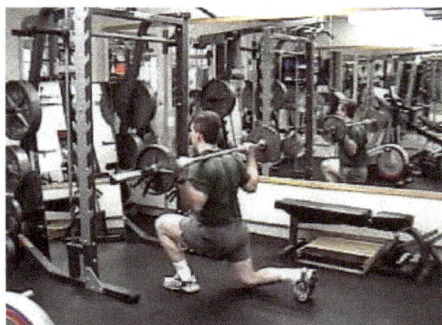
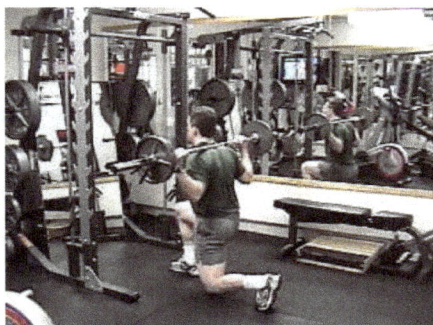

Alternating Bar Lunge (Extend Toes & Foot, Balancing: 1-3 Sets 7-10 Reps)

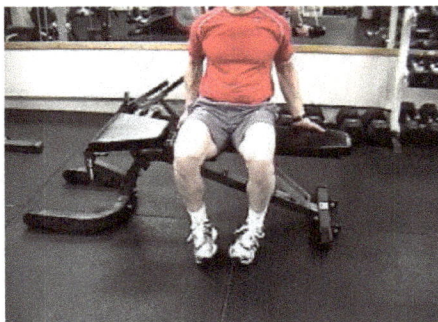

Definition: Inversion "Invert" (Lift Inside of Foot)

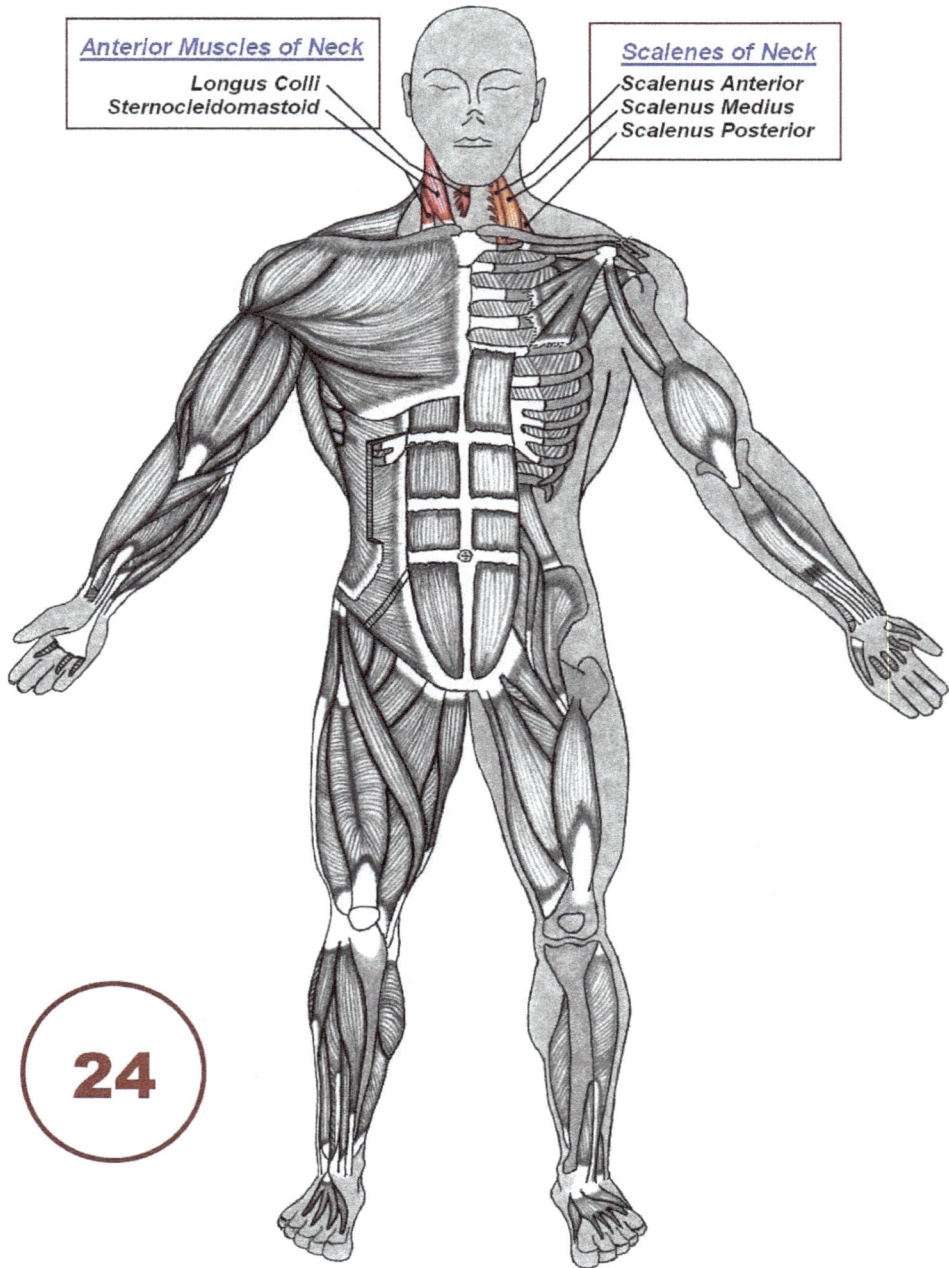

Anterior Muscles of Neck

Anterior Muscles of Neck
Longus Colli
Sternocleidomastoid

Scalenes of Neck
Scalenus Anterior
Scalenus Medius
Scalenus Posterior

24

Neck - Longus Colli

Anterior Muscles of Neck

Longus Colli
Sternocleidomastoid

Primary Function

Flexion - Flexes cervical spine
and tilts head forward.

Rotation - Rotates cervical
spine and turns head
side to side.

Scalenes of Neck

Scalenus Anterior
Scalenus Medius
Scalenus Posterior

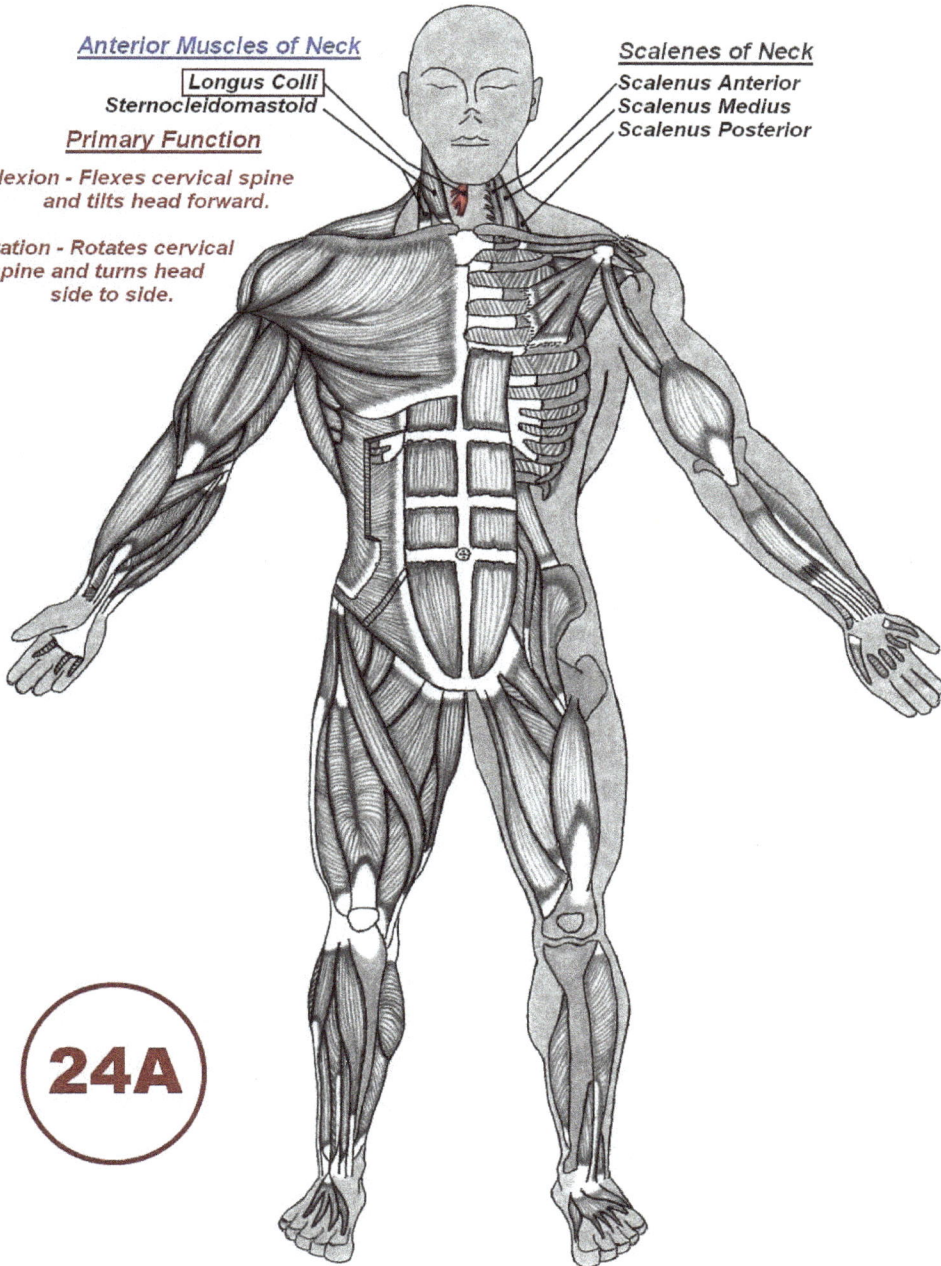

24A

Neck - Sternocleidomastoid

Anterior Muscles of Neck

Longus Colli

Sternocleidomastoid

Primary Function at Neck

Flexion - *Flexes cervical spine and tilts head forward.*

Lateral Flexion - *Flexes cervical spine and head to the side.*

Rotation - *Rotates cervical spine and turns head side to side.*

Scalenes of Neck

Scalenus Anterior
Scalenus Medius
Scalenus Posterior

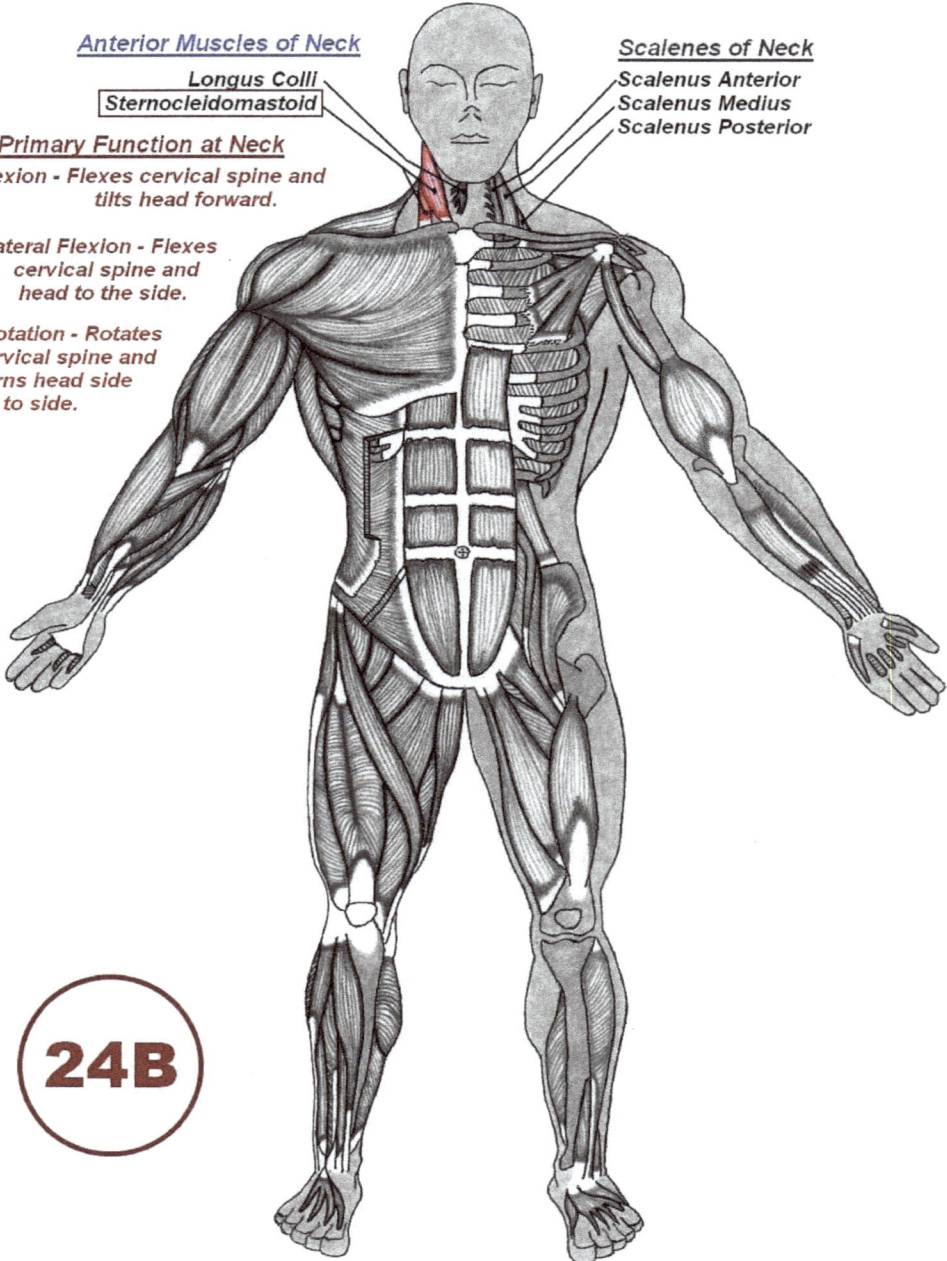

24B

24A and B - Exercises

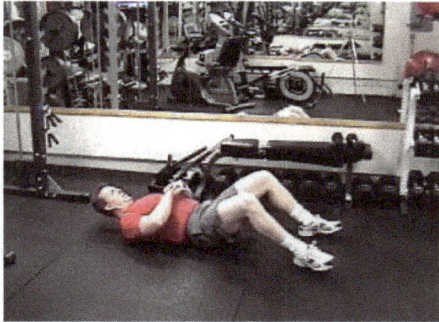

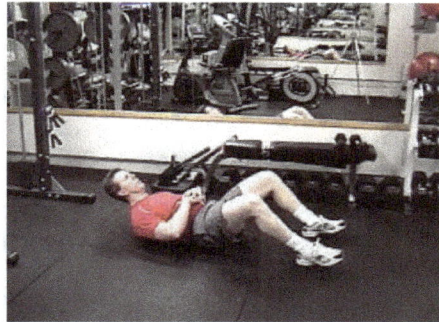

Ab Crunch on Floor (Supports Head: 1-3 Sets 10-30 Reps)

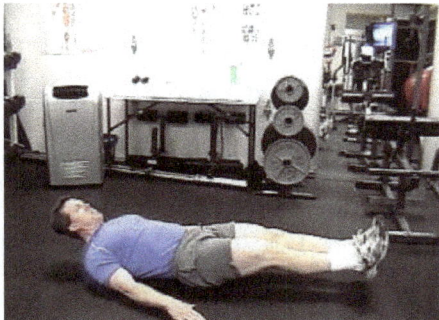

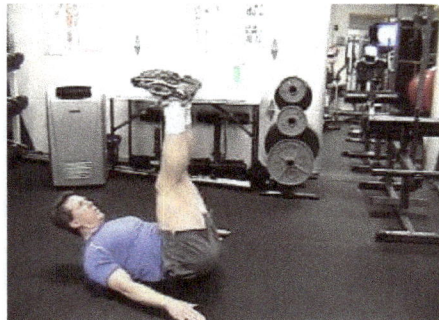

Leg Lift on Floor (Supports Head: 1-3 Sets 10-15 Reps)

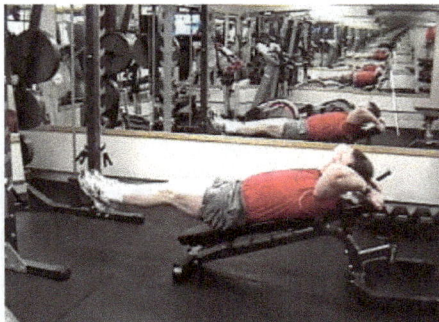

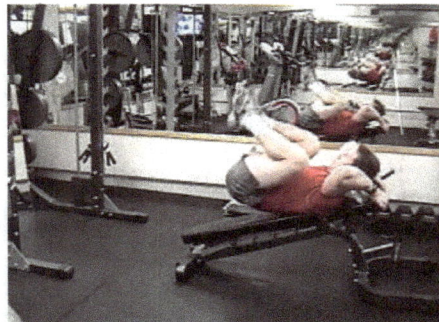

Reverse Crunch on Incline Bench (Supports Head: 1-3 Sets 10-15 Reps)

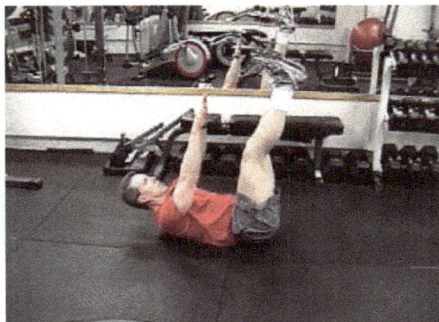

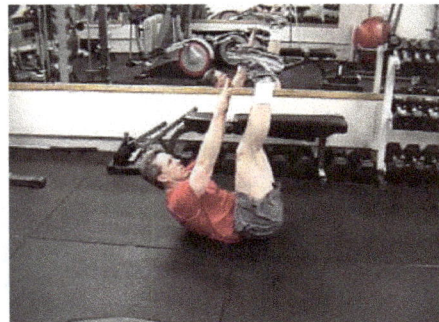

Partial V-Ups (Supports Head: 1-3 Sets 10-15 Reps)

24A and B - Exercises

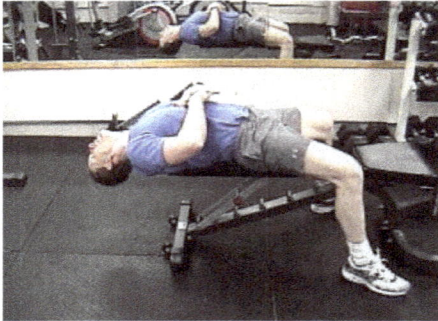

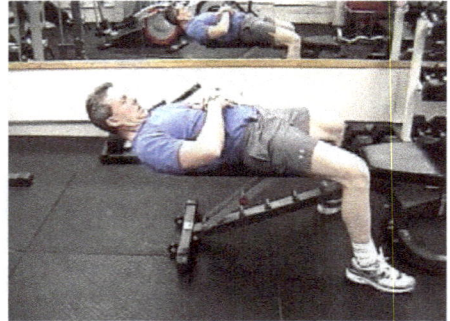

Lying Supine Neck Flex (Weighted or No Weight: 1 Set 7-10 Reps)

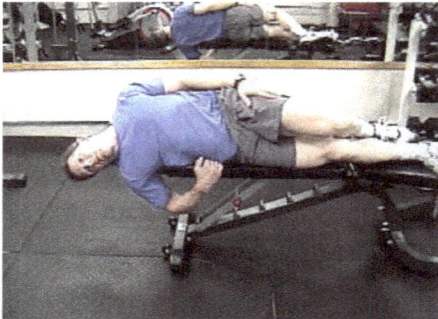

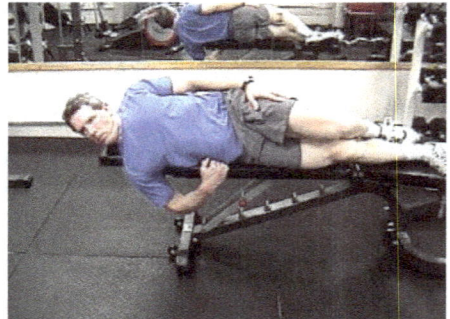

Side Lying Lateral Neck Flex (Weighted or No Weight: 1 Set 7-10 Reps Each Side)

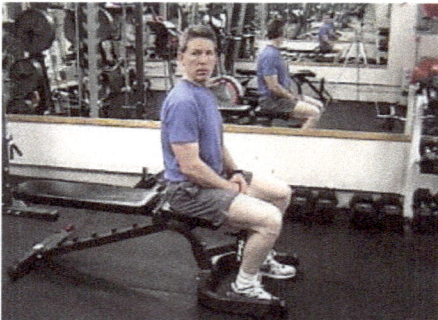

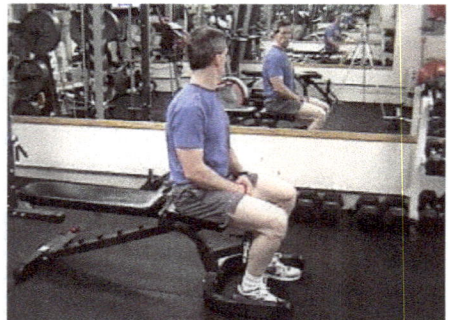

Head Rotation (1 Set 7-10 Reps Each Side)

Neck - Scalenus Anterior

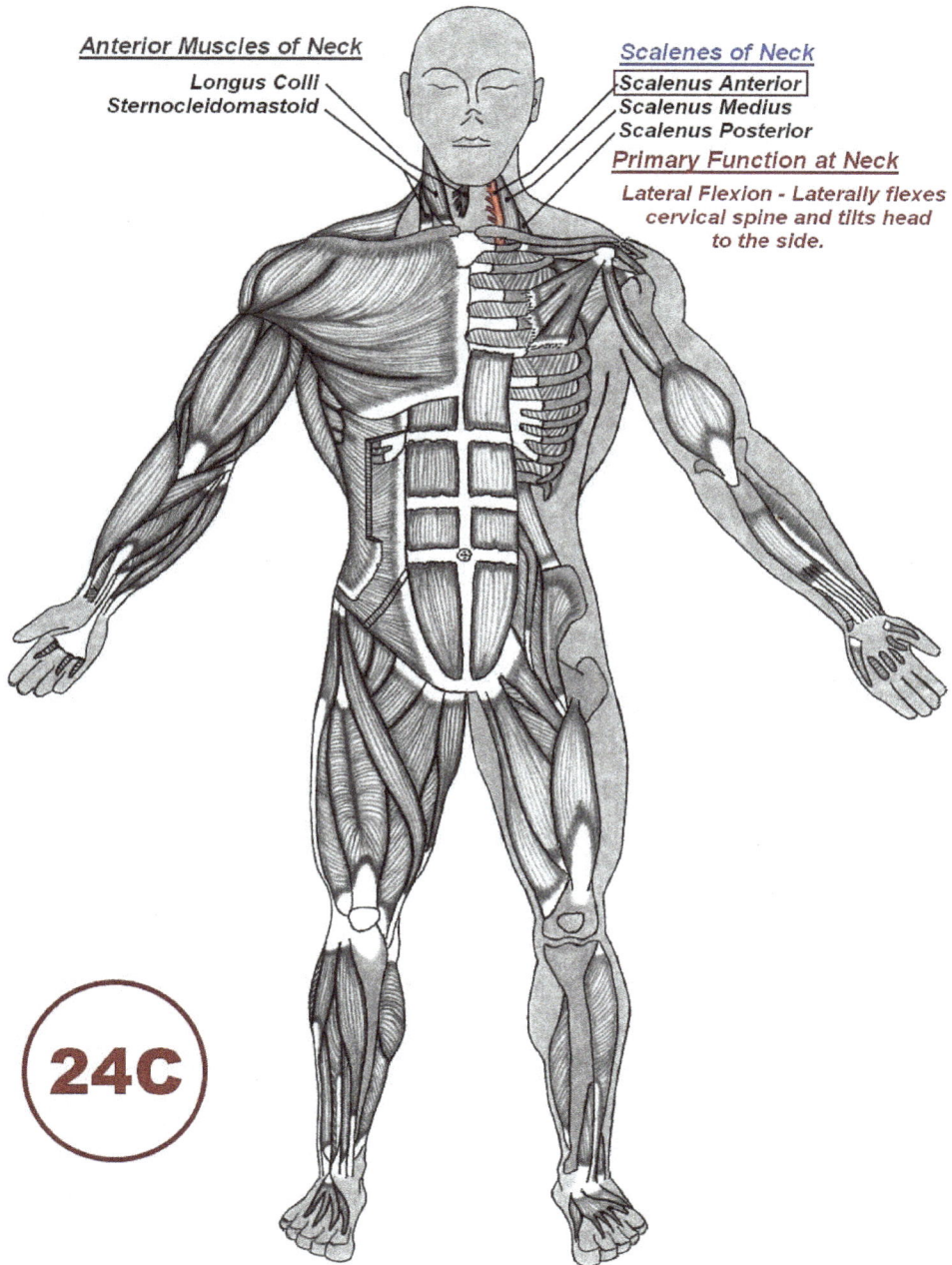

Anterior Muscles of Neck
Longus Colli
Sternocleidomastoid

Scalenes of Neck
Scalenus Anterior
Scalenus Medius
Scalenus Posterior

Primary Function at Neck
Lateral Flexion - Laterally flexes
cervical spine and tilts head
to the side.

24C

Neck - Scalenus Medius

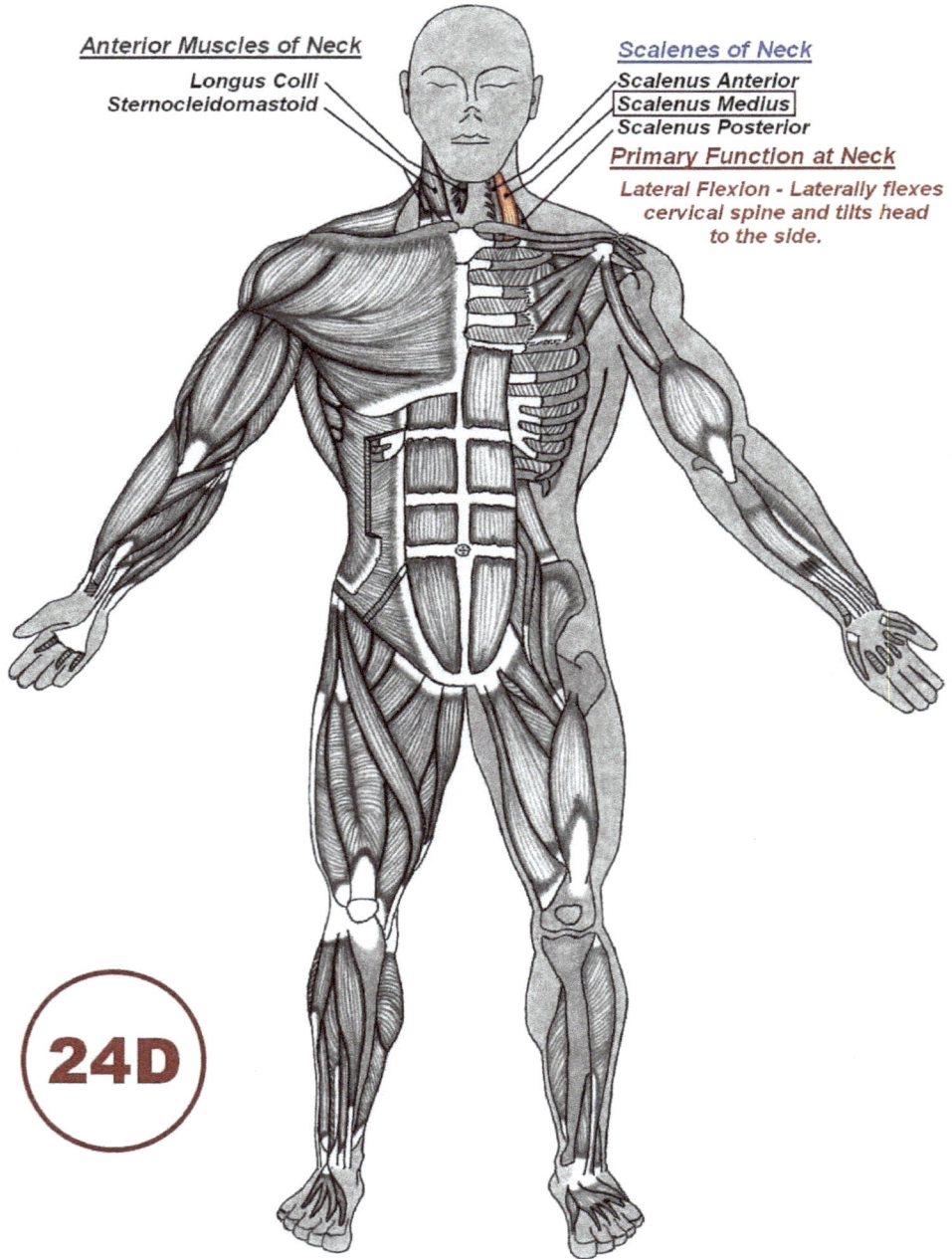

Anterior Muscles of Neck
Longus Colli
Sternocleidomastoid

Scalenes of Neck
Scalenus Anterior
Scalenus Medius
Scalenus Posterior

Primary Function at Neck
Lateral Flexion - Laterally flexes cervical spine and tilts head to the side.

24D

Neck - Scalenus Posterior

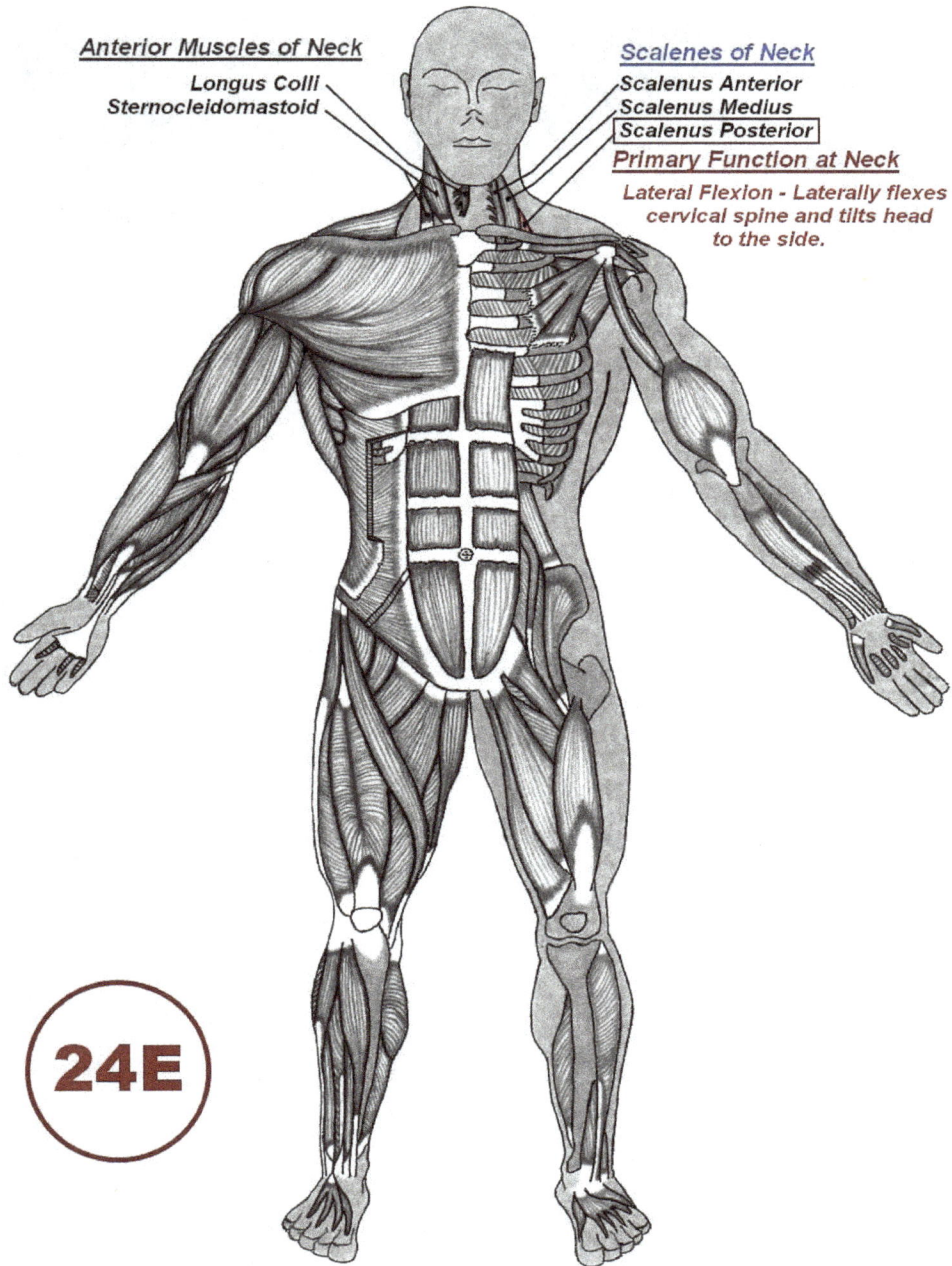

Anterior Muscles of Neck
Longus Colli
Sternocleidomastoid

Scalenes of Neck
Scalenus Anterior
Scalenus Medius
Scalenus Posterior

Primary Function at Neck
Lateral Flexion - Laterally flexes cervical spine and tilts head to the side.

24E

24C, D and E - Exercises

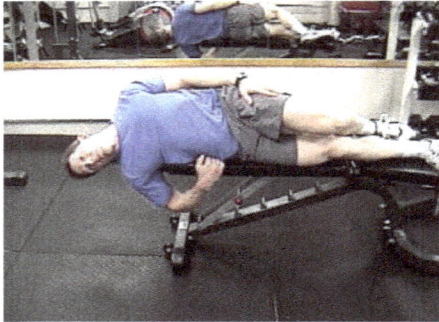
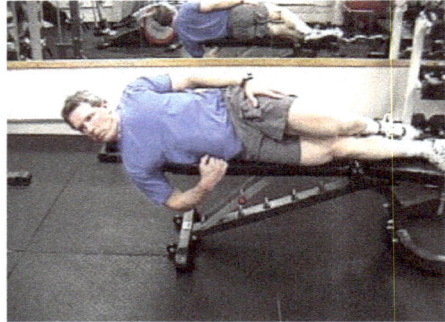

Side-Lying Lateral Neck Flex (Weighted or No Weight: 1 Set 7-10 Reps Each Side)

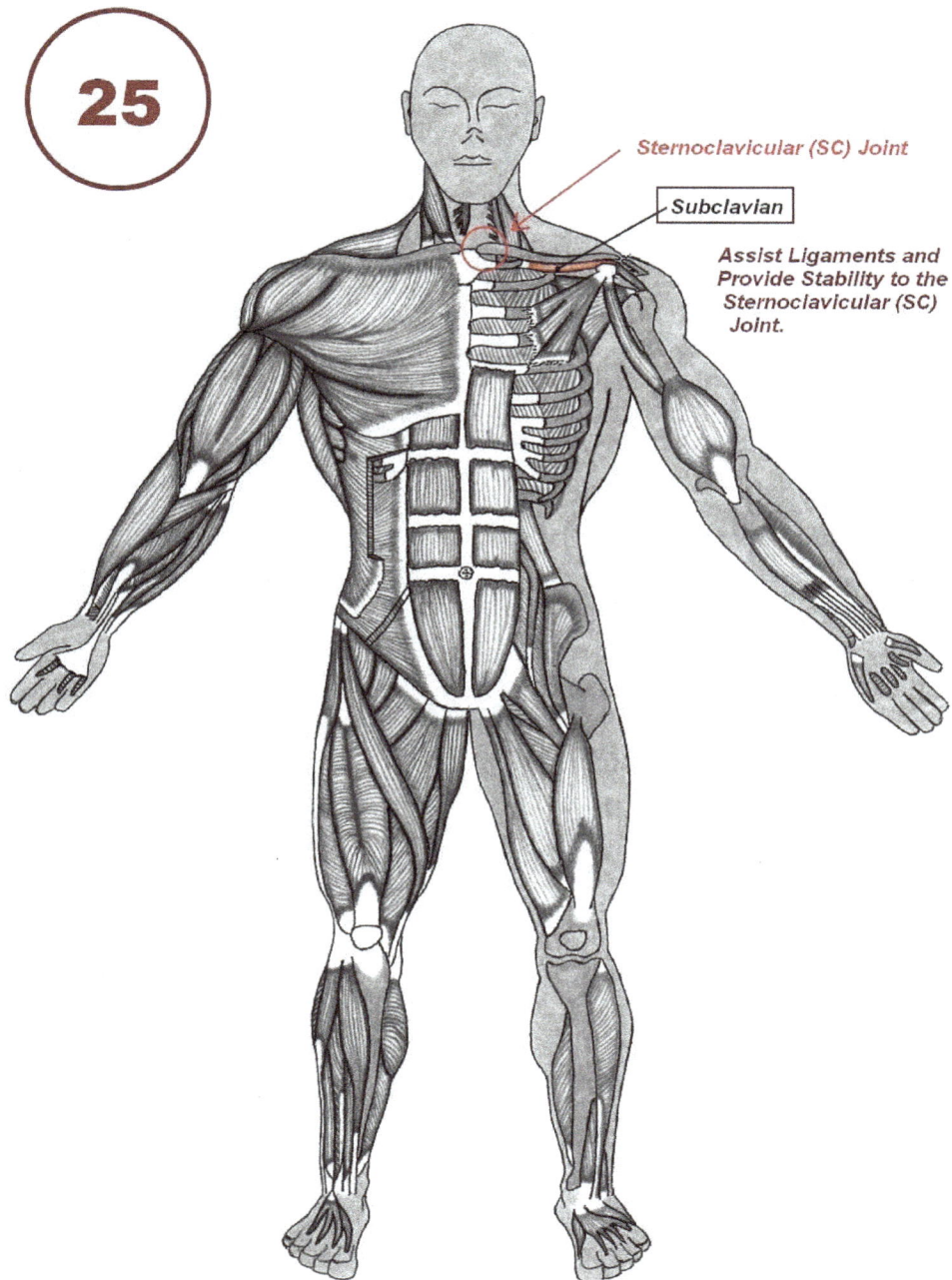

Subclavian

25

Sternoclavicular (SC) Joint

Subclavian

Assist Ligaments and Provide Stability to the Sternoclavicular (SC) Joint.

Muscles of Hands

26

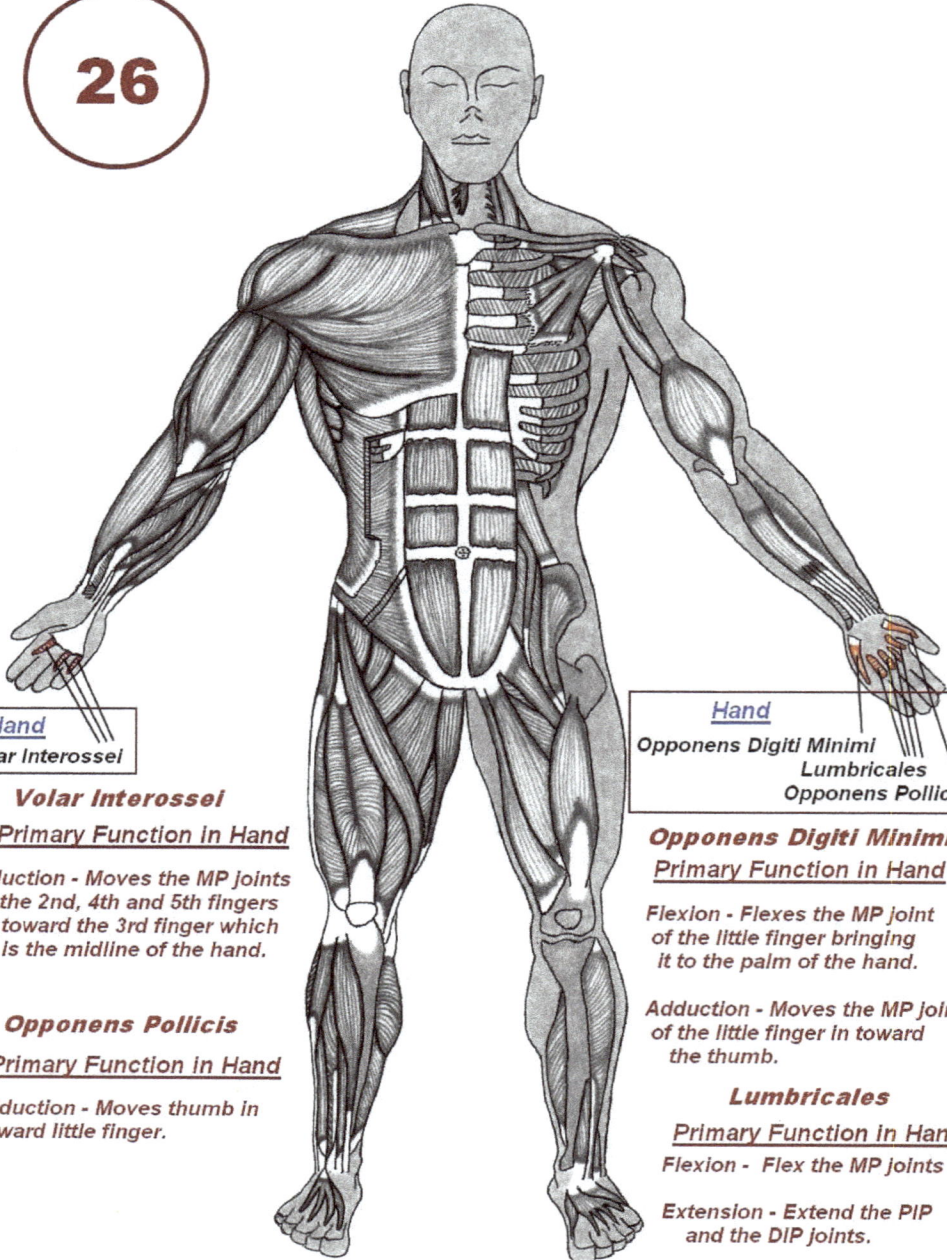

Hand
Volar Interossei

Volar Interossei

Primary Function in Hand

Adduction - Moves the MP joints
of the 2nd, 4th and 5th fingers
in toward the 3rd finger which
is the midline of the hand.

Opponens Pollicis

Primary Function in Hand

Adduction - Moves thumb in
toward little finger.

Hand
Opponens Digiti Minimi
Lumbricales
Opponens Pollicis

Opponens Digiti Minimi

Primary Function in Hand

Flexion - Flexes the MP joint
of the little finger bringing
it to the palm of the hand.

Adduction - Moves the MP joint
of the little finger in toward
the thumb.

Lumbricales

Primary Function in Hand
Flexion - Flex the MP joints

Extension - Extend the PIP
and the DIP joints.

26 - Exercises

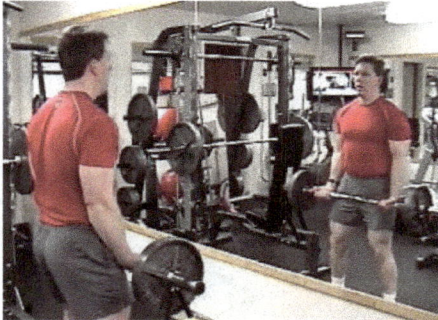

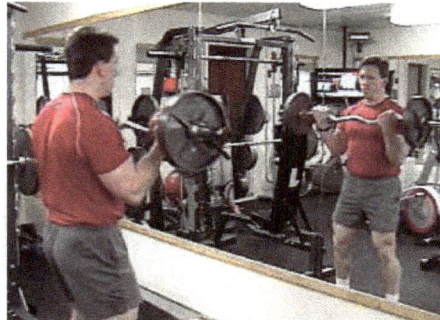

Biceps Standing EZ-Bar Curl (Hand Grip: 1-3 Sets 7-15 Reps)

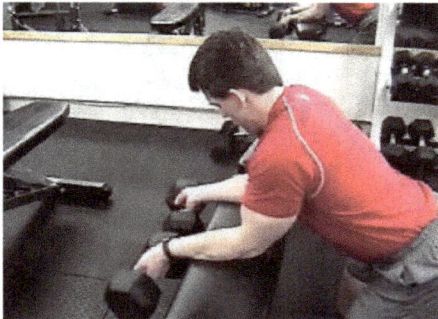

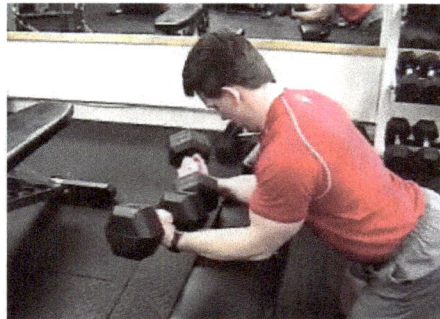

Wrist Curls on Bench (Hand Grip: 1-3 Sets 7-10 Reps)

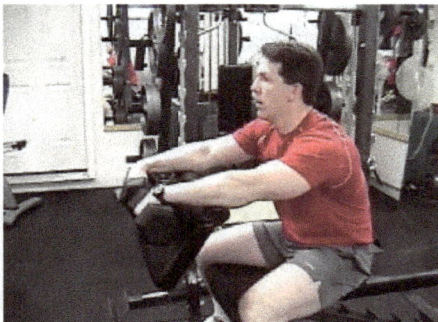

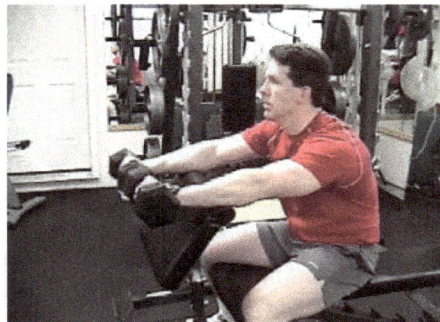

Forearm Extension "Reverse Wrist Curl" (Hand Grip: 1-3 Sets 7-10 Reps)

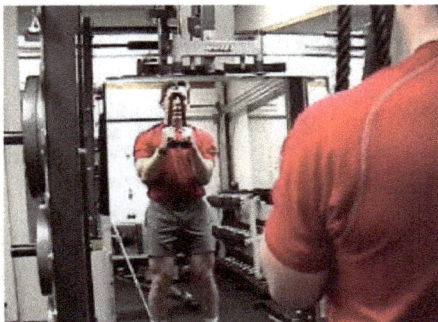

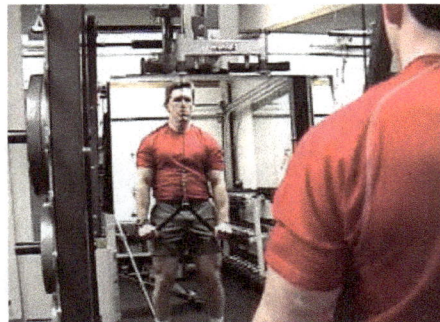

Triceps Cable Push Down (Hand Grip: 1-3 Sets 7-15 Reps)

26 - Exercises

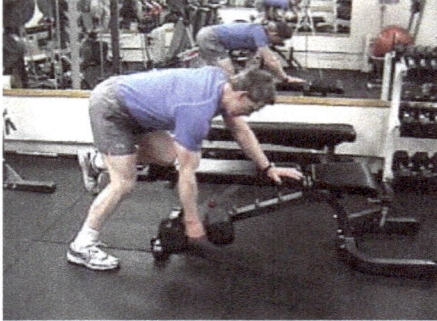

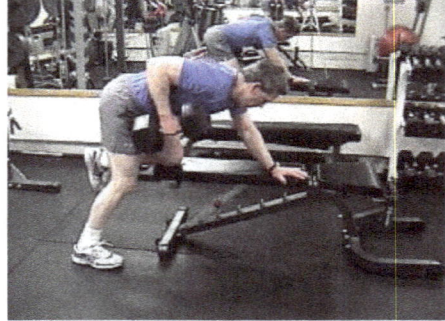

Kneeling Dumbbell Row (Hand Grip: 1-3 Sets 7-15 Reps)

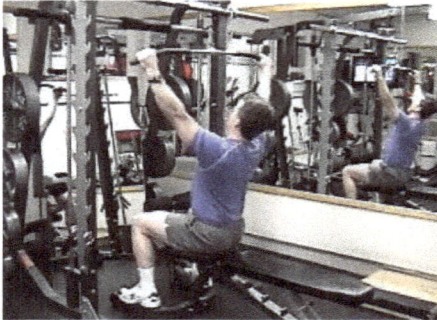

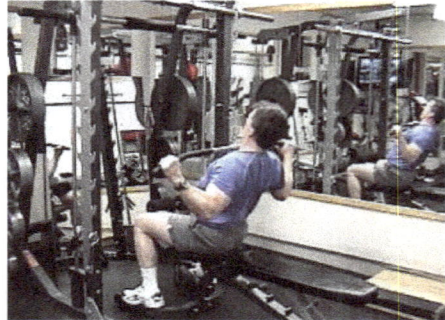

Lat Wide Grip Front Pull Down (Hand Grip: 1-3 Sets 7-15 Reps)

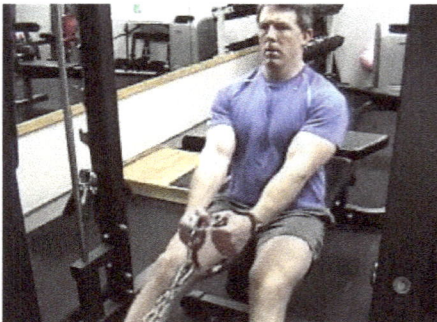

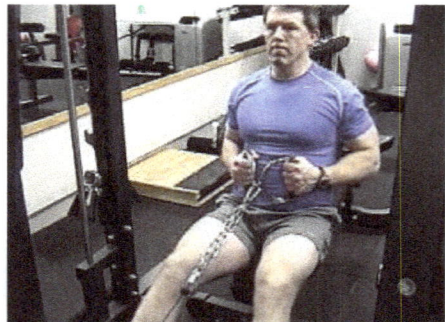

Seated Close Grip Cable Row (Hand Grip: 1-3 Sets 7-15 Reps)

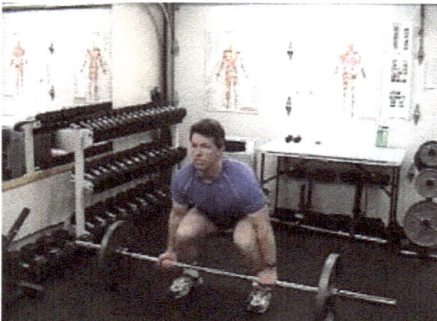

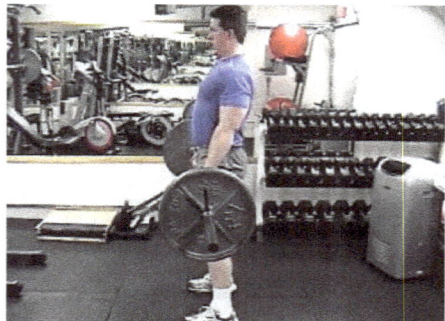

Dead-Lift (Hand Grip: 1-3 Sets 7-10 Reps)

Muscles of Foot

27

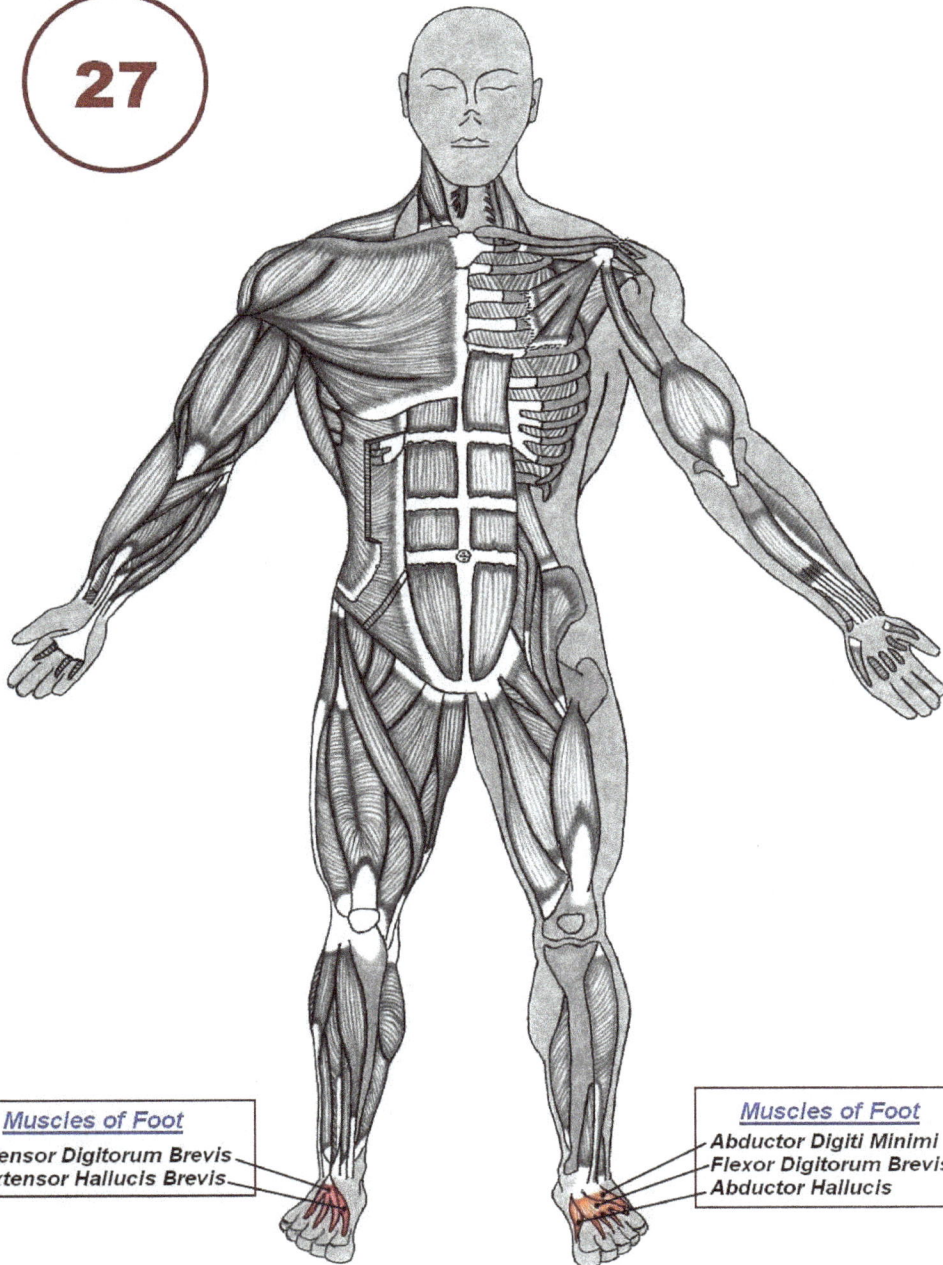

Muscles of Foot
Extensor Digitorum Brevis
Extensor Hallucis Brevis

Muscles of Foot
Abductor Digiti Minimi
Flexor Digitorum Brevis
Abductor Hallucis

Foot - Extensor Digitorum Brevis

27A

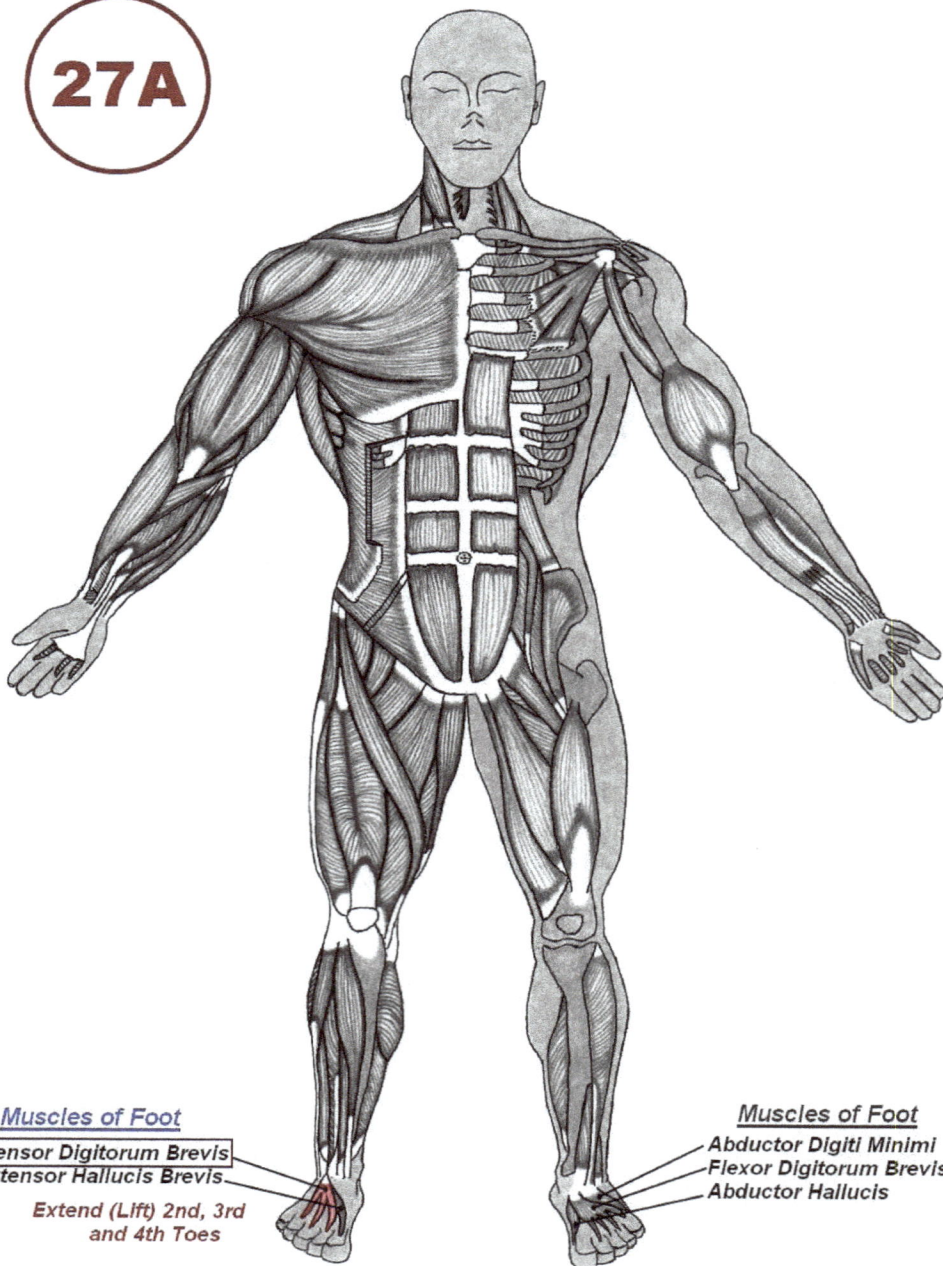

Muscles of Foot

Extensor Digitorum Brevis
Extensor Hallucis Brevis

Extend (Lift) 2nd, 3rd and 4th Toes

Muscles of Foot

Abductor Digiti Minimi
Flexor Digitorum Brevis
Abductor Hallucis

Foot - Extensor Hallucis Brevis

27B

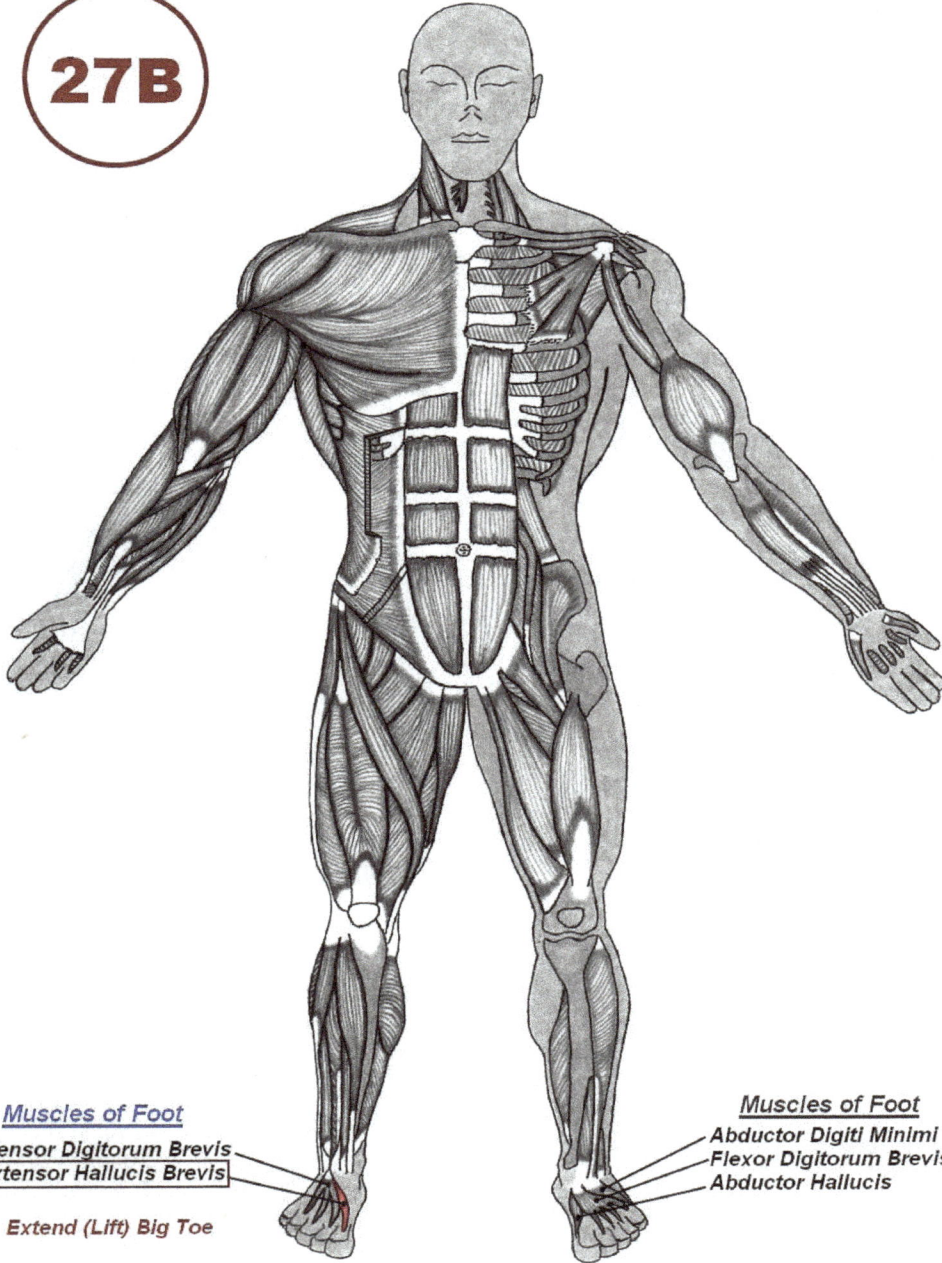

Muscles of Foot

Extensor Digitorum Brevis
Extensor Hallucis Brevis

Extend (Lift) Big Toe

Muscles of Foot

Abductor Digiti Minimi
Flexor Digitorum Brevis
Abductor Hallucis

Foot - Abductor Digiti Minimi

27C

Muscles of Foot

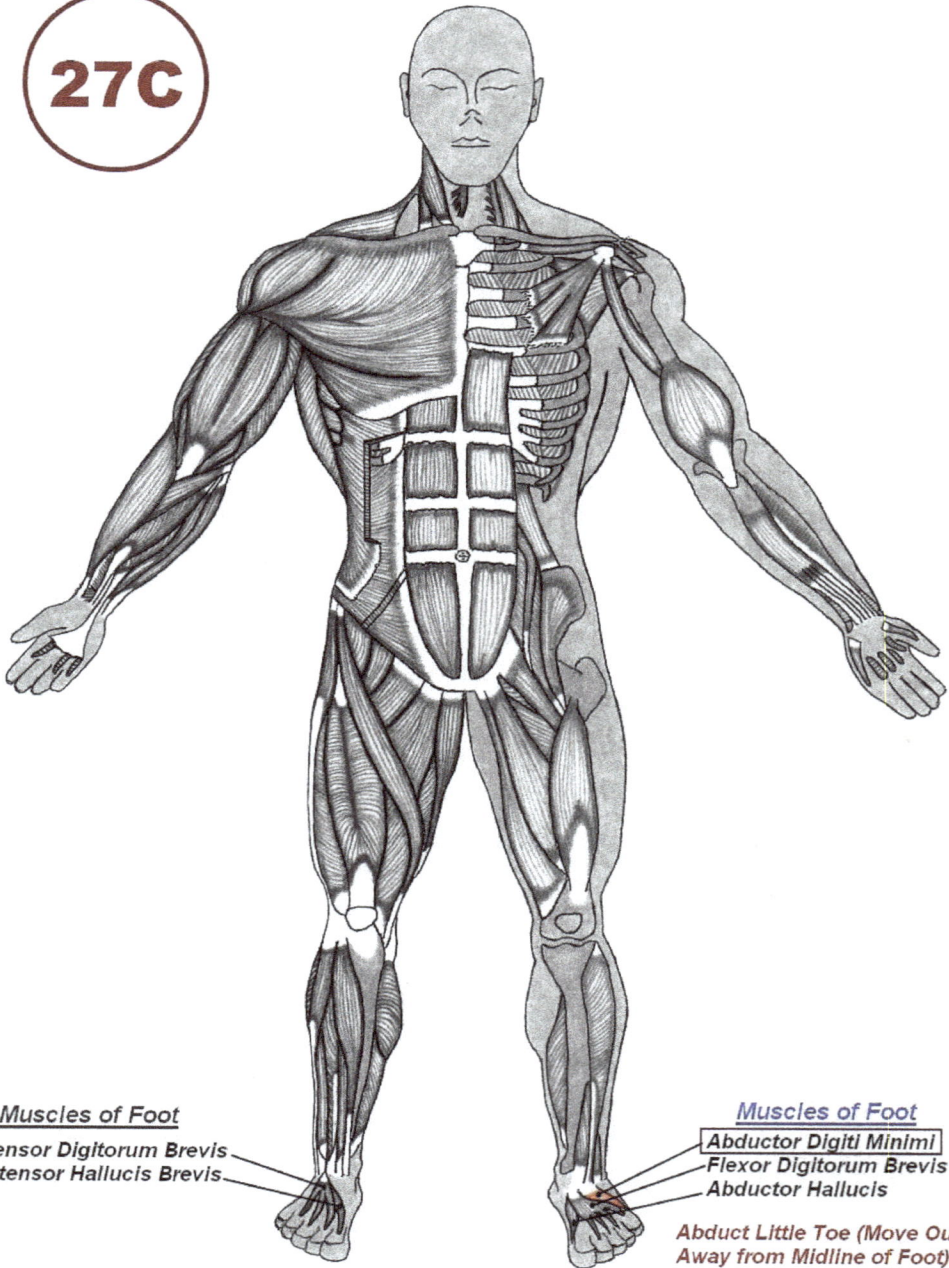

Extensor Digitorum Brevis
Extensor Hallucis Brevis

Muscles of Foot

Abductor Digiti Minimi
Flexor Digitorum Brevis
Abductor Hallucis

Abduct Little Toe (Move Out Away from Midline of Foot)

100

Foot - Abductor Hallucis

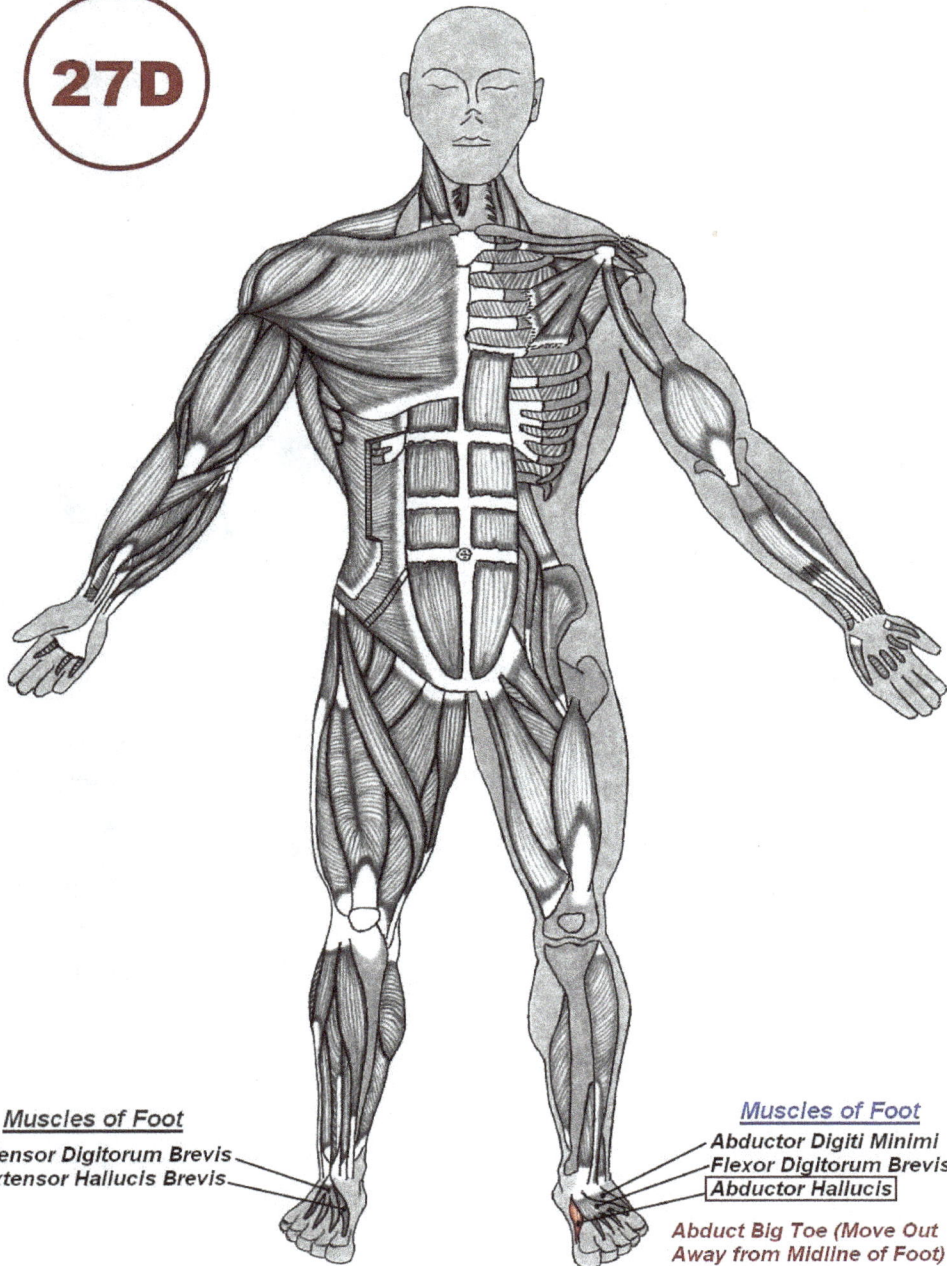

27D

Muscles of Foot

Extensor Digitorum Brevis
Extensor Hallucis Brevis

Muscles of Foot

Abductor Digiti Minimi
Flexor Digitorum Brevis
Abductor Hallucis

*Abduct Big Toe (Move Out
Away from Midline of Foot)*

27A, B, C and D - Exercises

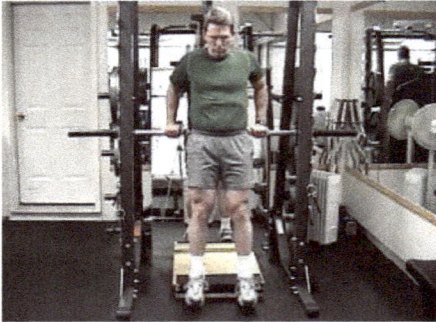

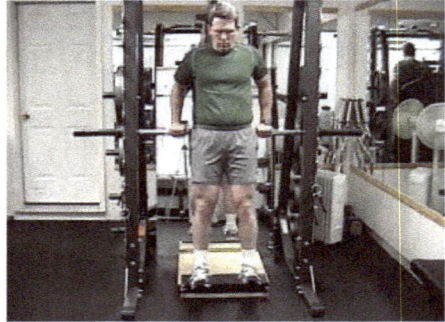

Tibialis Crunch (While Flexing Foot Up, Toes May Abduct Out)

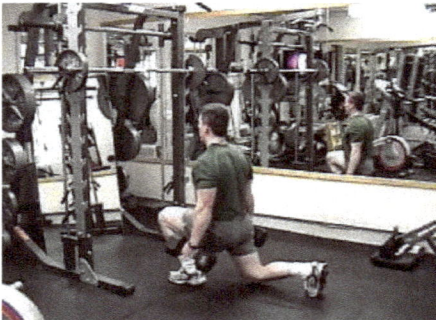

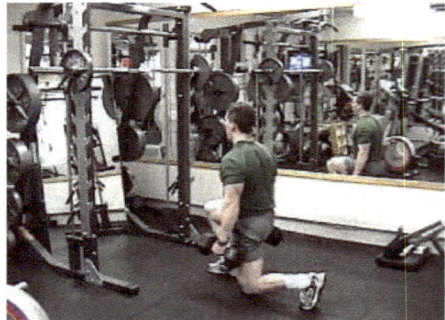

Alternating Dumbbell Lunge (Toes May Abduct Out While Stepping Out)

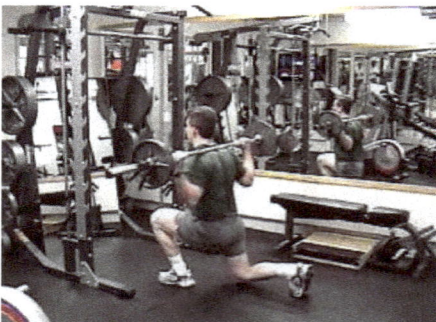

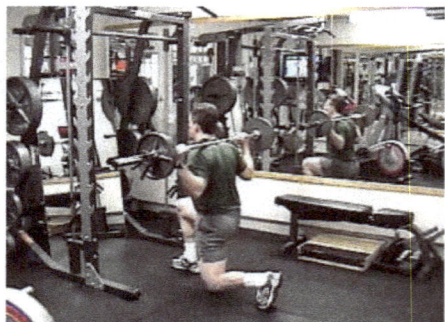

Alternating Bar Lunge (Toes May Abduct Out While Stepping Out)

Foot - Flexor Digitorum Brevis

27E

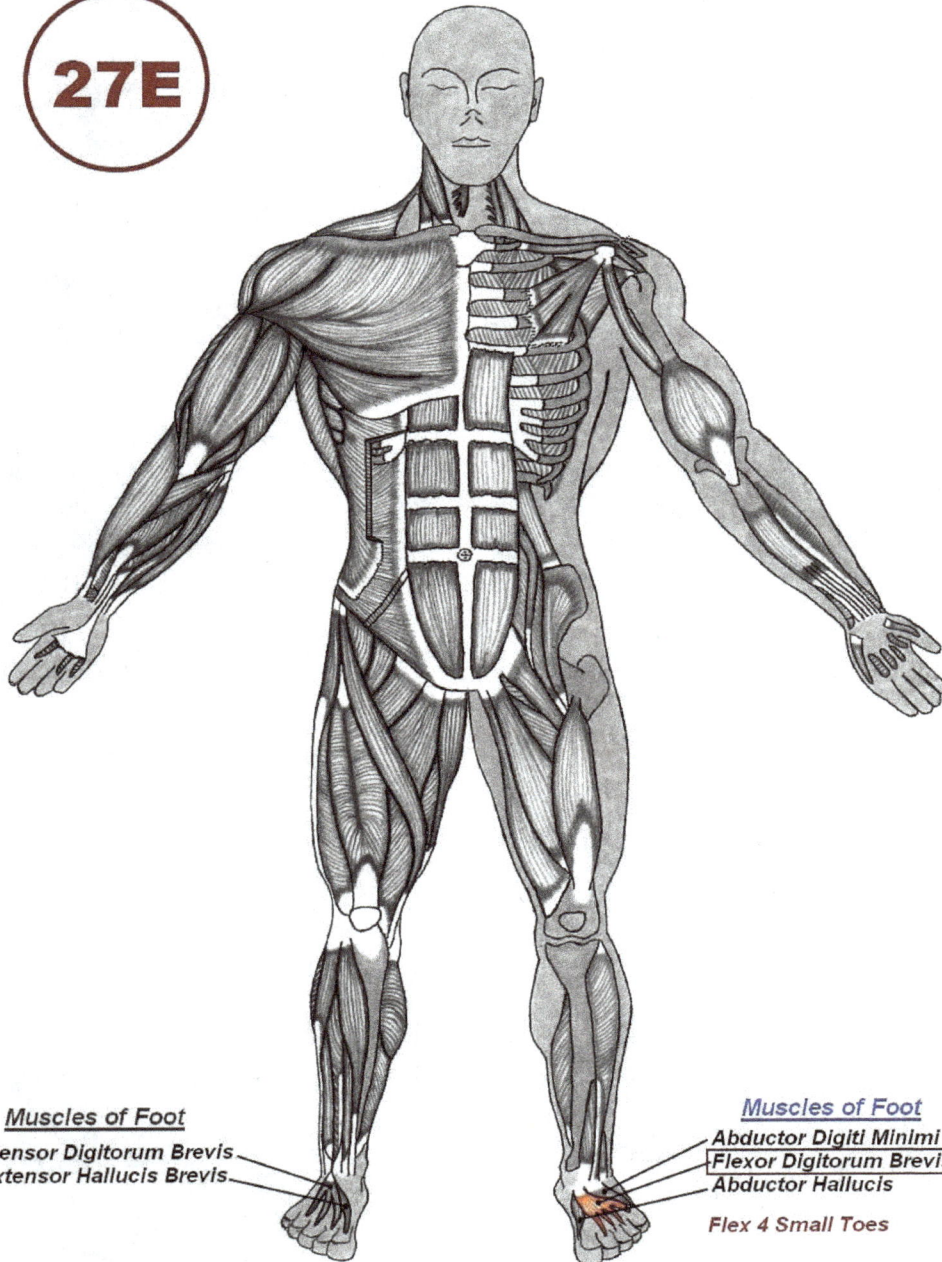

Muscles of Foot

Extensor Digitorum Brevis
Extensor Hallucis Brevis

Muscles of Foot

Abductor Digiti Minimi
Flexor Digitorum Brevis
Abductor Hallucis

Flex 4 Small Toes

103

27E - Exercises

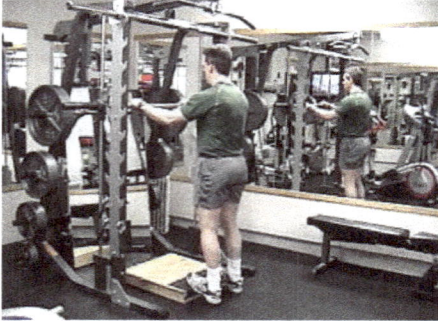
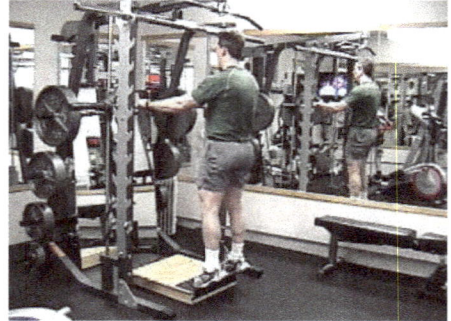

Standing Calve Raise - High Rep (Flex Bottom of Foot: 1-3 Sets 10-30 Reps)

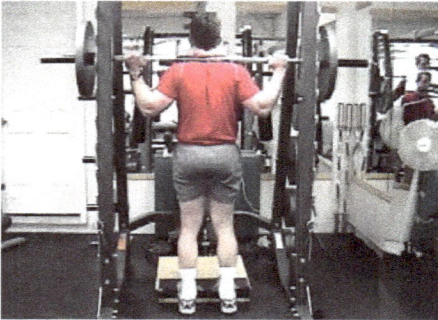
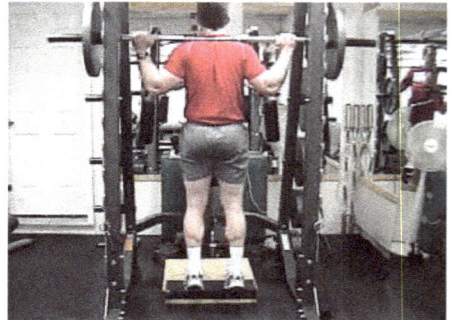

Standing Calve Raise - Weighted (Flex Bottom of Foot: 1-3 Sets 10-15 Reps)

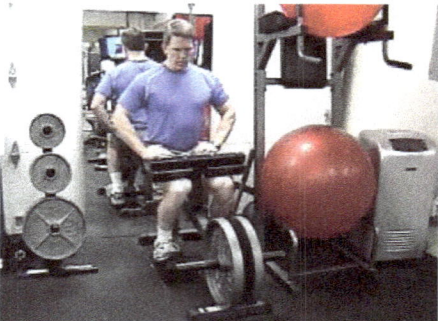
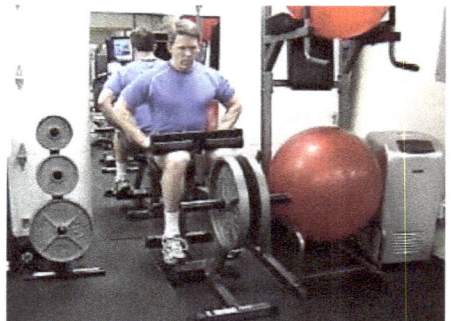

Seated Calve Raise (Flex Bottom of Foot: 1-3 Sets 10-15 Reps)

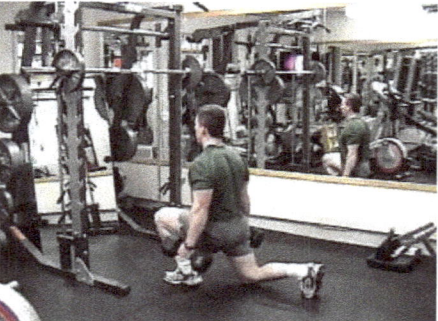
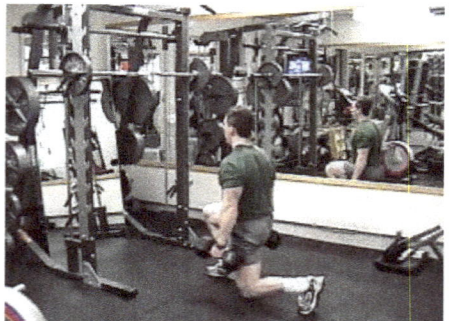

Dumbbell Lunge (Flex Bottom of Foot Pushing Back: 1-3 Sets 7-10 Reps)

Major Muscles (Posterior) - Male

Superficial / Intermediate   **Intermediate / Deep**

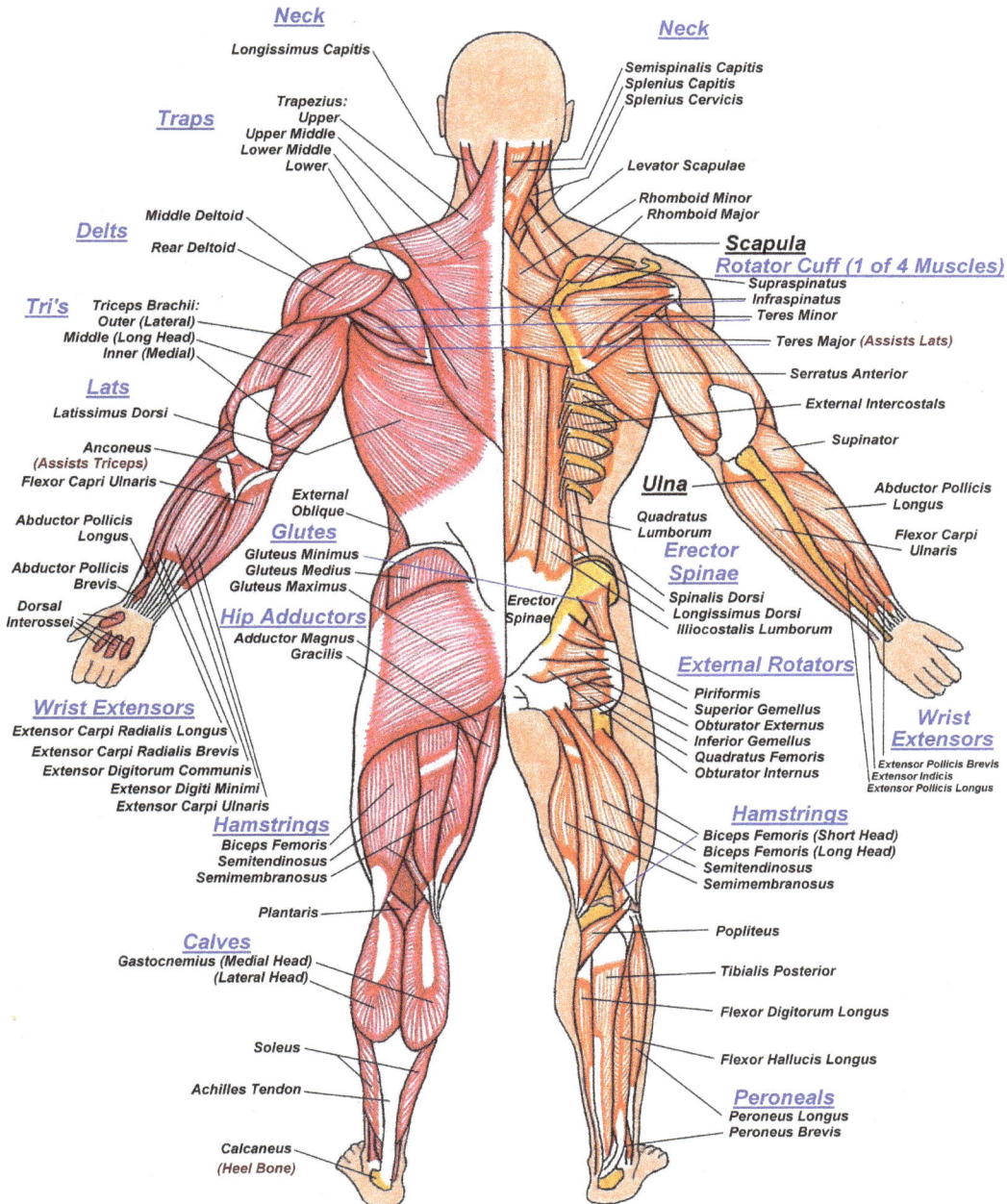

Neck
Longissimus Capitis

Traps
Trapezius:
Upper
Upper Middle
Lower Middle
Lower

Delts
Middle Deltoid
Rear Deltoid

Tri's
Triceps Brachii:
Outer (Lateral)
Middle (Long Head)
Inner (Medial)

Lats
Latissimus Dorsi

Anconeus
(Assists Triceps)
Flexor Capri Ulnaris

Abductor Pollicis
Longus

Abductor Pollicis
Brevis

Dorsal
Interossei

External
Oblique

Glutes
Gluteus Minimus
Gluteus Medius
Gluteus Maximus

Hip Adductors
Adductor Magnus
Gracilis

Wrist Extensors
Extensor Carpi Radialis Longus
Extensor Carpi Radialis Brevis
Extensor Digitorum Communis
Extensor Digiti Minimi
Extensor Carpi Ulnaris

Hamstrings
Biceps Femoris
Semitendinosus
Semimembranosus

Plantaris

Calves
Gastocnemius (Medial Head)
(Lateral Head)

Soleus

Achilles Tendon

Calcaneus
(Heel Bone)

Neck
Semispinalis Capitis
Splenius Capitis
Splenius Cervicis

Levator Scapulae

Rhomboid Minor
Rhomboid Major

Scapula
Rotator Cuff (1 of 4 Muscles)
Supraspinatus
Infraspinatus
Teres Minor

Teres Major (Assists Lats)

Serratus Anterior

External Intercostals

Supinator

Abductor Pollicis
Longus

Flexor Carpi
Ulnaris

Ulna
Quadratus
Lumborum

**Erector
Spinae**
Spinalis Dorsi
Longissimus Dorsi
Illiocostalis Lumborum

Erector
Spinae

External Rotators
Piriformis
Superior Gemellus
Obturator Externus
Inferior Gemellus
Quadratus Femoris
Obturator Internus

**Wrist
Extensors**
Extensor Pollicis Brevis
Extensor Indicis
Extensor Pollicis Longus

Hamstrings
Biceps Femoris (Short Head)
Biceps Femoris (Long Head)
Semitendinosus
Semimembranosus

Popliteus

Tibialis Posterior

Flexor Digitorum Longus

Flexor Hallucis Longus

Peroneals
Peroneus Longus
Peroneus Brevis

105

Trapezius (Trap's)

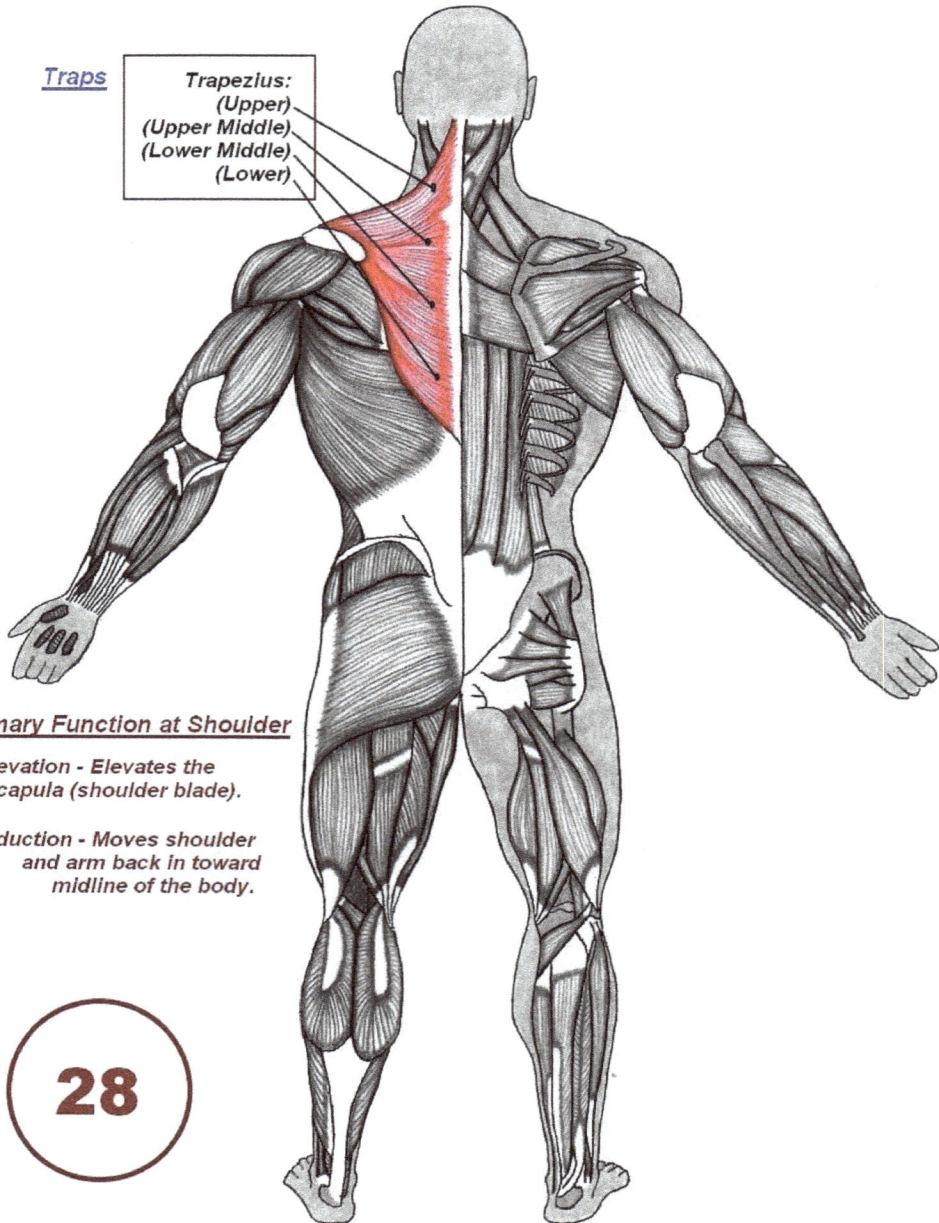

Traps

Trapezius:
(Upper)
(Upper Middle)
(Lower Middle)
(Lower)

Primary Function at Shoulder

Elevation - Elevates the Scapula (shoulder blade).

Adduction - Moves shoulder and arm back in toward midline of the body.

28

28 - Exercises

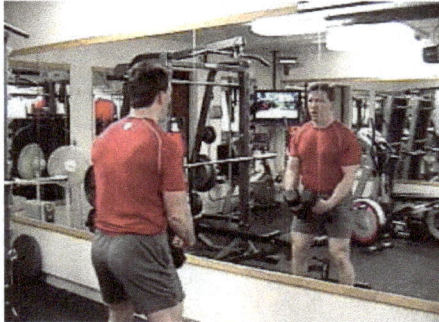

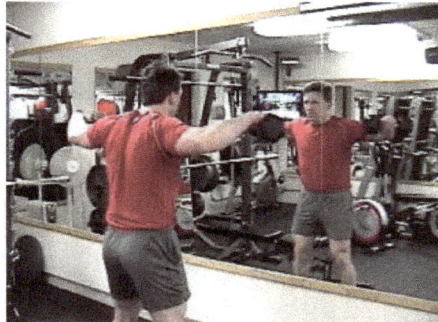

Shoulder Upright Lateral DB Raise (Front Start Position: 1-3 Sets 7-10 Reps)

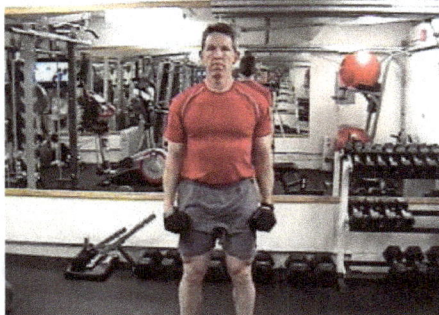

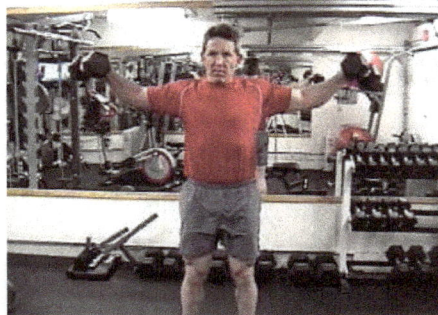

Shoulder Upright Lateral DB Raise (Side Start Position: 1-3 Sets 7-10 Reps)

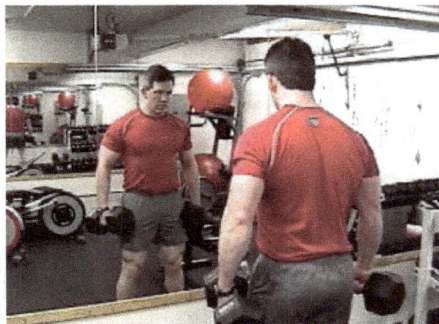

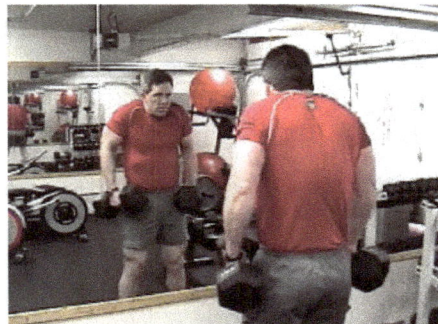

Standing Dumbbell Shrugs (1-3 Sets 7-10 Reps)

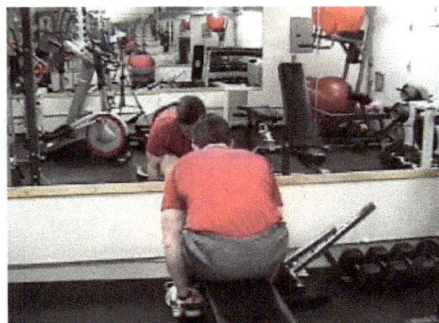

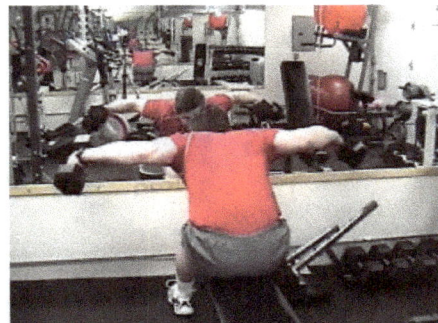

Shoulder Seated Bent Lateral Dumbbell Raise (1-3 Sets 7-10 Reps)

28 - Exercises

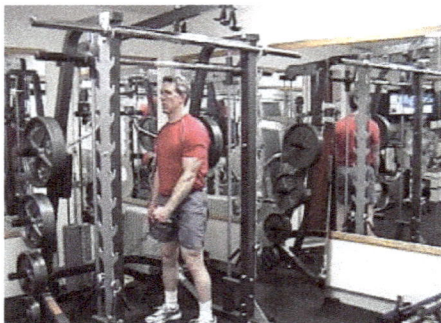

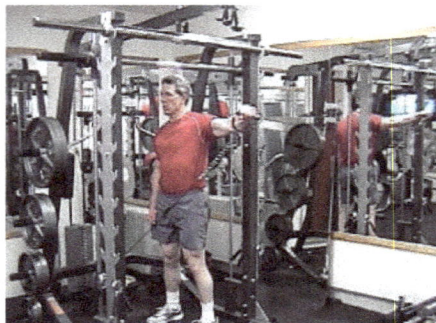

Shoulder Standing Cable Lateral Raise (1-3 Sets 7-10 Reps)

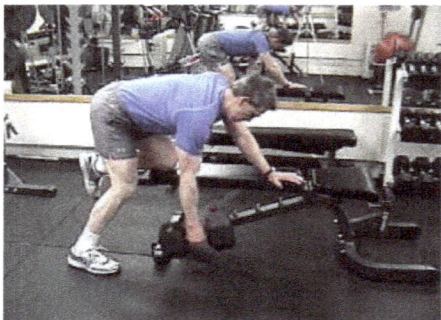

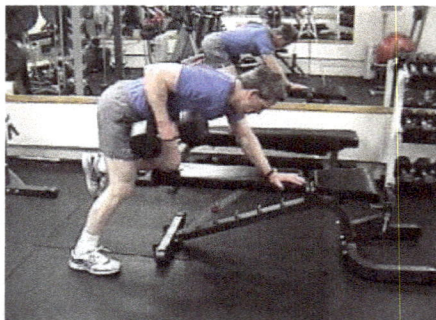

Kneeling Dumbbell Row (1-3 Sets 7-15 Reps)

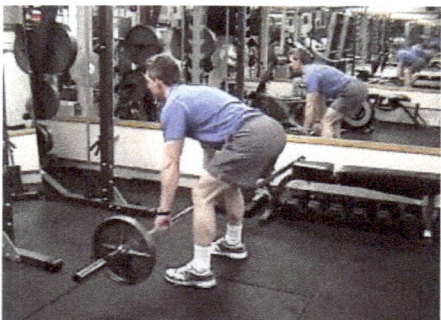

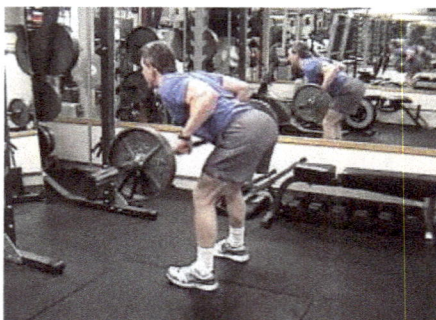

Standing Bent Bar Row (1-3 Sets 7-10 Reps)

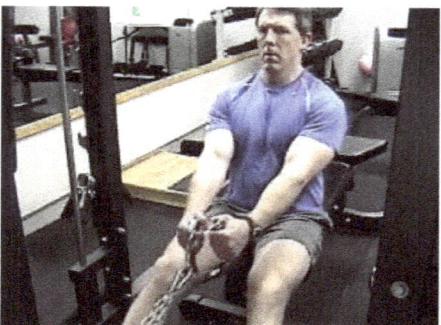

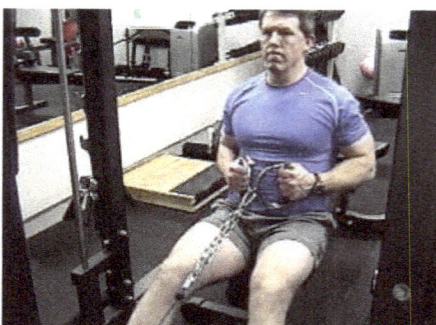

Seated Close Grip Cable Row (1-3 Sets 7-15 Reps)

28 - Exercises

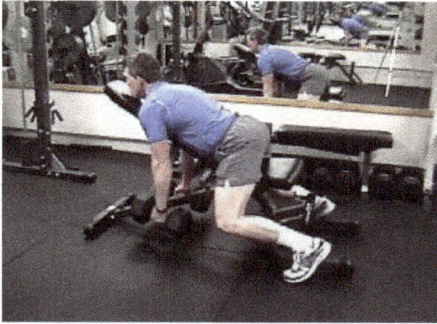

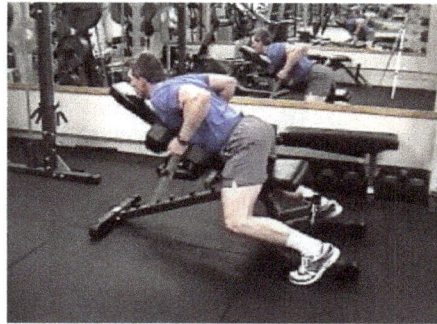

Seated Incline Double Dumbbell Row (1-3 Sets 7-15 Reps)

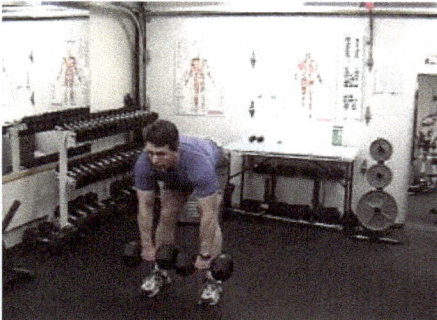

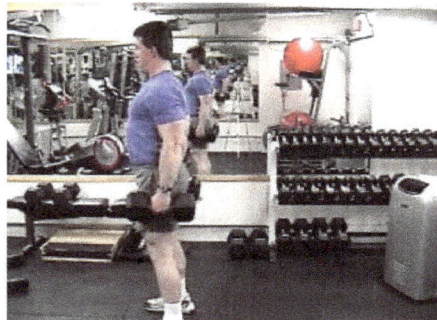

Straight Leg Dumbbell Dead-Lift (1-3 Sets 7-10 Reps)

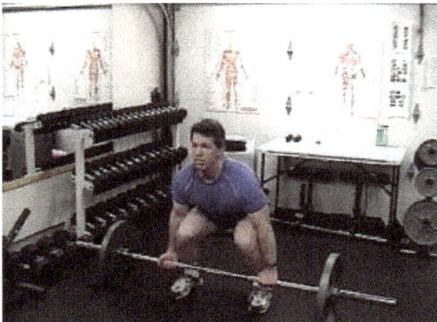

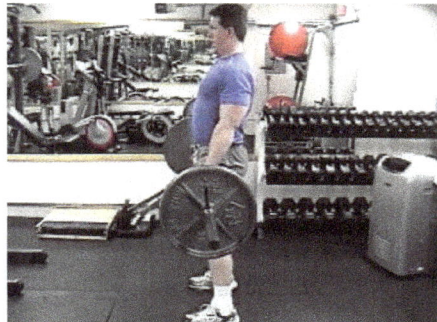

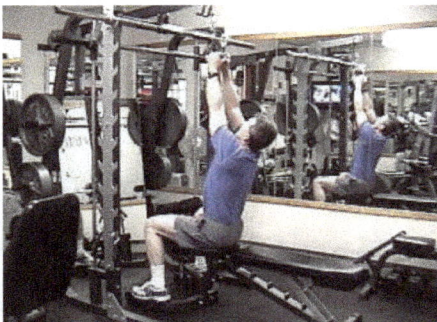

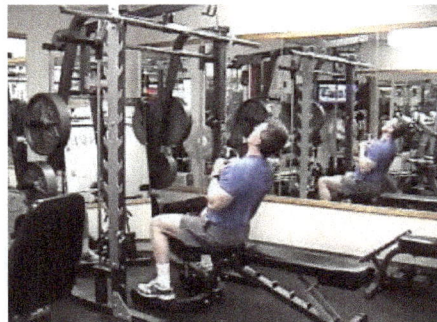

Dead-Lift (1-3 Sets 7-10 Reps)

Lat Close Grip Pull Down (1-3 Sets 7-15 Reps)

28 - Exercises

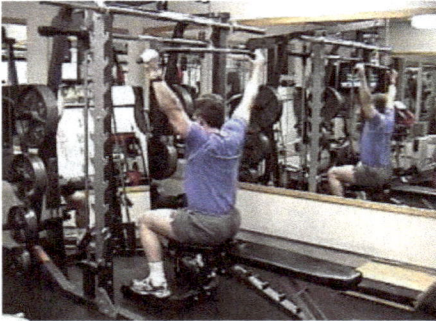

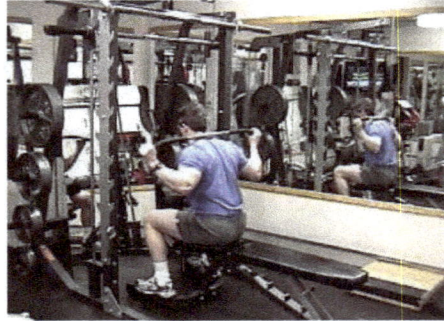

Lat Wide Grip Behind Head Pull Down (1-3 Sets 7-10 Reps)

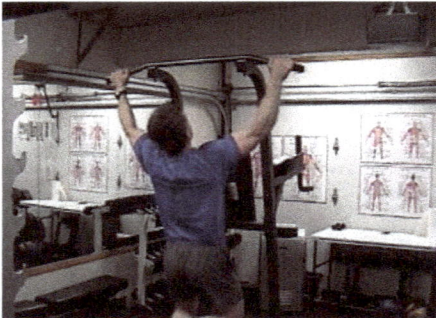

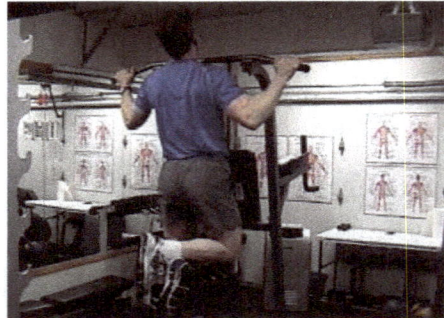

Chin Ups (1-3 Sets 7-15 Reps)

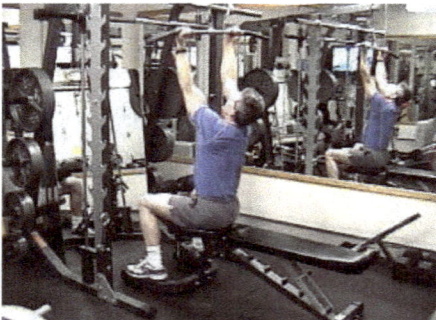

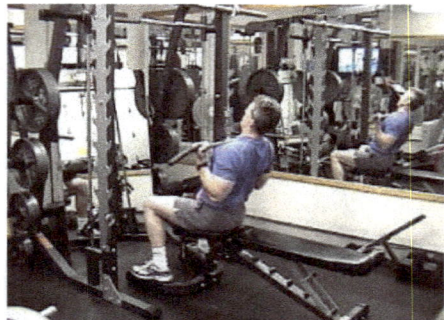

Lat Reverse Grip Pull Down (1-3 Sets 7-15 Reps)

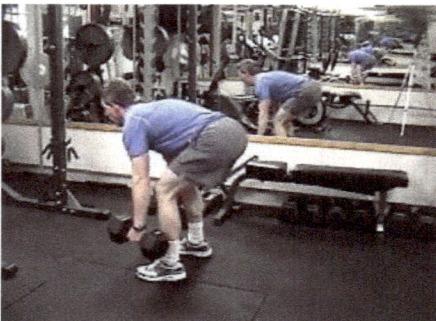

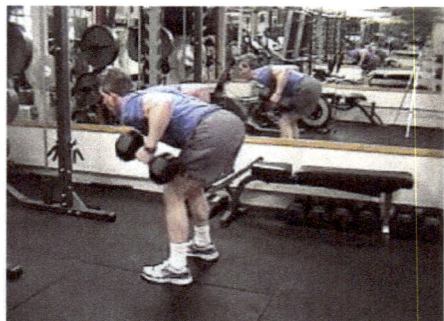

Standing Bent Double Dumbbell Row (1-3 Sets 7-10 Reps)

Levator Scapulae

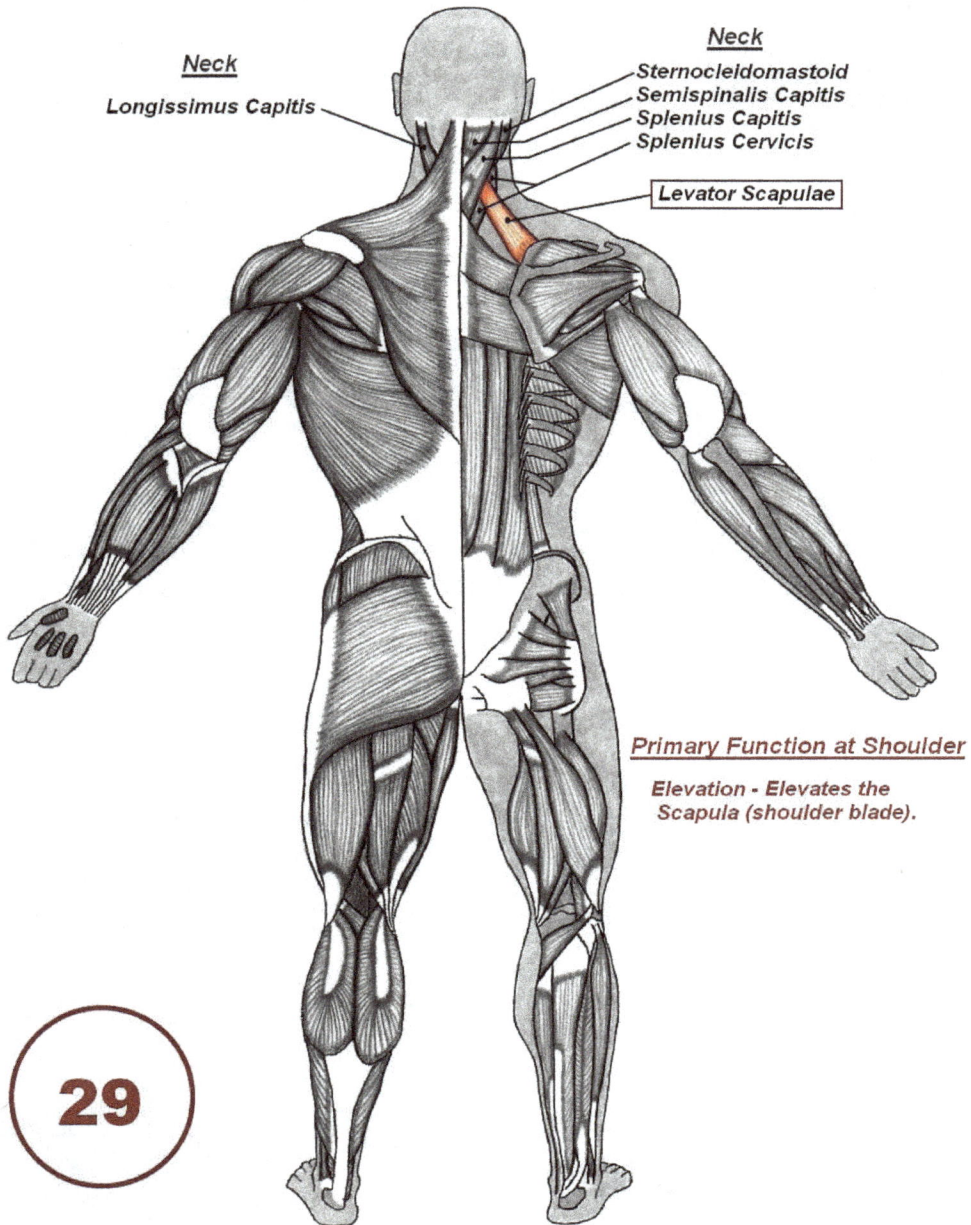

Neck

Longissimus Capitis

Neck

Sternocleidomastoid
Semispinalis Capitis
Splenius Capitis
Splenius Cervicis

Levator Scapulae

Primary Function at Shoulder

Elevation - Elevates the
Scapula (shoulder blade).

29

29 - Exercises

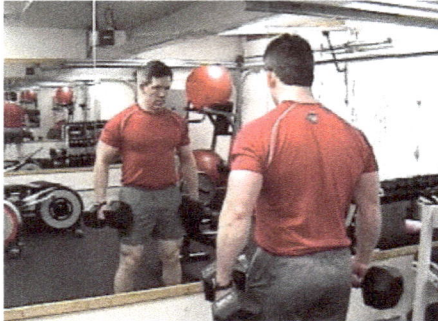

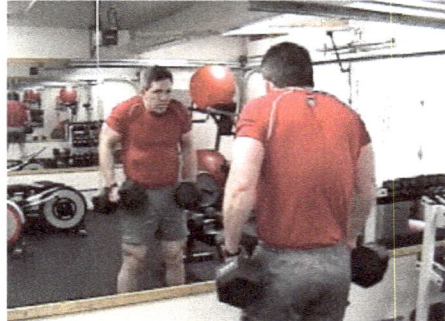

Standing Dumbbell Shrugs (1-3 Sets 7-10 Reps)

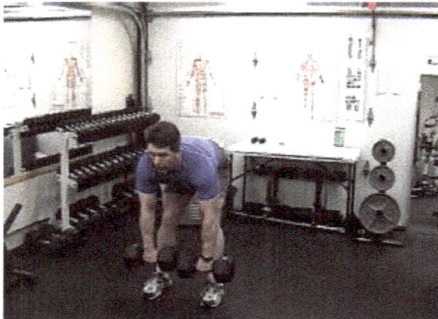

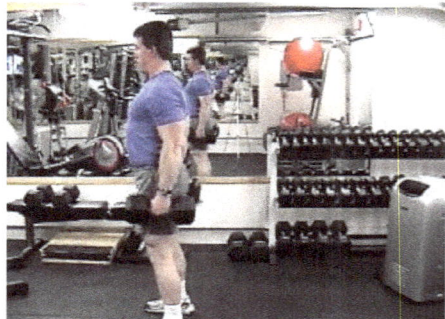

Straight Leg Dumbbell Dead-Lift (1-3 Sets 7-10 Reps)

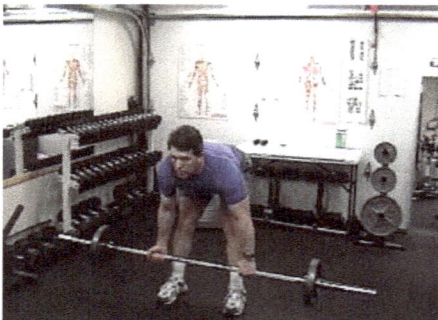

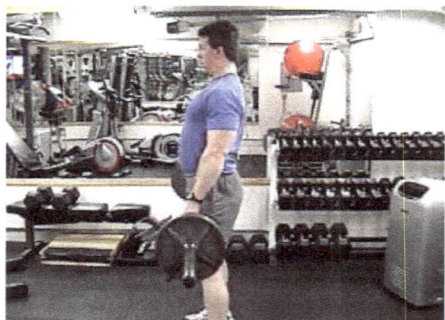

Straight Leg Bar Dead-Lift (1-3 Sets 7-10 Reps)

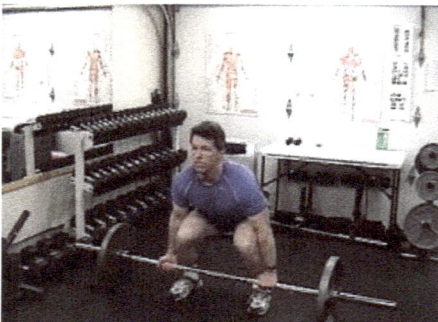

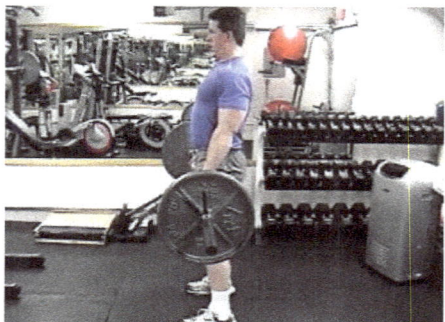

Dead-Lift (1-3 Sets 7-10 Reps)

Latissimus Dorsi (Lat's)

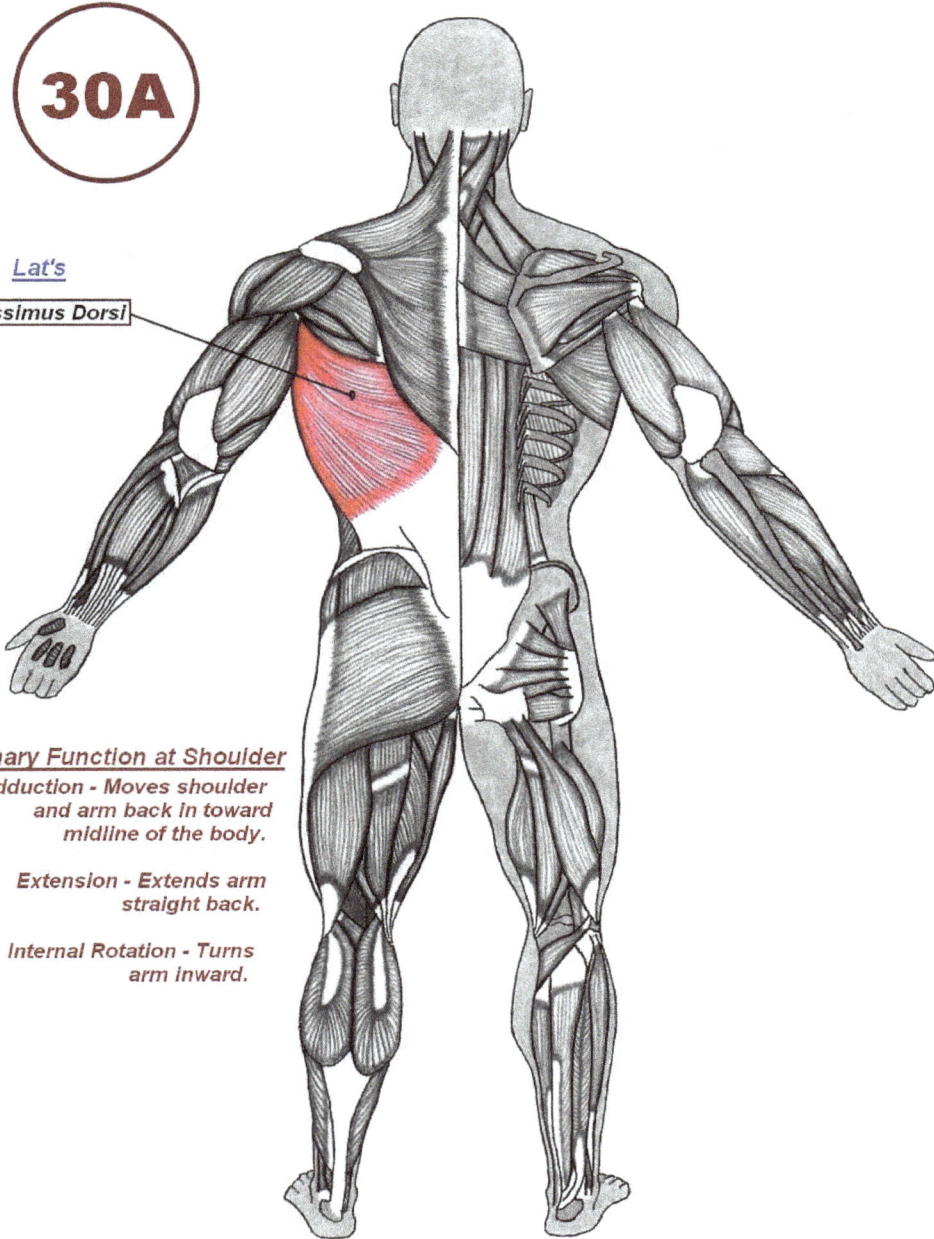

30A

Lat's

Latissimus Dorsi

Primary Function at Shoulder
*Adduction - Moves shoulder
and arm back in toward
midline of the body.*

*Extension - Extends arm
straight back.*

*Internal Rotation - Turns
arm inward.*

Teres Major

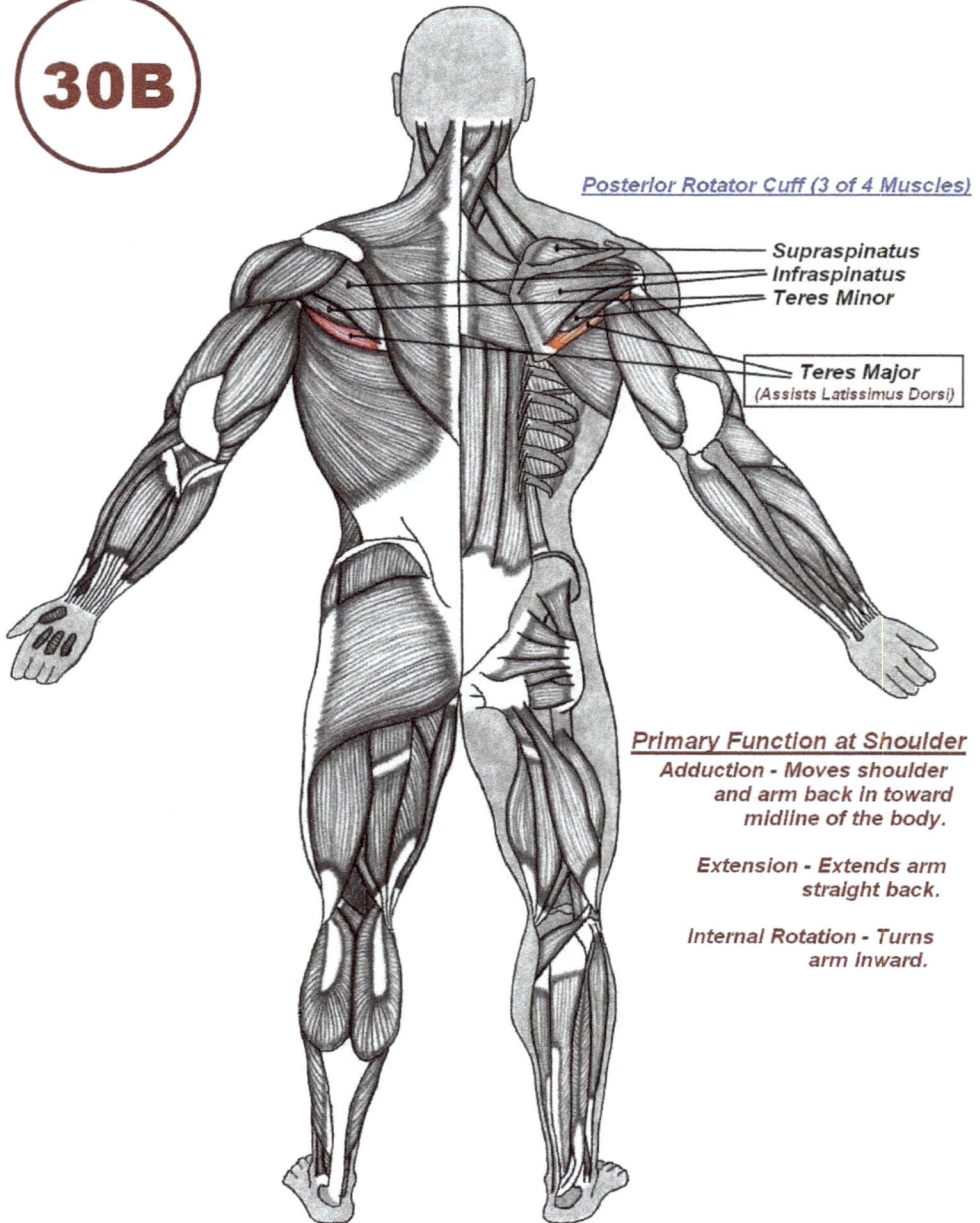

30B

Posterior Rotator Cuff (3 of 4 Muscles)

Supraspinatus
Infraspinatus
Teres Minor

Teres Major
(Assists Latissimus Dorsi)

Primary Function at Shoulder
Adduction - Moves shoulder and arm back in toward midline of the body.

Extension - Extends arm straight back.

Internal Rotation - Turns arm inward.

30A and B - Exercises

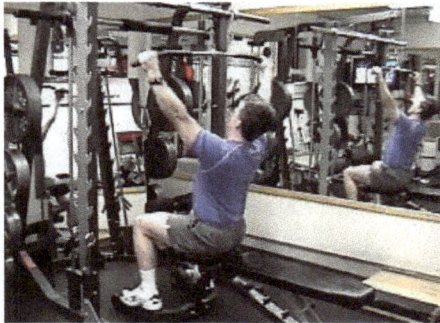

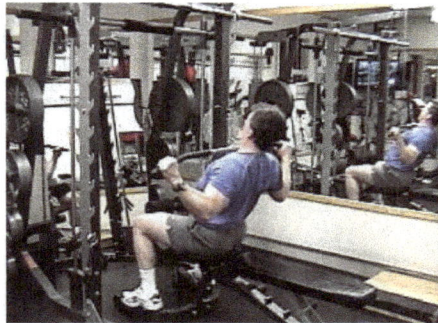

Lat Wide Grip Front Pull Down (1-3 Sets 7-15 Reps)

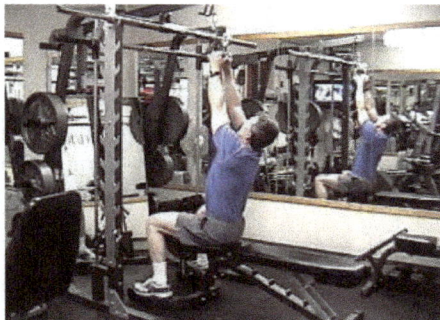

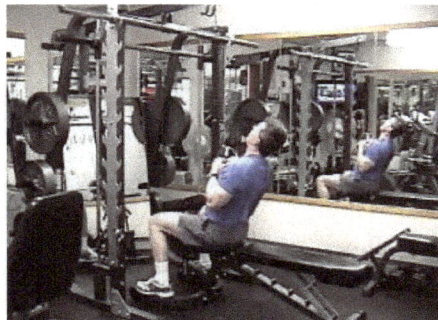

Lat Close Grip Pull Down (1-3 Sets 7-15 Reps)

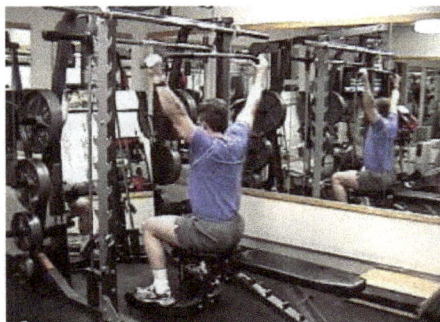

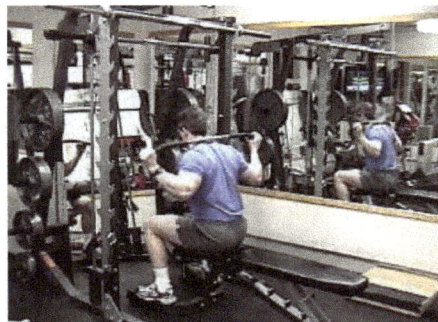

Lat Wide Grip Behind Head Pull Down (1-3 Sets 7-10 Reps)

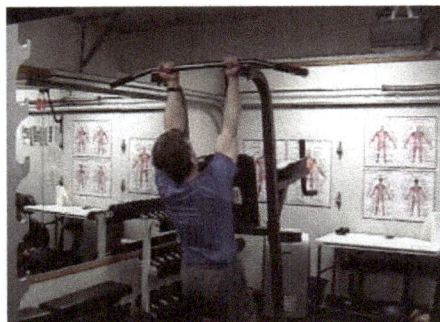

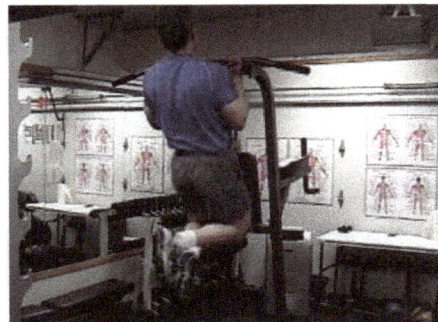

Reverse Chin Ups (1-3 Sets 7-15 Reps)

30A and B - Exercises

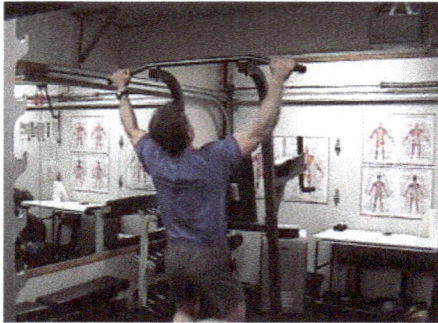

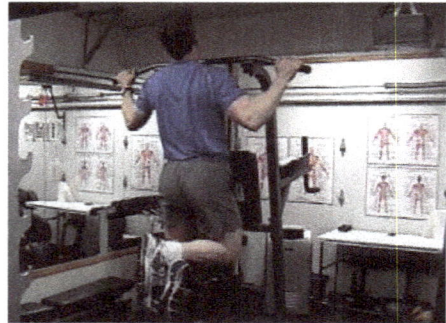

Chin Ups (1-3 Sets 7-15 Reps)

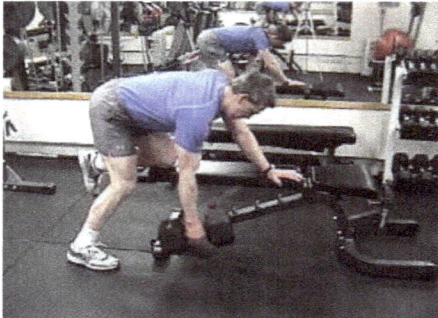

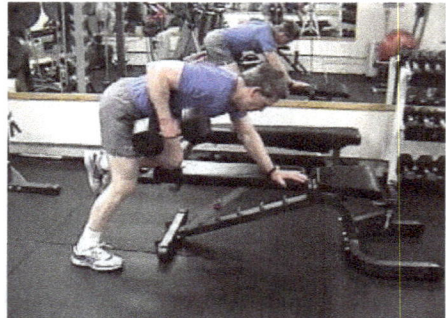

Kneeling Dumbbell Row (1-3 Sets 7-15 Reps)

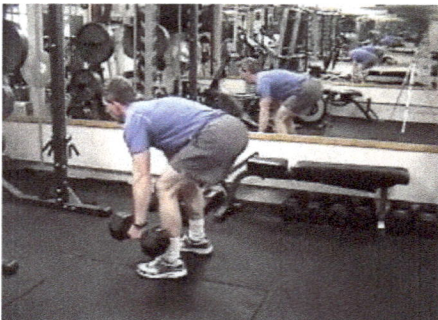

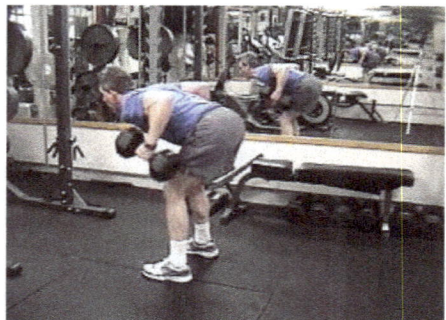

Standing Bent Double Dumbbell Row (1-3 Sets 7-10 Reps)

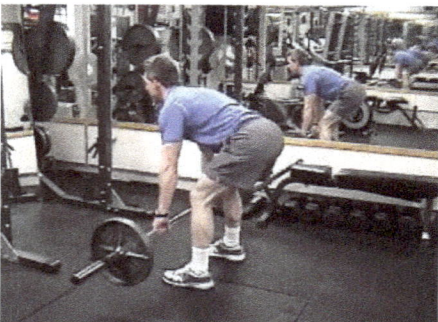

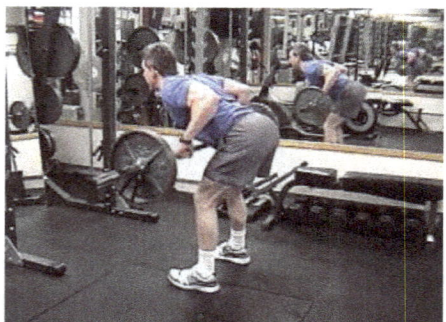

Standing Bent Bar Row (1-3 Sets 7-10 Reps)

30A and B - Exercises

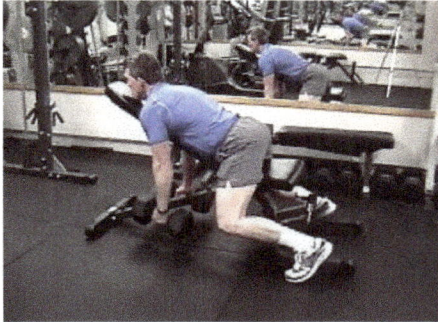

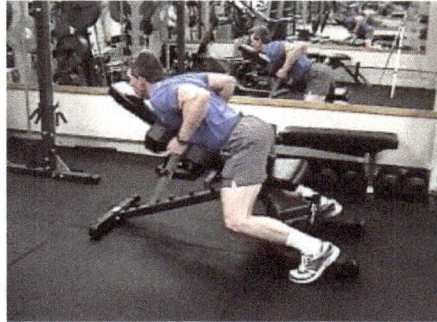

Seated Incline Double Dumbbell Row (1-3 Sets 7-15 Reps)

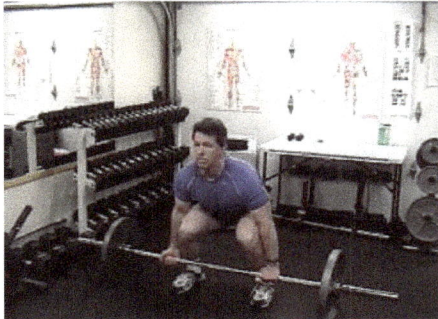

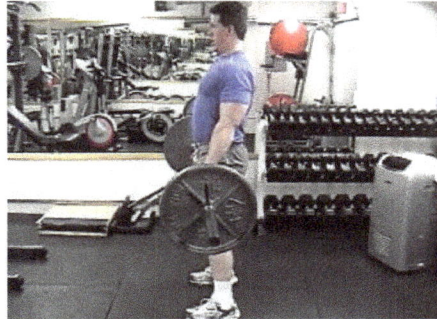

Dead-Lift (1-3 Sets 7-10 Reps)

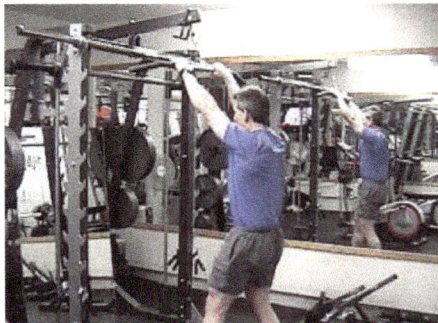

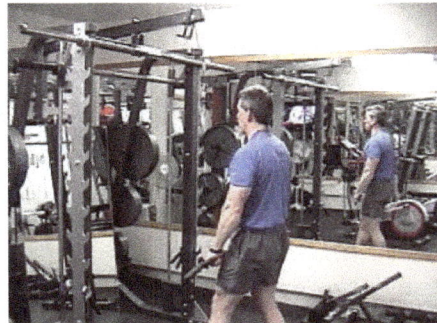

Straight Arm Narrow Grip Cable Pull Down (1-3 Sets 7-15 Reps)

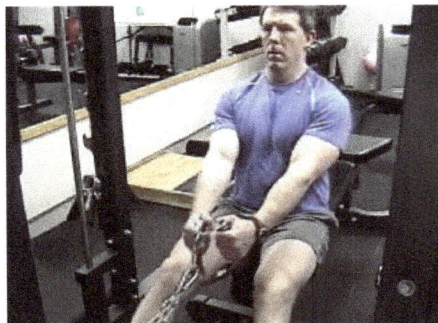

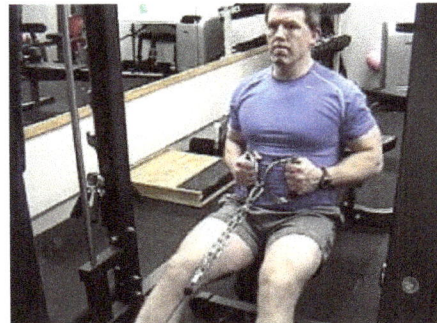

Seated Close Grip Cable Row (1-3 Sets 7-15 Reps)

Rhomboid Muscles of Back

31

Rhomboids
- Rhomboid Minor
- Rhomboid Major

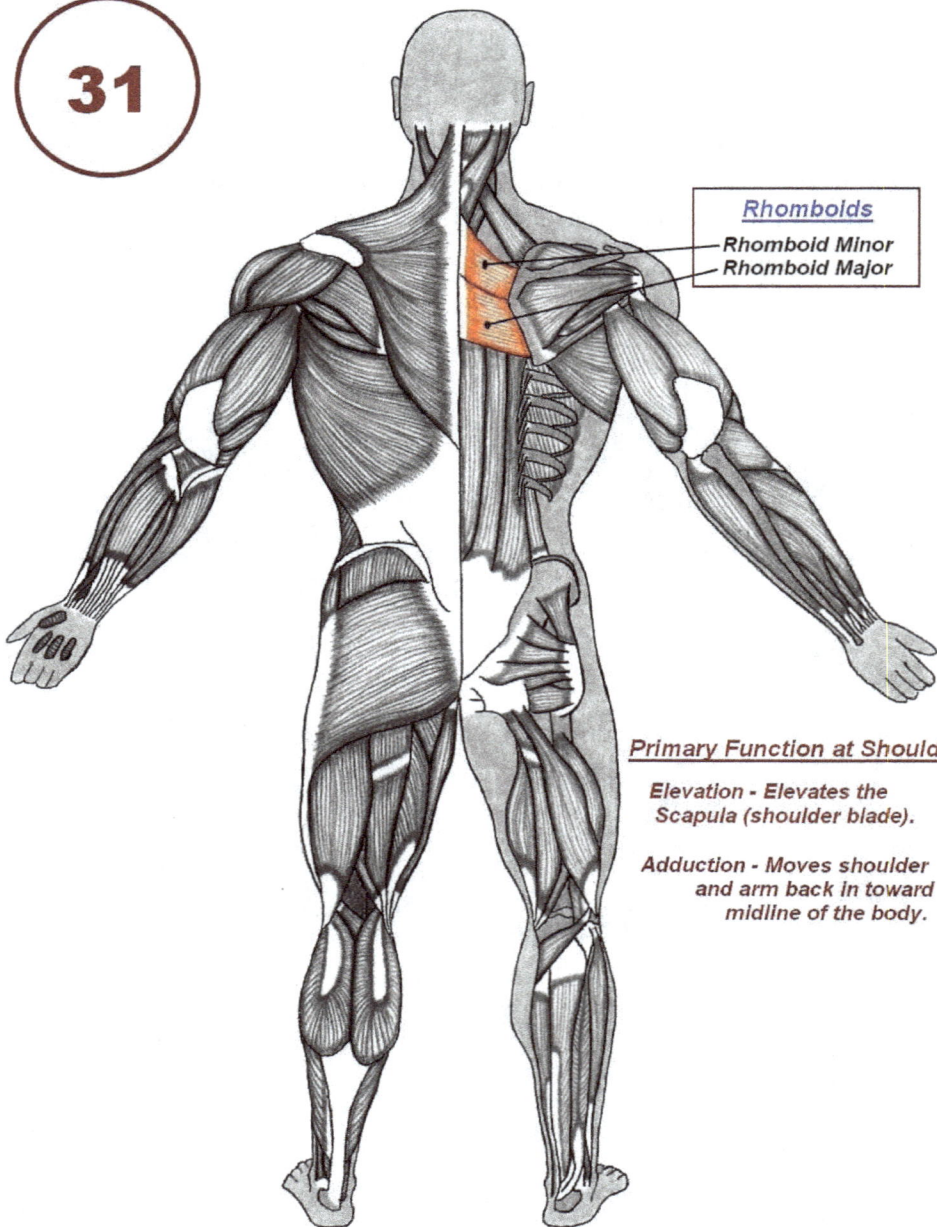

Primary Function at Shoulder

Elevation - Elevates the Scapula (shoulder blade).

Adduction - Moves shoulder and arm back in toward midline of the body.

31 - Exercises

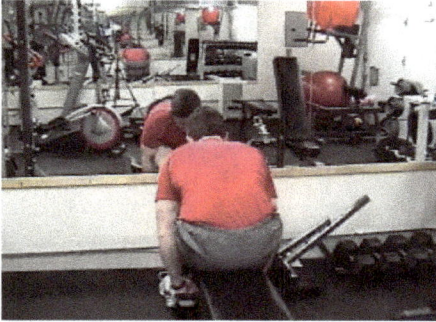

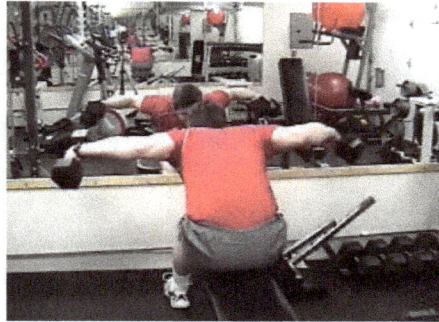

Shoulder Seated Bent Lateral Dumbbell Raise (1-3 Sets 7-10 Reps)

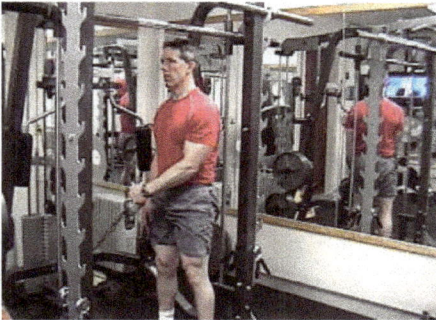

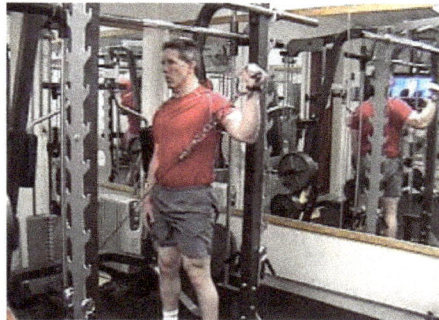

Shoulder Standing Cable External Rotation (1-3 Sets 7-10 Reps)

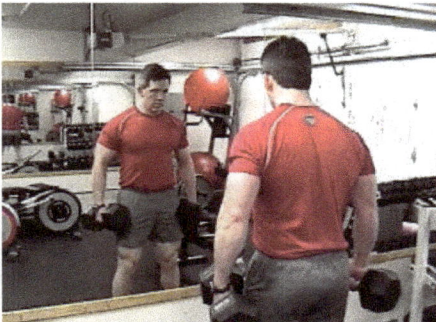

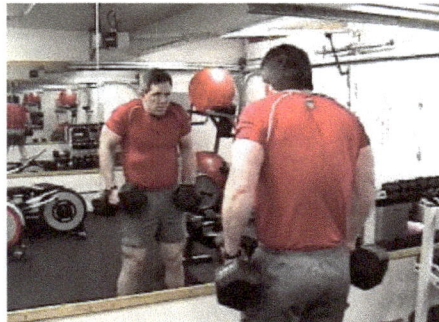

Standing Dumbbell Shrugs (1-3 Sets 7-10 Reps)

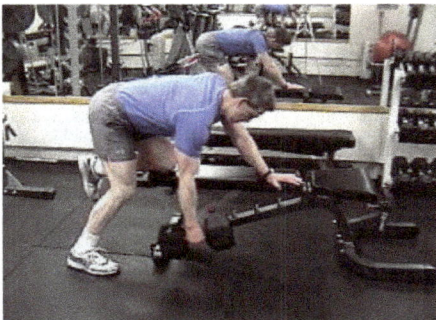

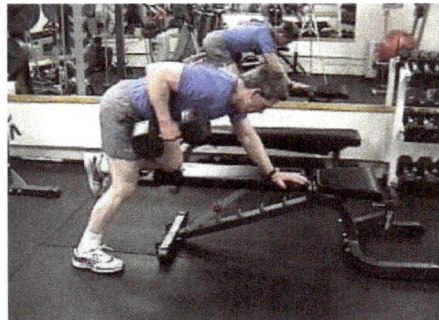

Kneeling Dumbbell Row (1-3 Sets 7-15 Reps)

31 - Exercises

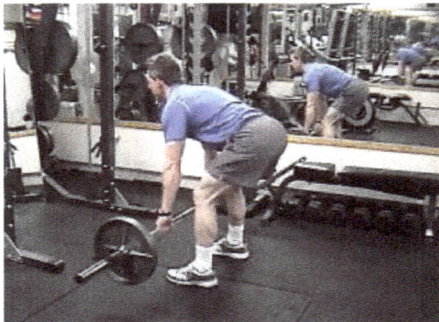

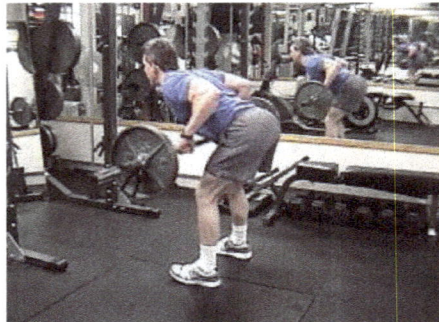

Standing Bent Bar Row (1-3 Sets 7-10 Reps)

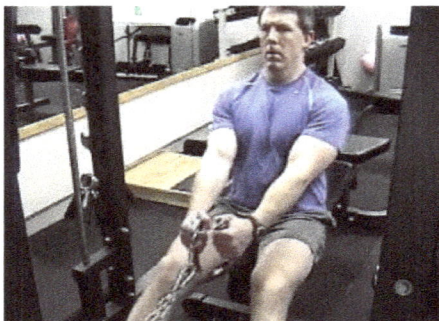

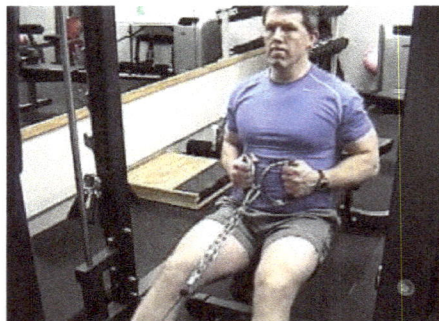

Seated Close Grip Cable Row (1-3 Sets 7-15 Reps)

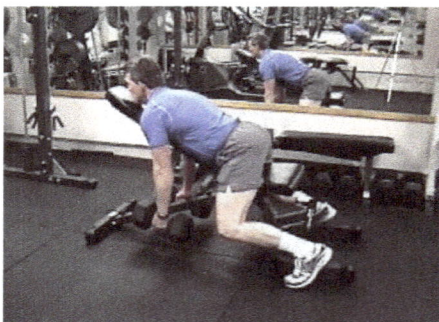

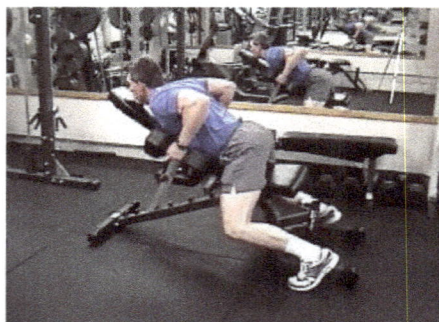

Seated Incline Double Dumbbell Row (1-3 Sets 7-15 Reps)

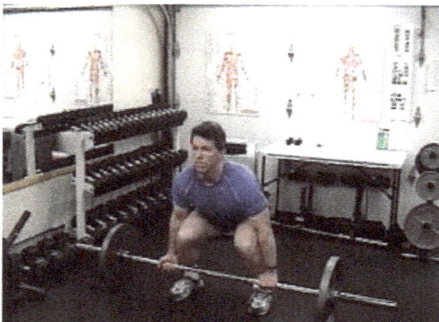

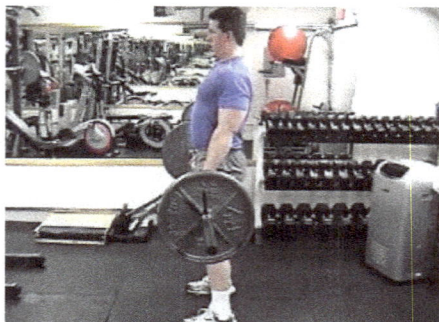

Dead-Lift (1-3 Sets 7-10 Reps)

Erector Spinae Muscles of Back

32

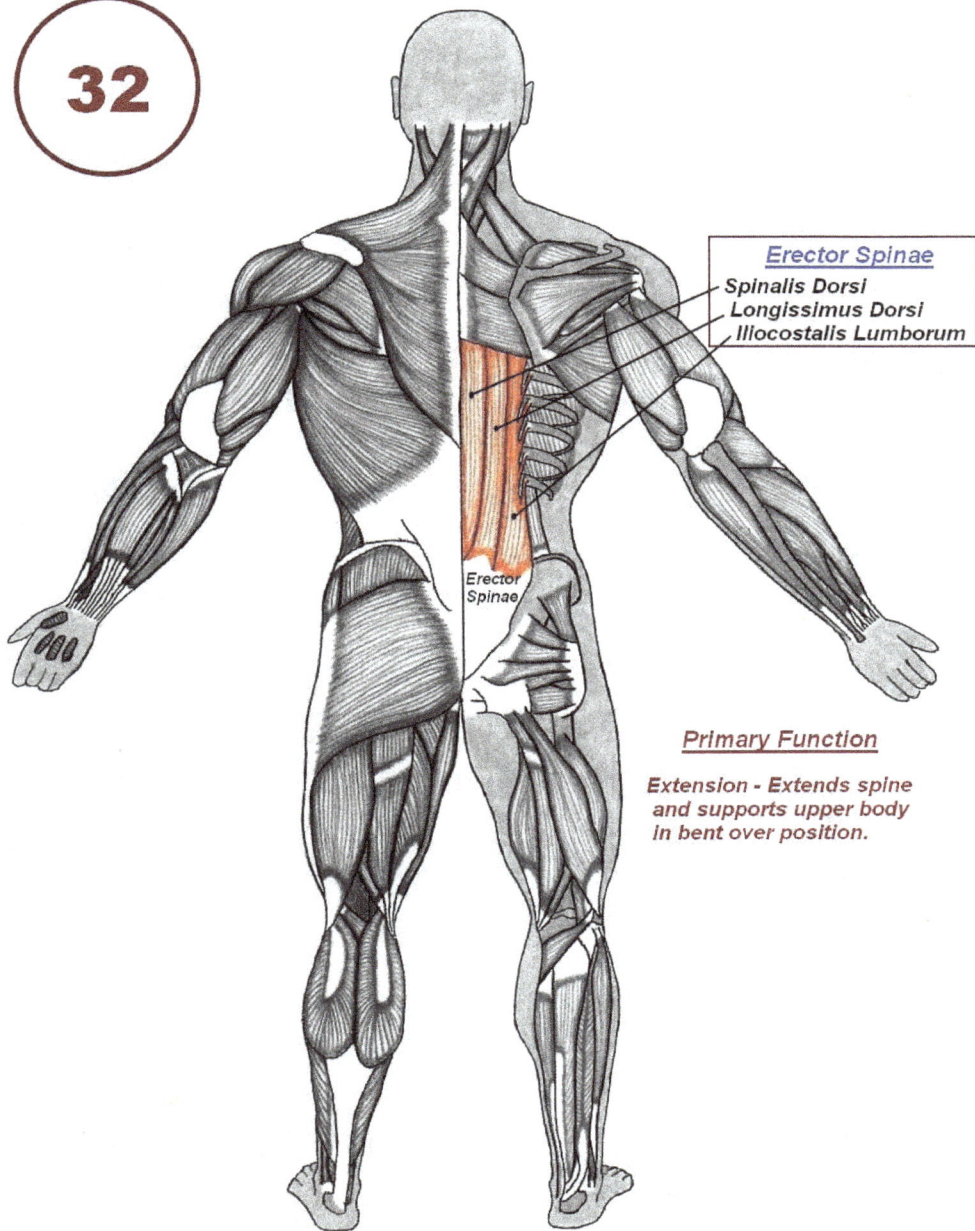

Erector Spinae
Spinalis Dorsi
Longissimus Dorsi
Iliocostalis Lumborum

Erector
Spinae

Primary Function

*Extension - Extends spine
and supports upper body
in bent over position.*

121

32 - Exercises

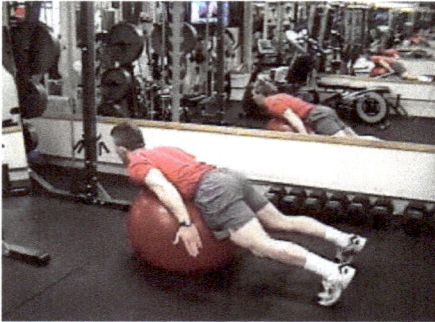

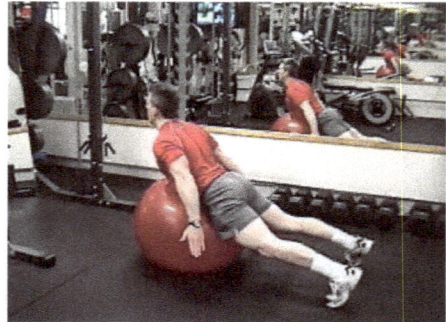

Back Extension on Stability Ball (1-3 Sets 7-15 Reps)

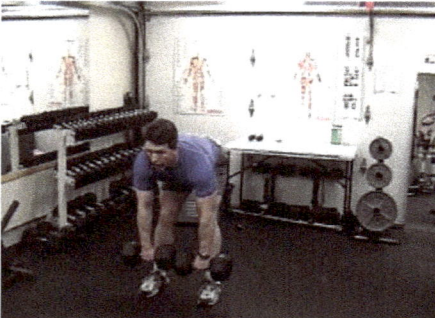

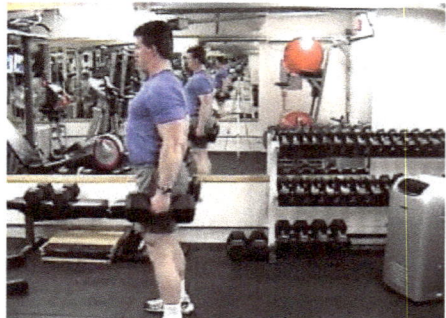

Straight Leg Dumbbell Dead-Lift (1-3 Sets 7-10 Reps)

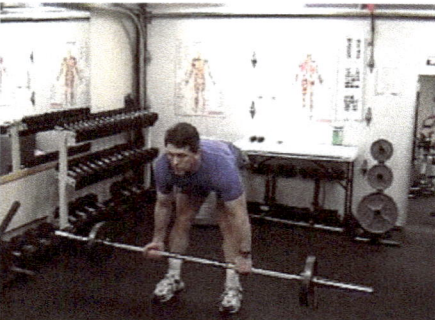

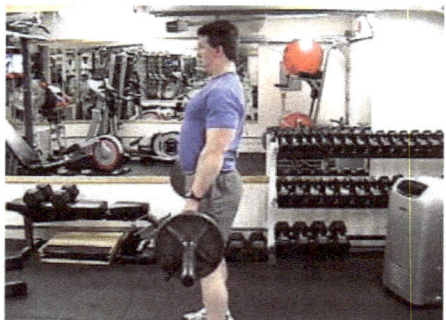

Straight Leg Bar Dead-Lift (1-3 Sets 7-10 Reps)

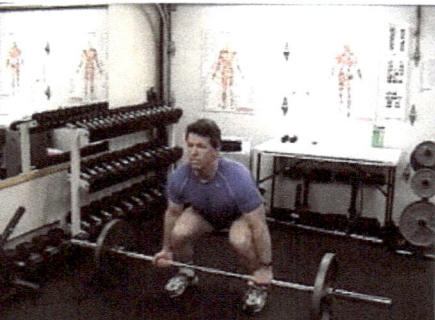

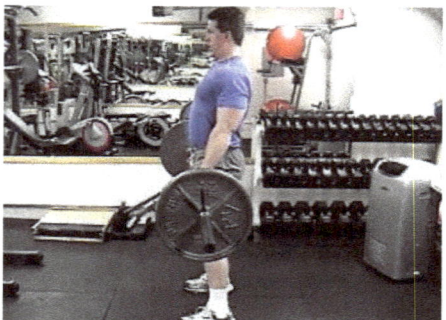

Dead-Lift (1-3 Sets 7-10 Reps)

32 - Exercises

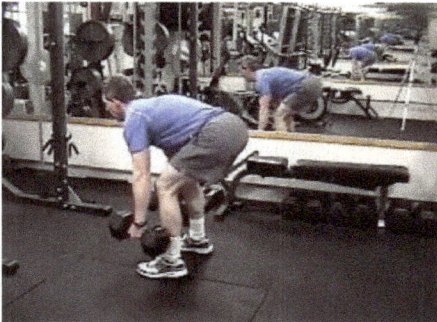
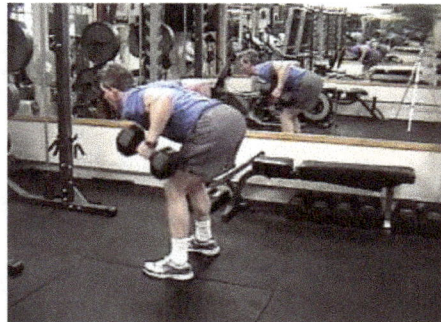

Standing Bent Double Dumbbell Row (Bent Position: 1-3 Sets 7-10 Reps)

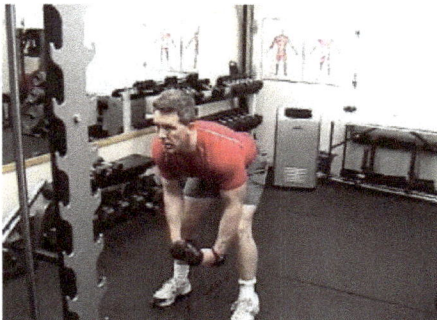
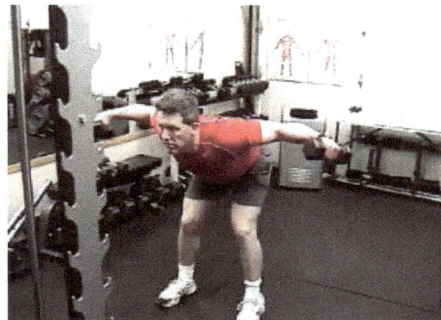

Standing Bent Lateral Dumbbell Raise (Bent Position: 1-3 Sets 7-10 Reps)

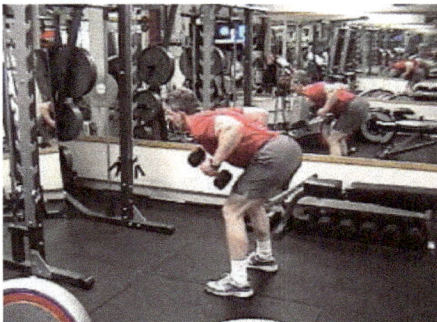
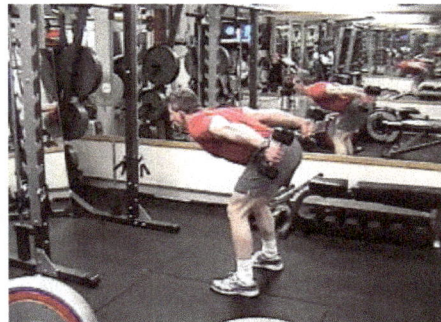

Triceps Double Dumbbell Kickback (Bent Position: 1-3 Sets 7-10 Reps)

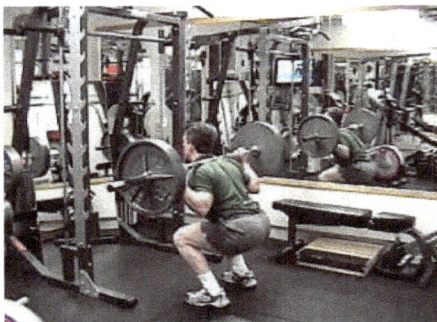
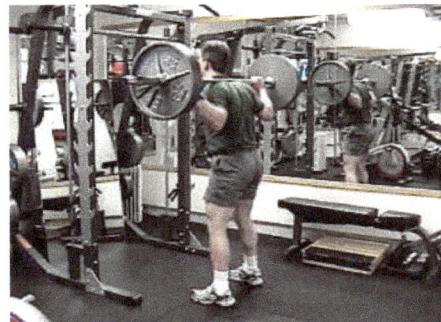

Free Weight Squats (Bent Position: 1-5 Sets 7-10 Reps)

Serratus Anterior (Posterior View)

33

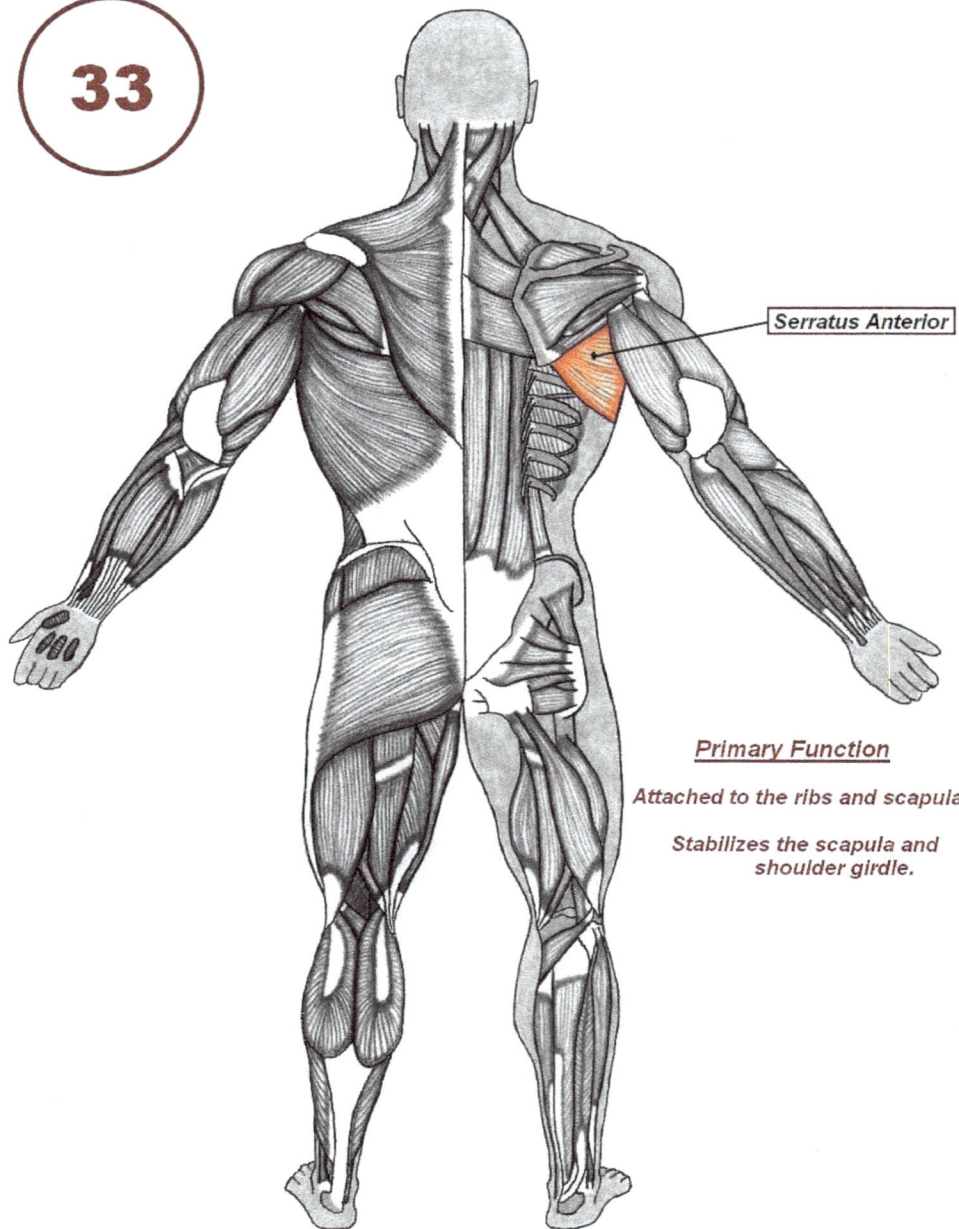

Serratus Anterior

Primary Function

Attached to the ribs and scapula.

Stabilizes the scapula and shoulder girdle.

33 - Exercises

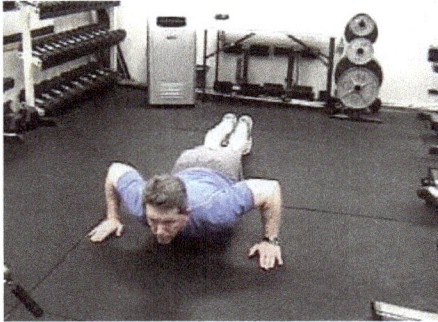

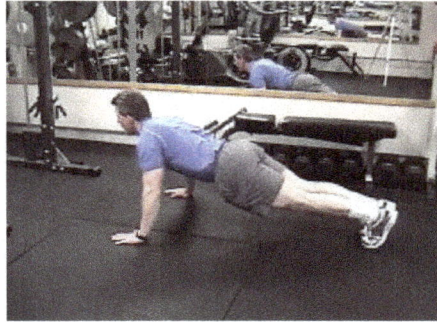

Push Ups (1-3 Sets 10-50 Reps)

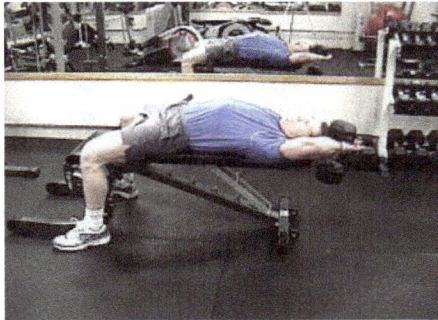

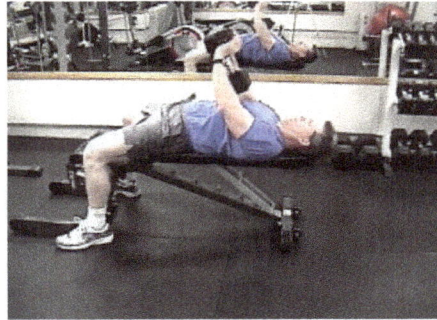

Lying Dumbbell Pull Over (1-3 Sets 7-15 Reps)

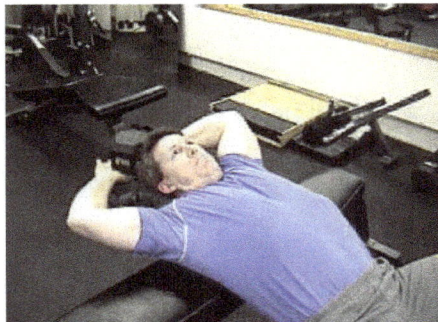

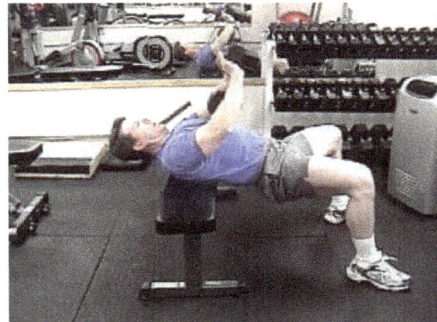

Lying Dumbbell Pull Over - Bridge Position (1-3 Sets 7-15 Reps)

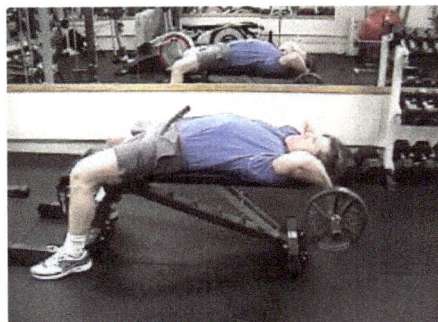

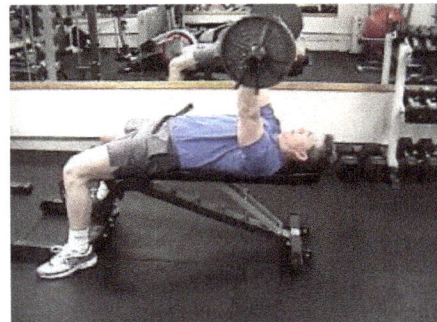

Lying EZ-Bar Pull Over (1-3 Sets 7-15 Reps)

33 - Exercises

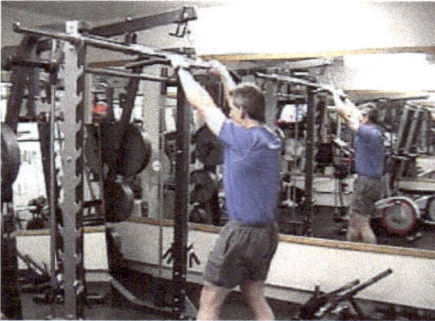

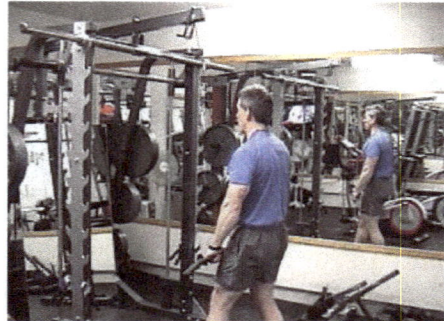

Staight Arm Narrow Grip Cable Pull Down (1-3 Sets 7-15 Reps)

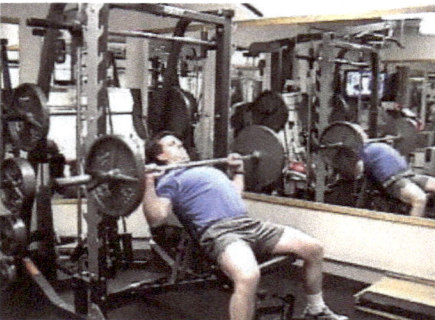

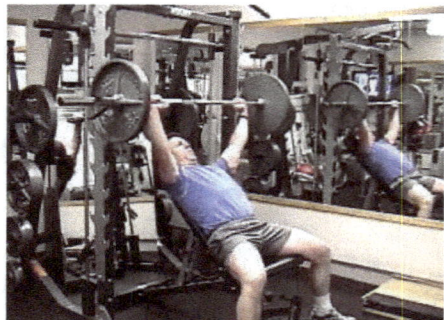

Chest Incline Bar Press (1-3 Sets 7-10 Reps)

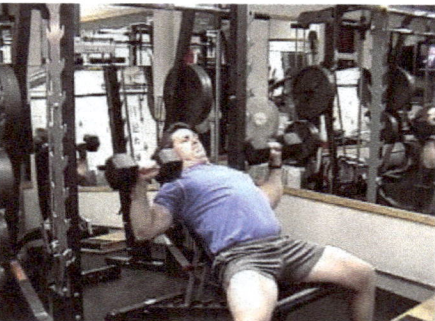

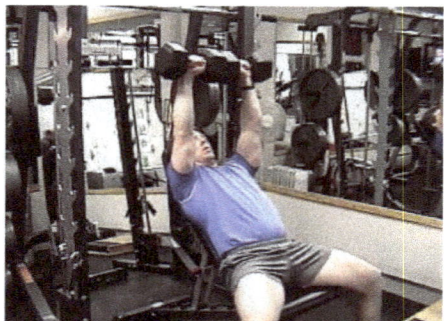

Chest Incline Dumbbell Press (1-3 Sets 7-10 Reps)

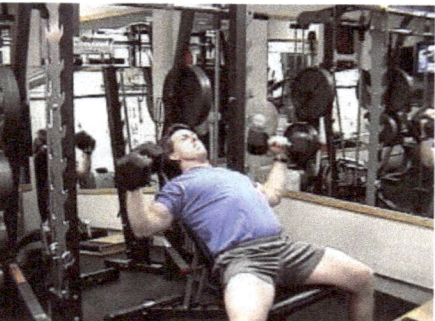

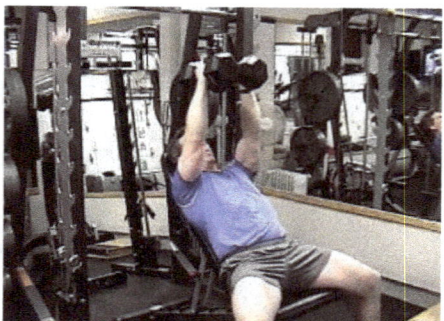

Chest Incline Flye (1-3 Sets 7-10 Reps)

External Intercostals

34

Intercostals
External Intercostals

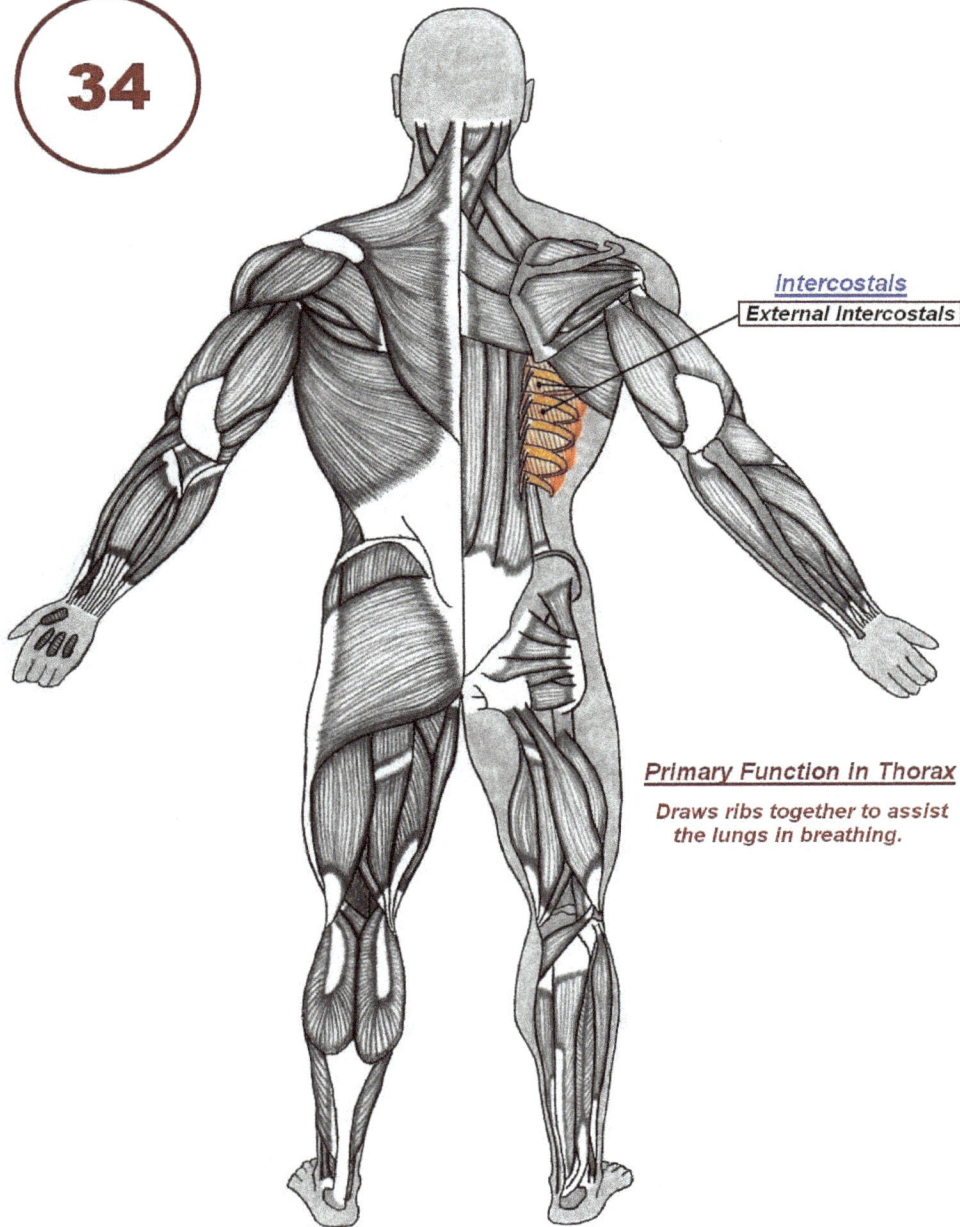

Primary Function in Thorax

*Draws ribs together to assist
the lungs in breathing.*

Rear Deltoid

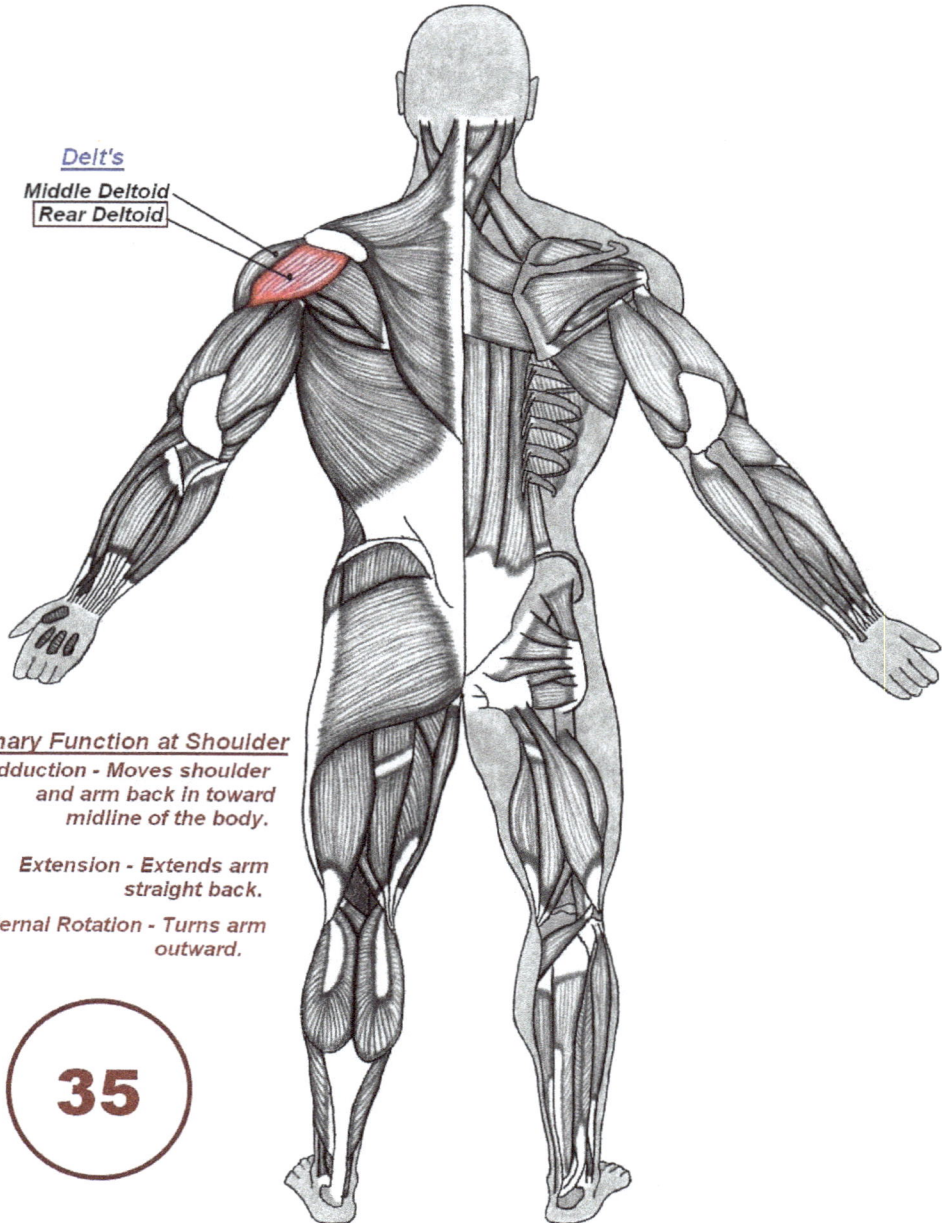

Delt's
Middle Deltoid
Rear Deltoid

Primary Function at Shoulder
*Adduction - Moves shoulder
and arm back in toward
midline of the body.*

*Extension - Extends arm
straight back.*

*External Rotation - Turns arm
outward.*

35

35 - Exercises

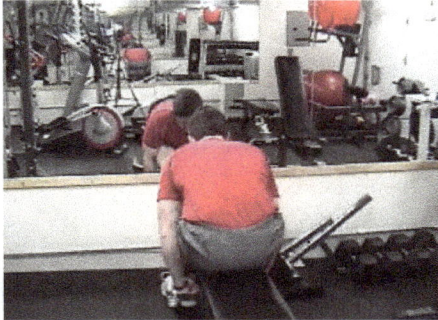

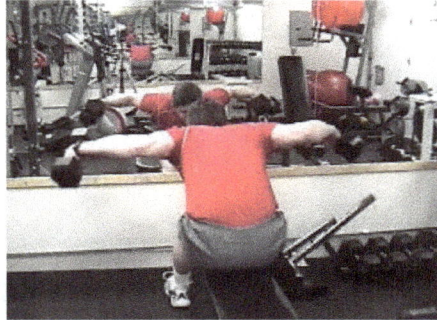

Shoulder Seated Bent Dumbbell Lateral Raise (1-3 Sets 7-10 Reps)

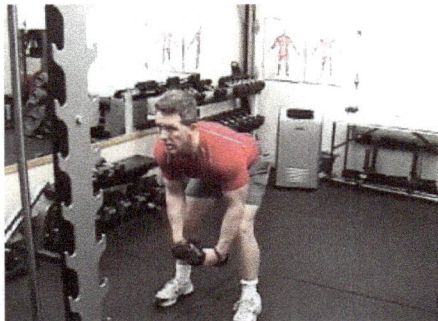

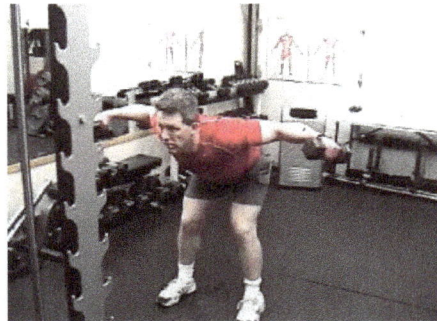

Shoulder Standing Bent Dumbbell Lateral Raise (1-3 Sets 7-10 Reps)

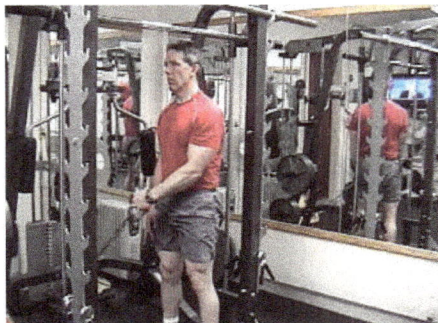

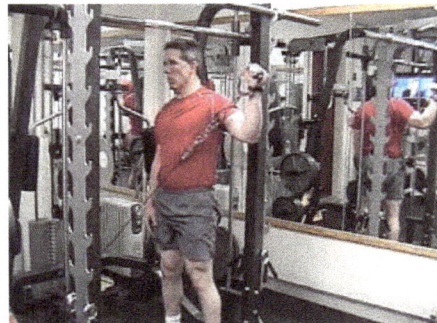

Shoulder Standing Cable External Rotation (1-3 Sets 7-10 Reps)

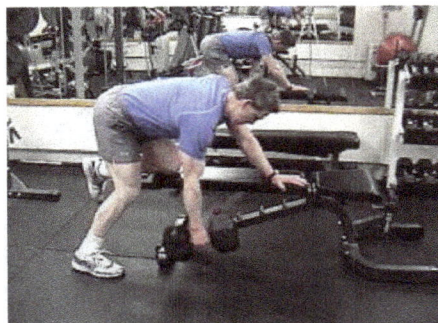

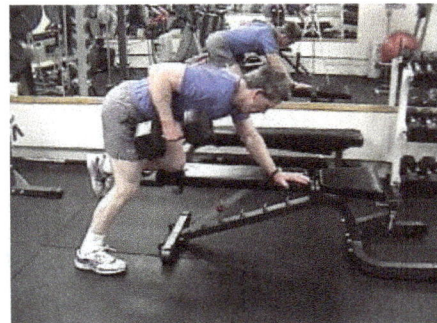

Kneeling Dumbbell Row (1-3 Sets 7-15 Reps)

35 - Exercises

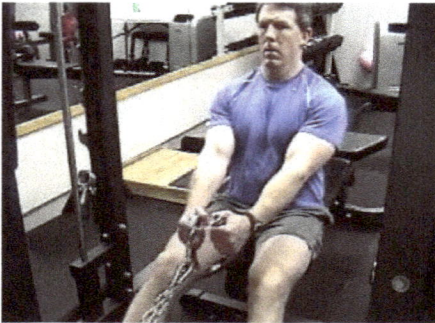

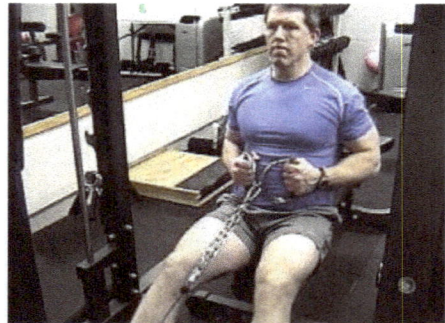

Seated Close Grip Cable Row (1-3 Sets 7-15 Reps)

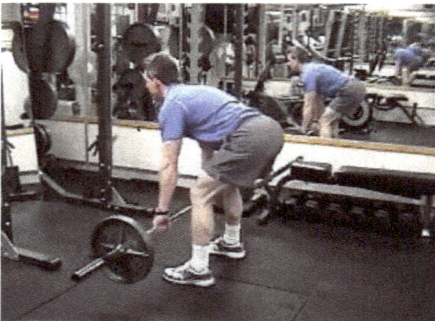

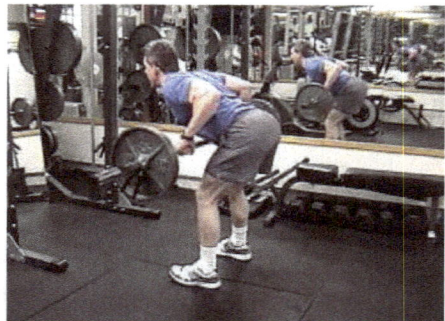

Standing Bent Bar Row (1-3 Sets 7-10 Reps)

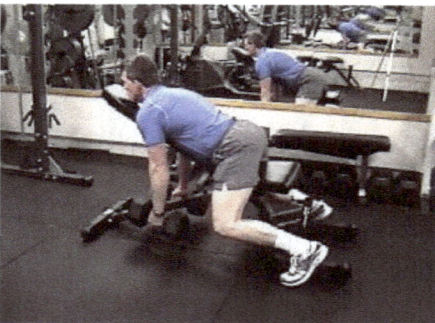

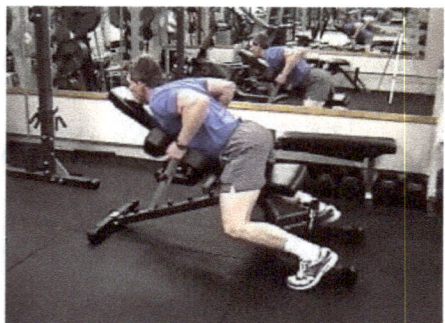

Seated Incline Double Dumbbell Row (1-3 Sets 7-15 Reps)

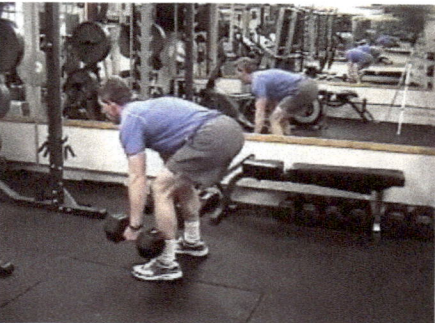

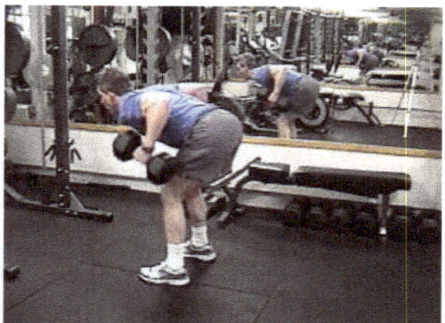

Standing Bent Double Dumbbell Row (1-3 Sets 7-10 Reps)

Middle Deltoid

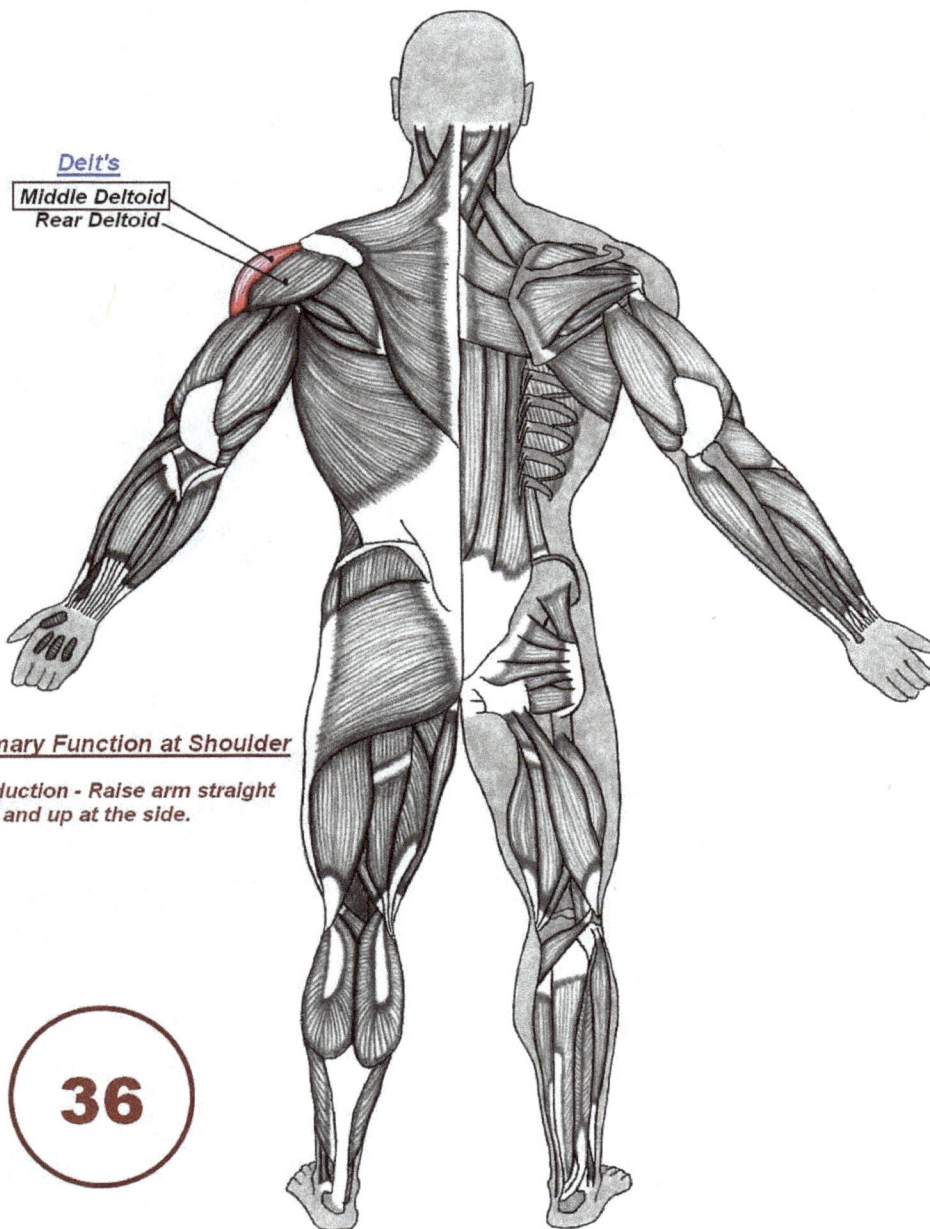

Delt's

Middle Deltoid
Rear Deltoid

Primary Function at Shoulder

Abduction - Raise arm straight out and up at the side.

36

36 - Exercises

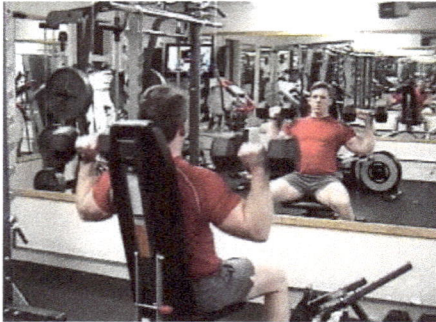

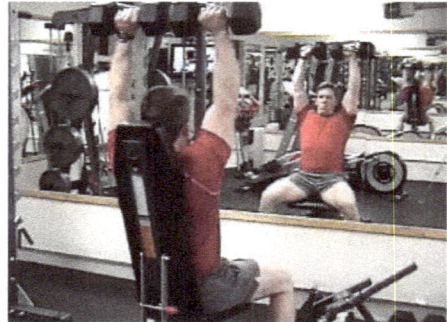

Shoulder Seated Dumbbell Press (1-5 Sets 7-10 Reps)

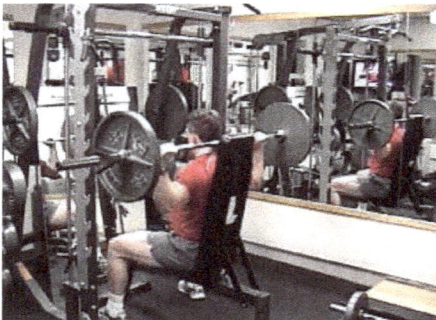

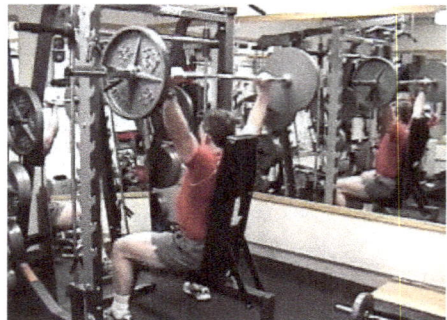

Shoulder Seated Bar Press "Military Press" (1-5 Sets 7-10 Reps)

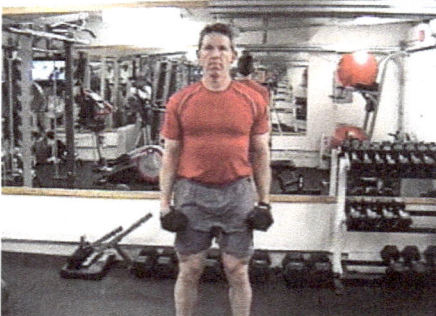

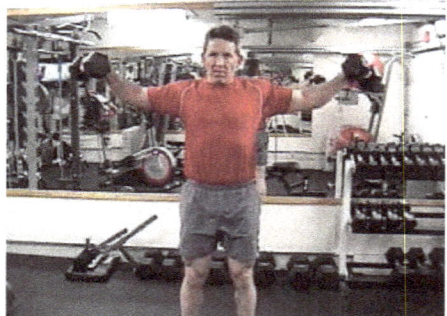

Shoulder Standing DB Lateral Raise (Side Start Position: 1-3 Sets 7-10 Reps)

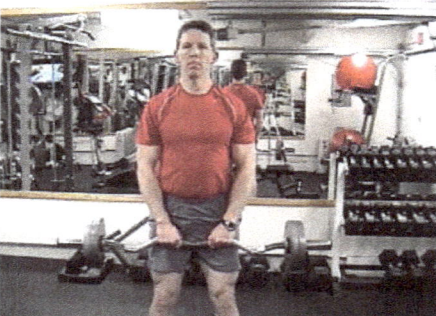

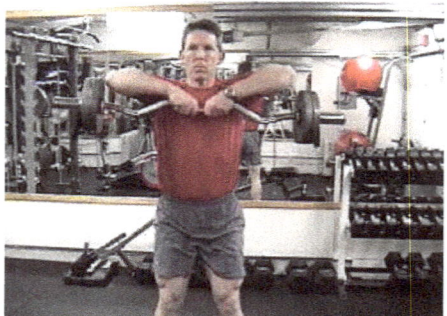

Standing Upright EZ-Bar Row (1-3 Sets 7-10 Reps)

36 - Exercises

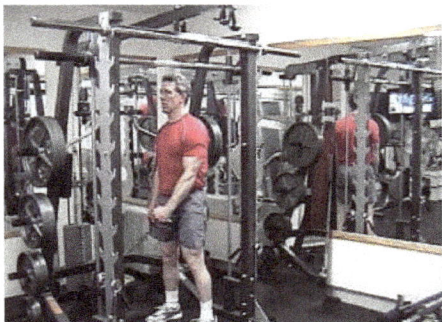
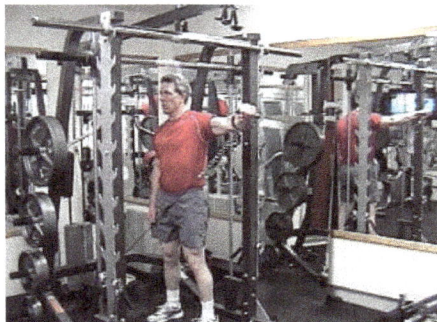

Shoulder Standing Cable Lateral Raise (1-3 Sets 7-10 Reps)

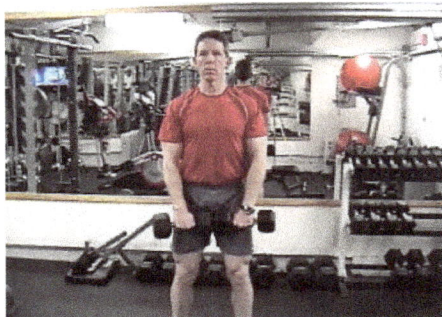
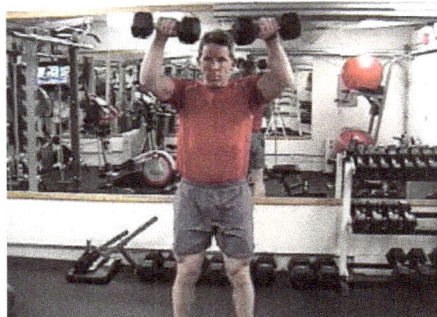

Shoulder Front Double Dumbbell Raise (1-3 Sets 7-10 Reps)

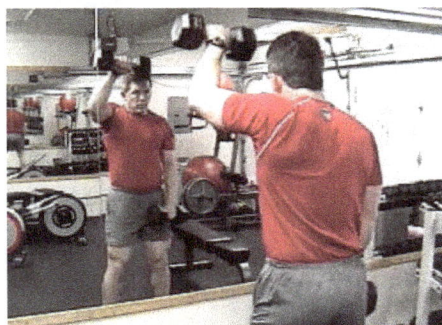
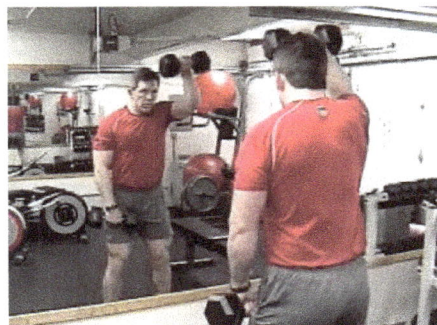

Shoulder Front Alternating Dumbbell Raise (1-3 Sets 7-10 Reps)

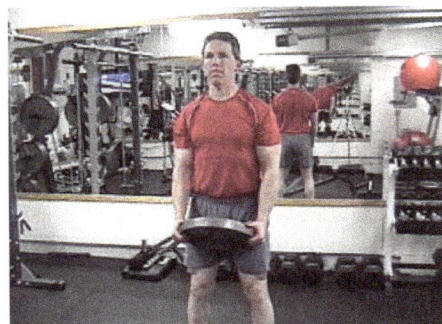
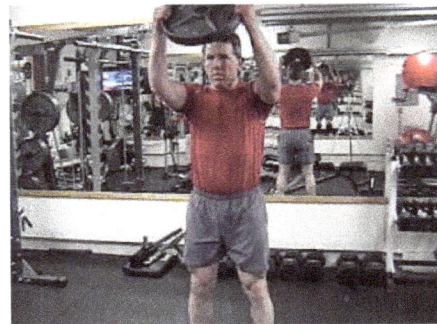

Shoulder Front Plate Raise (1-3 Sets 7-10 Reps)

Posterior Rotator Cuff Muscles

37

Posterior Rotator Cuff (3 of 4 Muscles)

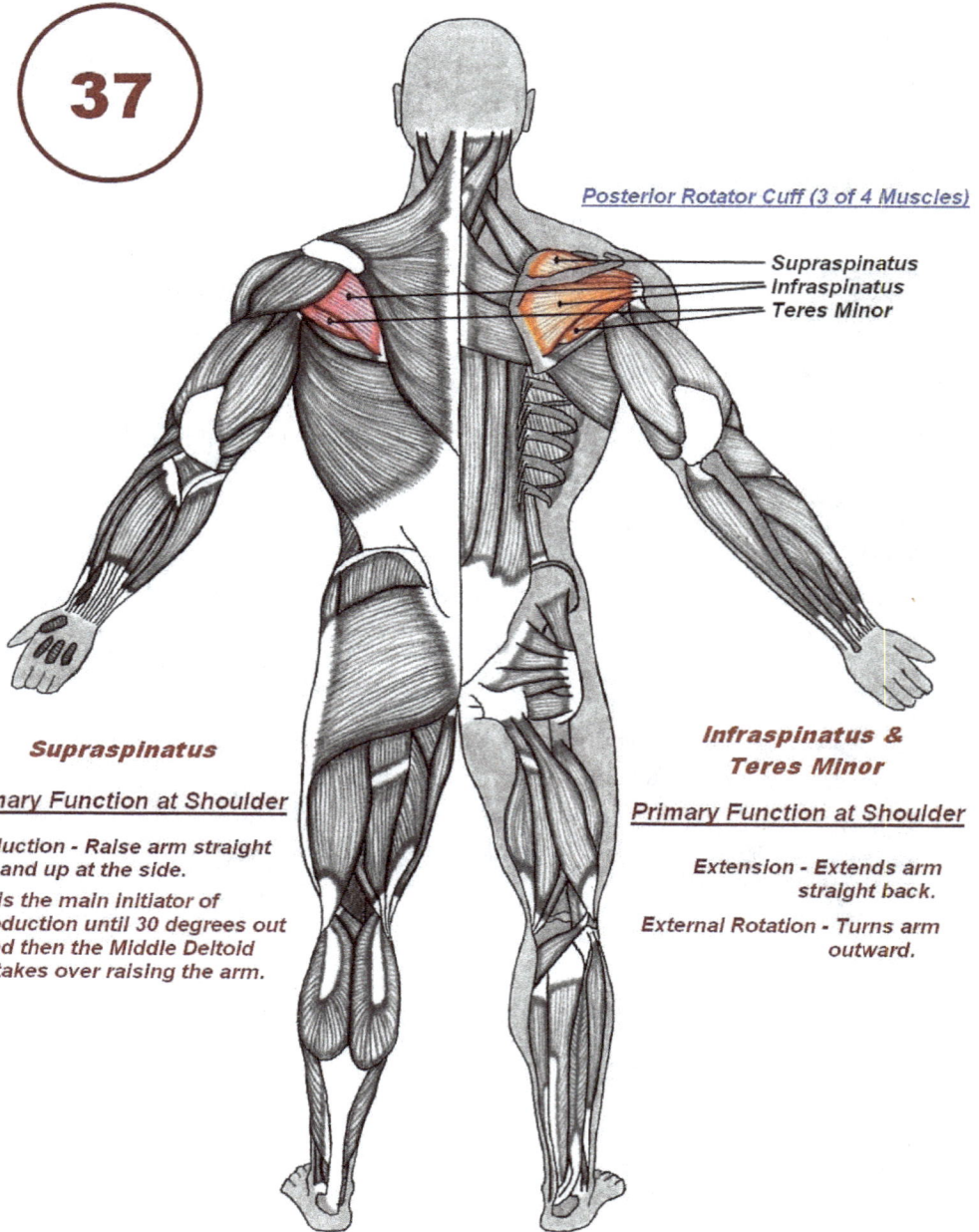

Supraspinatus
Infraspinatus
Teres Minor

Supraspinatus

Primary Function at Shoulder

Abduction - Raise arm straight out and up at the side.

- It is the main initiator of abduction until 30 degrees out and then the Middle Deltoid takes over raising the arm.

Infraspinatus & Teres Minor

Primary Function at Shoulder

Extension - Extends arm straight back.

External Rotation - Turns arm outward.

37 - Exercises

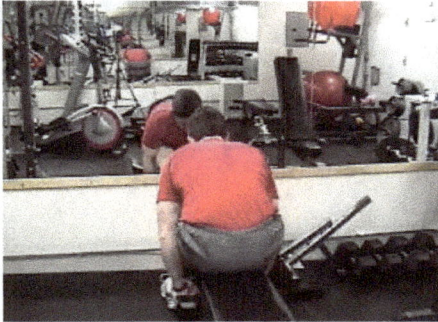

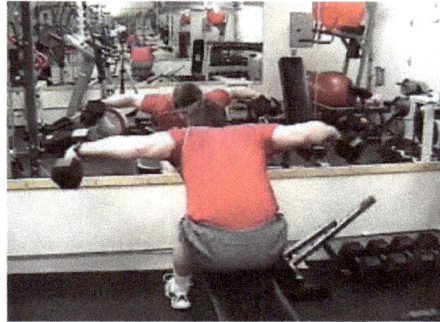

Shoulder Seated Bent Dumbbell Lateral Raise (1-3 Sets 7-10 Reps)

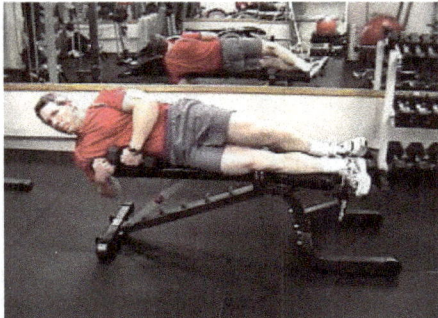

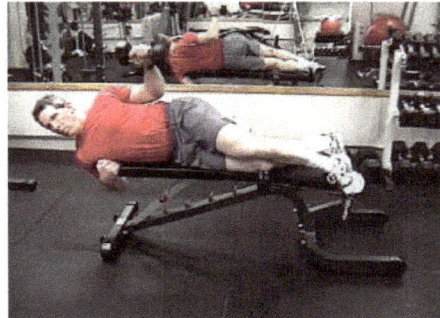

Shoulder Side-Lying External Rotation (1-3 Sets 7-10 Reps)

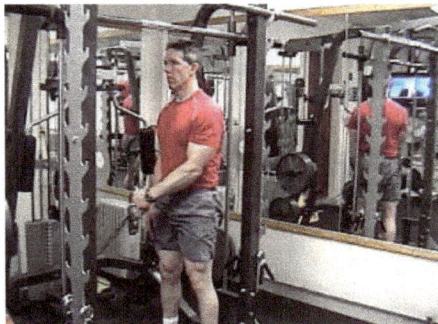

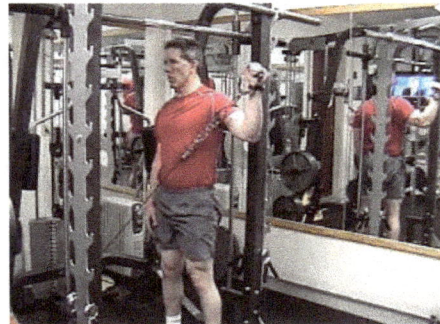

Shoulder Standing Cable External Rotation (1-3 Sets 7-10 Reps)

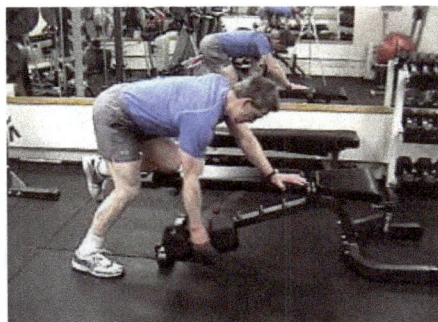

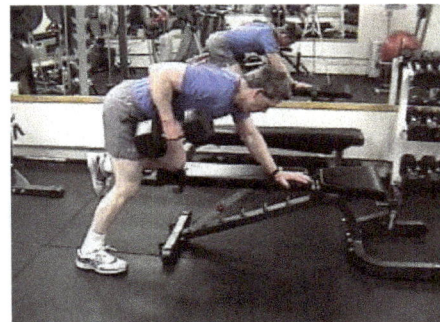

Kneeling Dumbbell Row (1-3 Set 7-15 Reps)

135

37 - Exercises

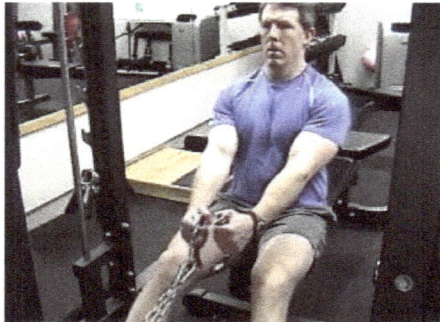

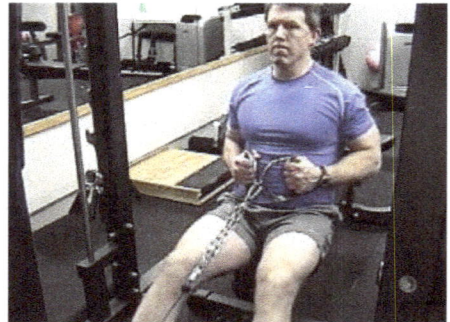

Seated Close Grip Cable Row (1-3 Sets 7-15 Reps)

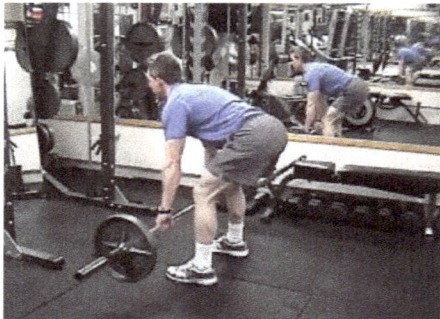

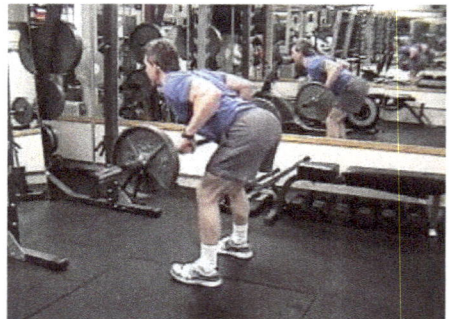

Standing Bent Bar Row (1-3 Sets 7-10 Reps)

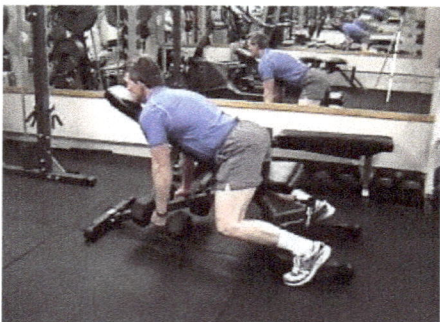

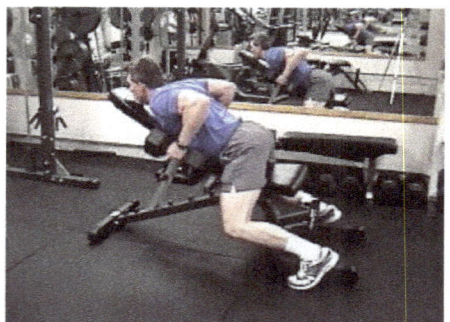

Seated Incline Double Dumbbell Row (1-3 Sets 7-15 Reps)

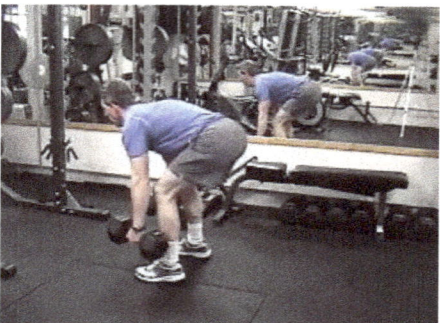

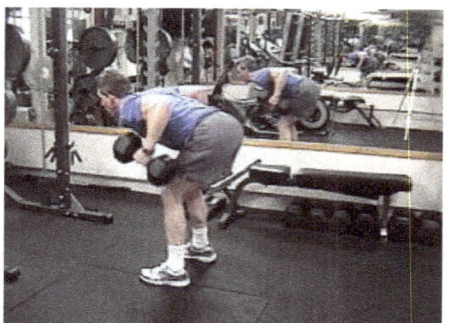

Standing Bent Double Dumbbell Row (1-3 Sets 7-10 Reps)

Quadratus Lumborum

38

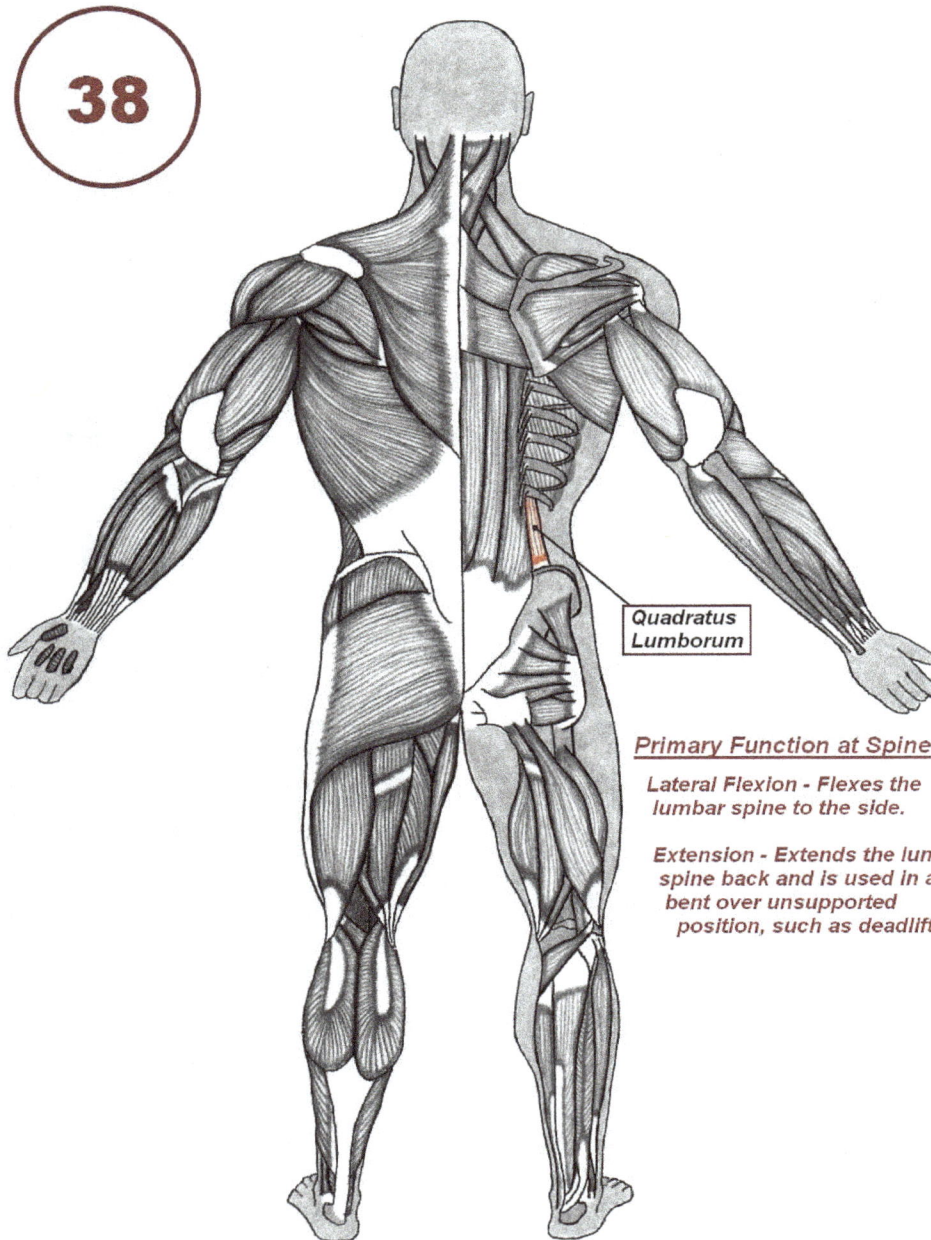

Quadratus
Lumborum

Primary Function at Spine

*Lateral Flexion - Flexes the
lumbar spine to the side.*

*Extension - Extends the lumbar
spine back and is used in a
bent over unsupported
position, such as deadlifts.*

38 - Exercises

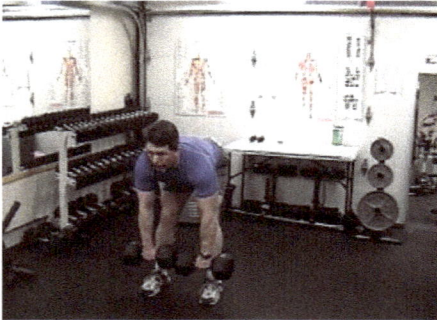
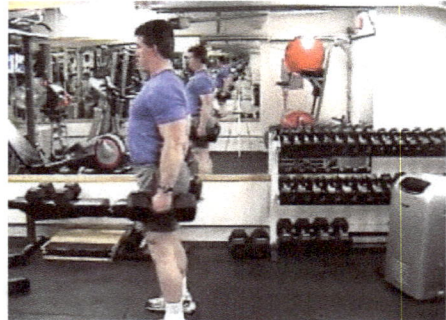

Straight Leg Dumbbell Dead-Lift (1-3 Sets 7-10 Reps)

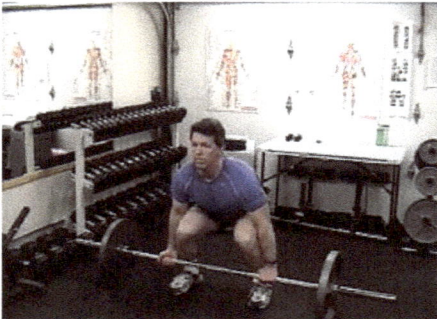
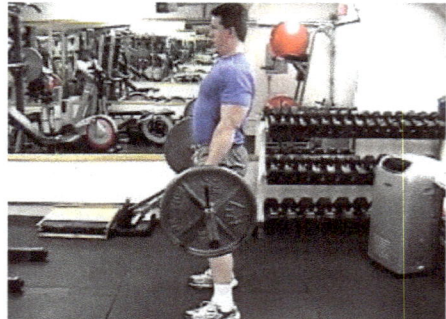

Dead-Lift (1-3 Sets 7-10 Reps)

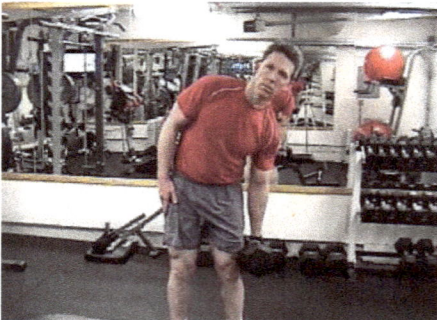
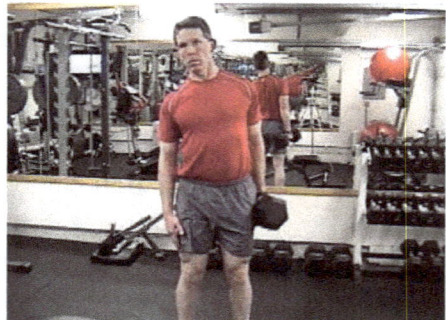

Standing Dumbbell Torso Lateral Raise (1-3 Sets 7-10 Reps)

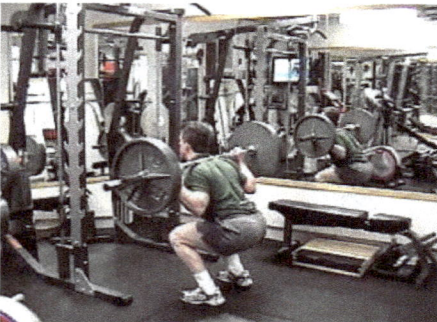
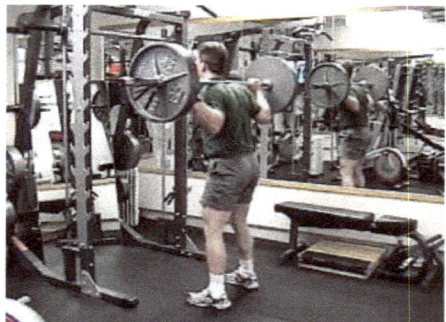

Free Weight Squat (1-5 Sets 7-10 Reps)

Obliques - External

39

External
Oblique

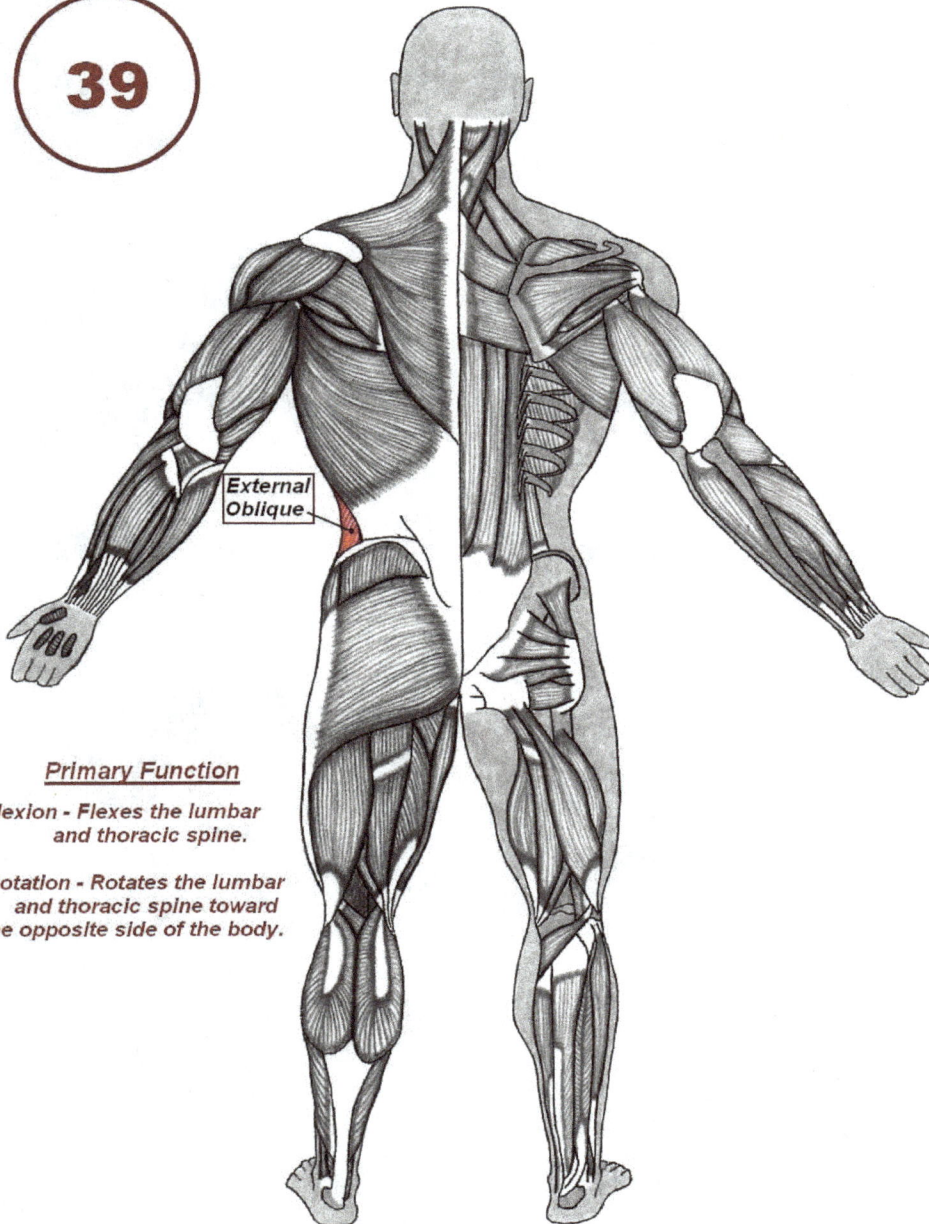

Primary Function

Flexion - Flexes the lumbar and thoracic spine.

Rotation - Rotates the lumbar and thoracic spine toward the opposite side of the body.

39 - Exercises

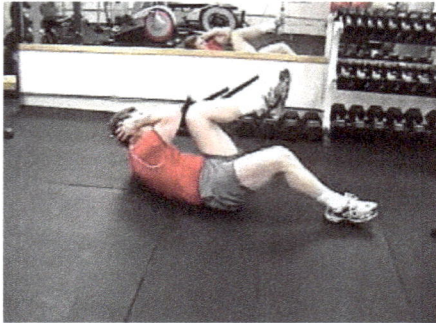

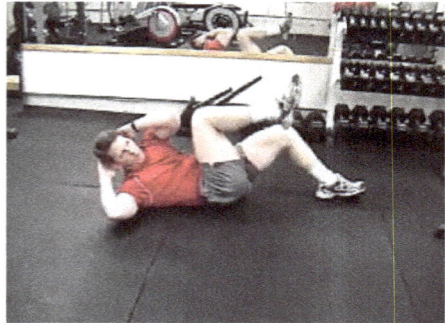

Lying Floor Twist "Bicycles" (1-3 Sets 10-15 Reps Each Side)

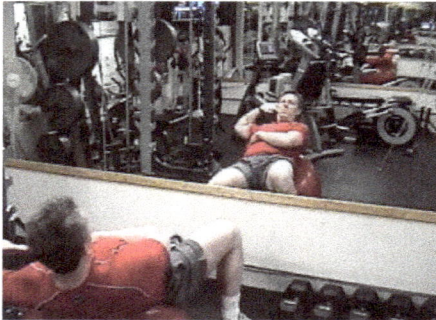

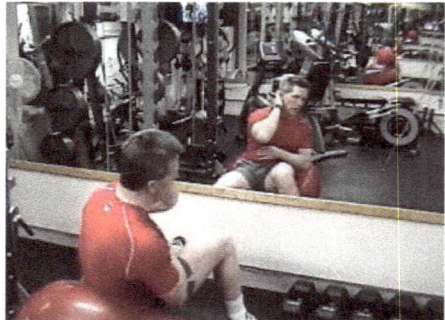

Stability Ball Twist (1-3 Sets 10-15 Reps Each Side)

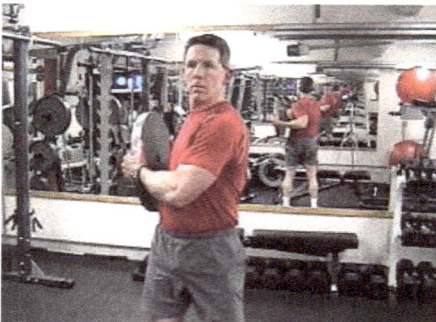

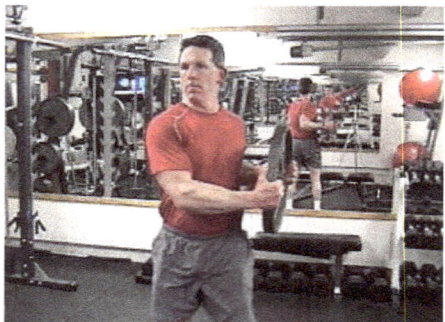

Standing Plate Twist (1-3 Sets 10-15 Reps Each Side)

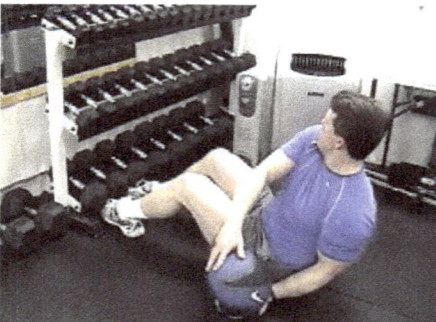

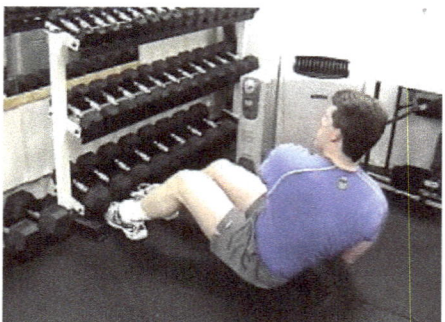

Seated Floor Twist With Medicine Ball (1-3 Sets 10-15 Reps Each Side)

39 - Exercises

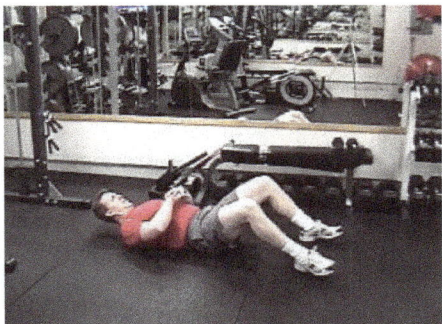

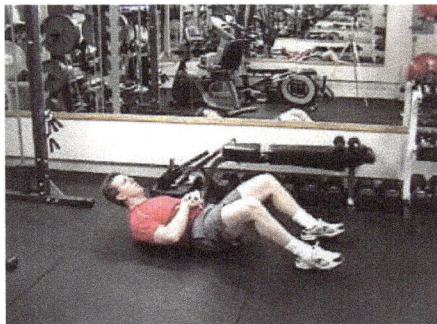

Ab Crunch on Floor (1-3 Sets 10-30 Reps)

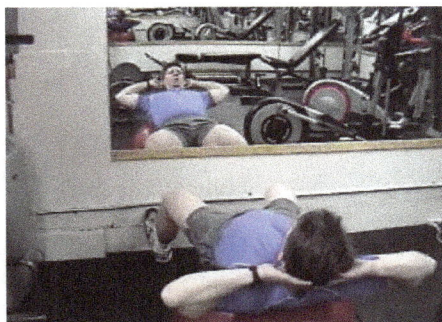

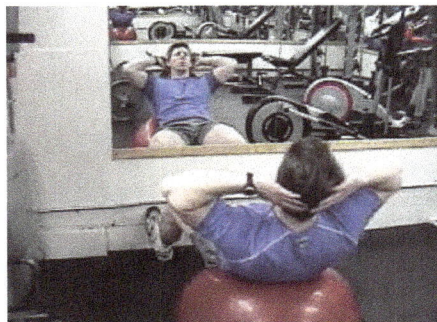

Ab Crunch on Stability Ball (1-3 Sets 10-30 Reps)

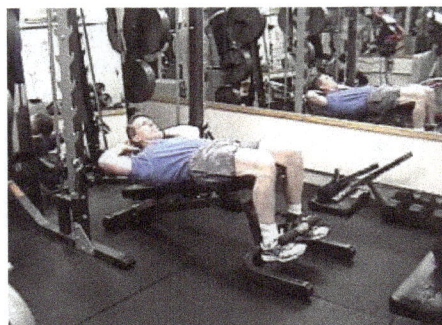

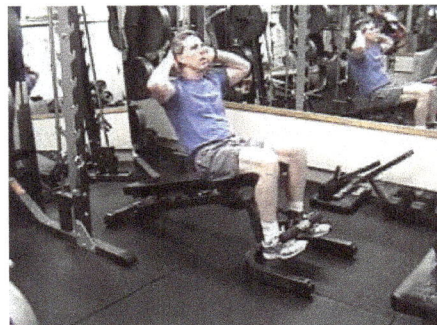

Decline Sit Ups (Hands support, but do not pull head: 1-3 Sets 10-30 Reps))

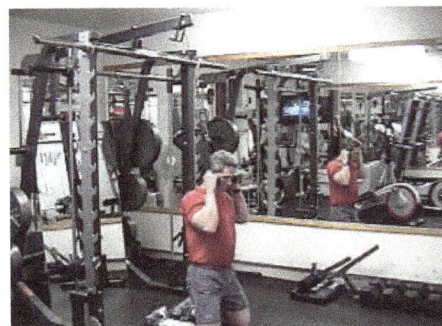

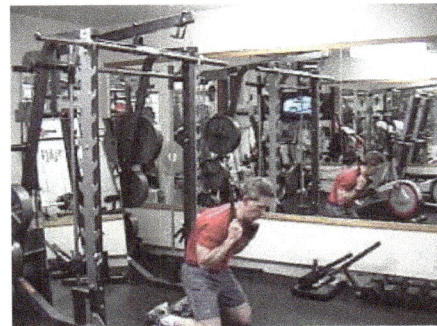

Kneeling Cable Crunch (1-3 Sets 10-30 Reps)

39 - Exercises

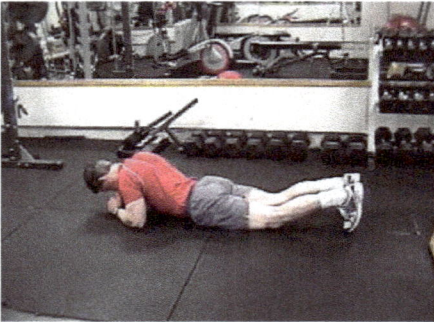

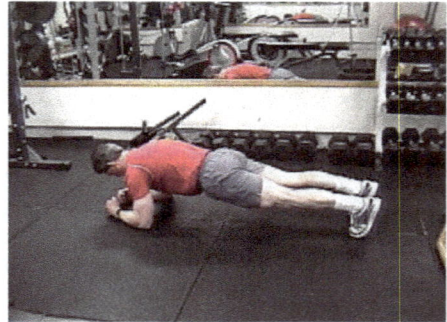

Prone Planks (1-3 Sets, Hold 30-60 Seconds/Set)

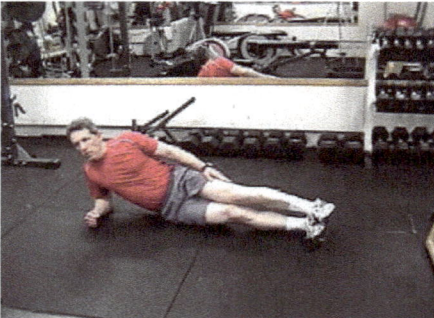

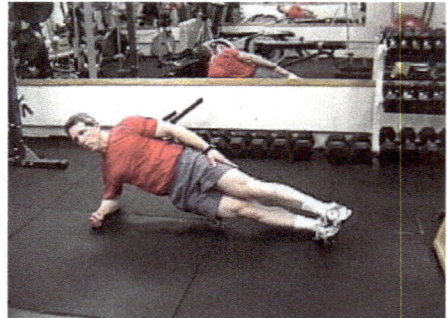

Side-Lying Planks (1-3 Sets, Hold 30-60 Seconds/Set Each Side)

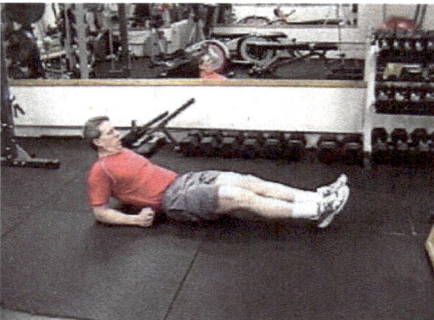

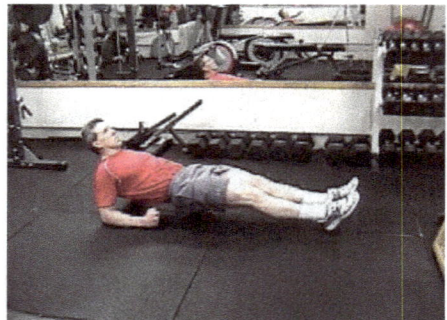

Supine Planks (1-3 Sets, Hold 30-60 Seconds/Set)

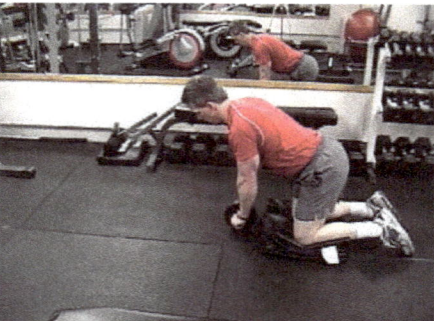

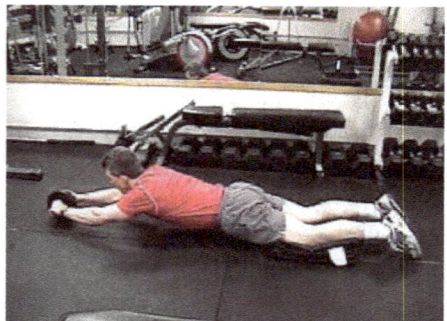

Ab Roller (1-3 Sets 7-10 Reps)

Triceps (Tri's)

40

Tri's

Triceps Brachii:
Outer (Lateral) Head
Middle (Long) Head
Inner (Medial) Head

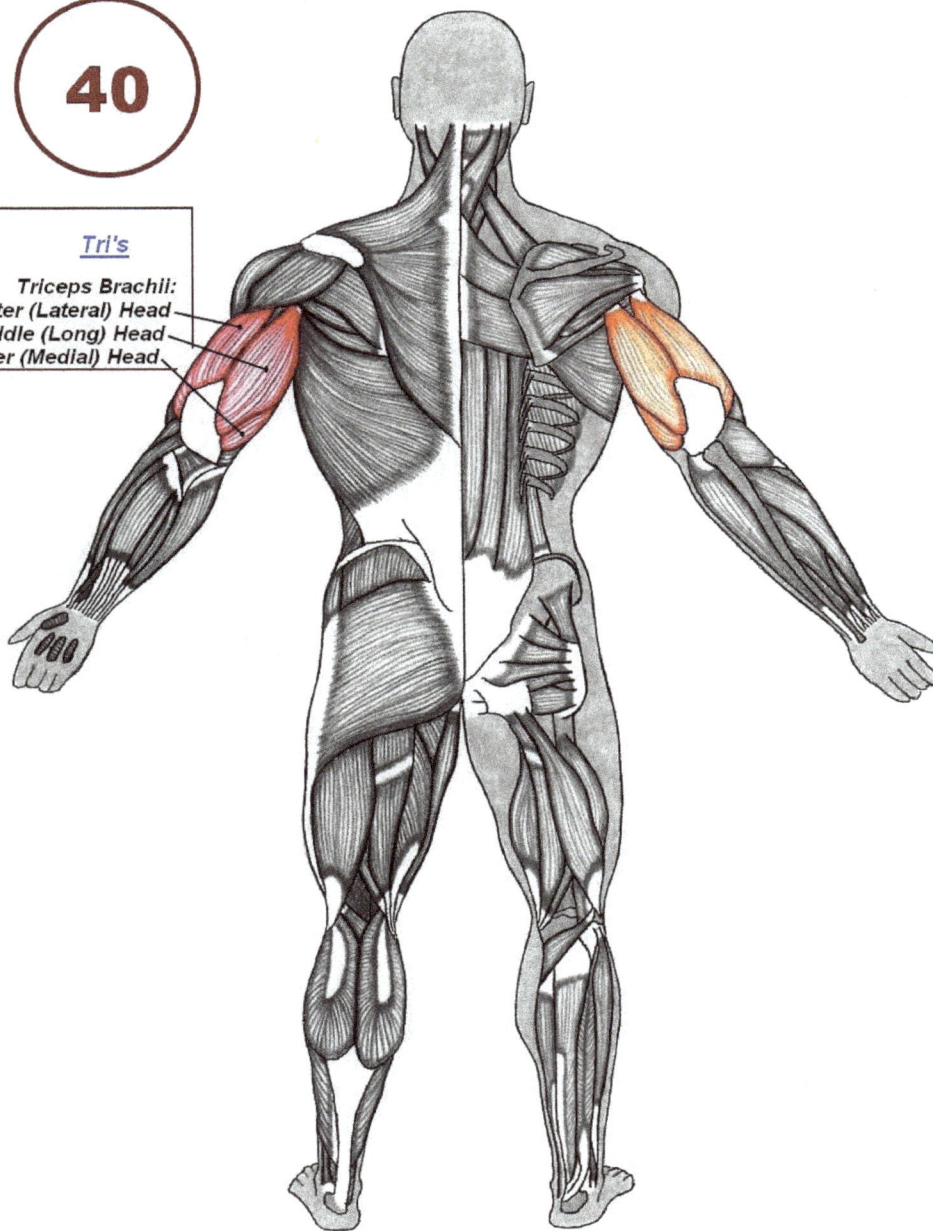

143

Tri's - Triceps Outer (Lateral) Head

40A

Tri's

Triceps Brachii:
Outer (Lateral) Head
Middle (Long) Head
Inner (Medial) Head

Primary Function at Elbow
Extension - Extends the elbow

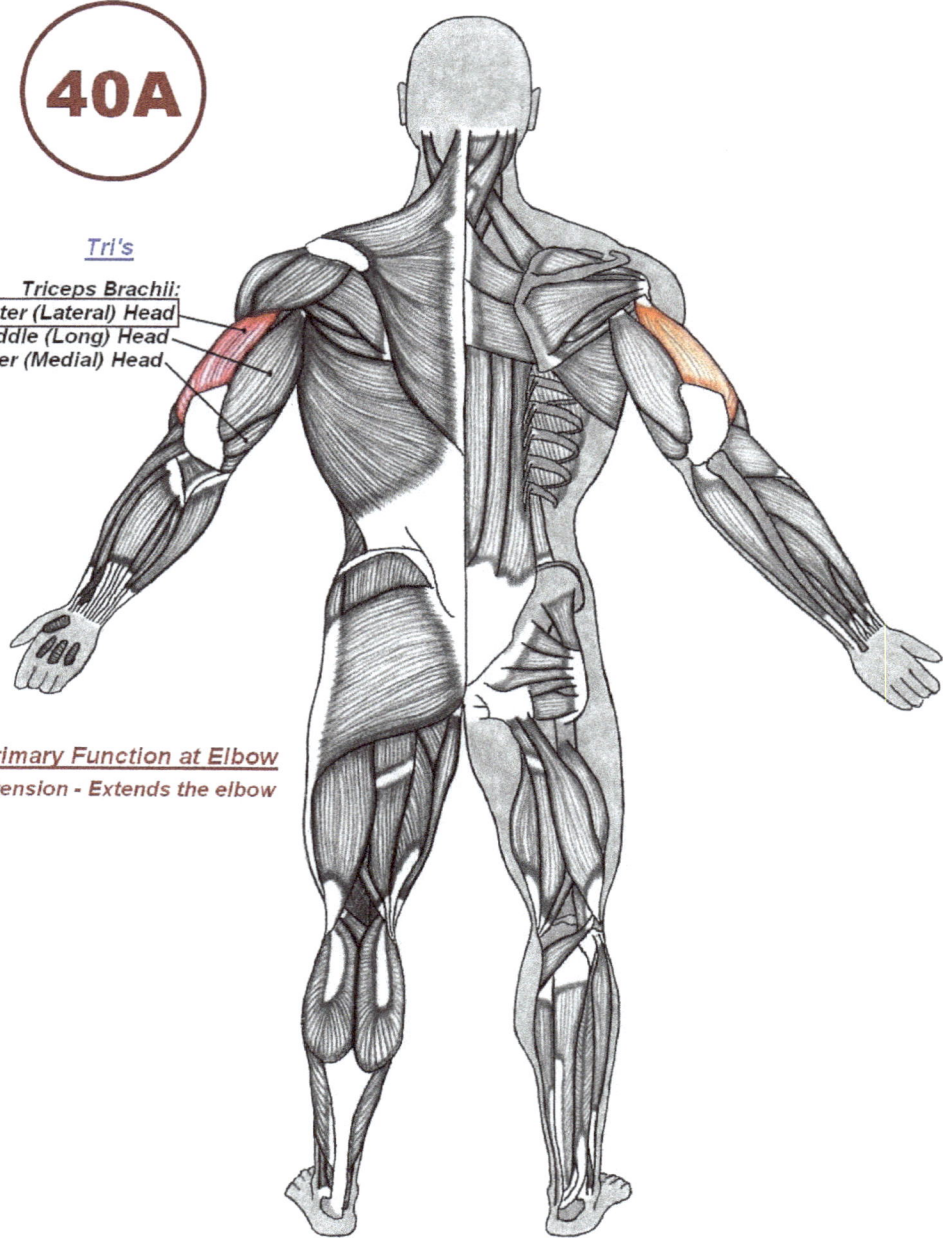

144

Tri's - Triceps Middle (Long) Head

40B

Tri's

Triceps Brachii:
Outer (Lateral) Head
Middle (Long) Head
Inner (Medial) Head

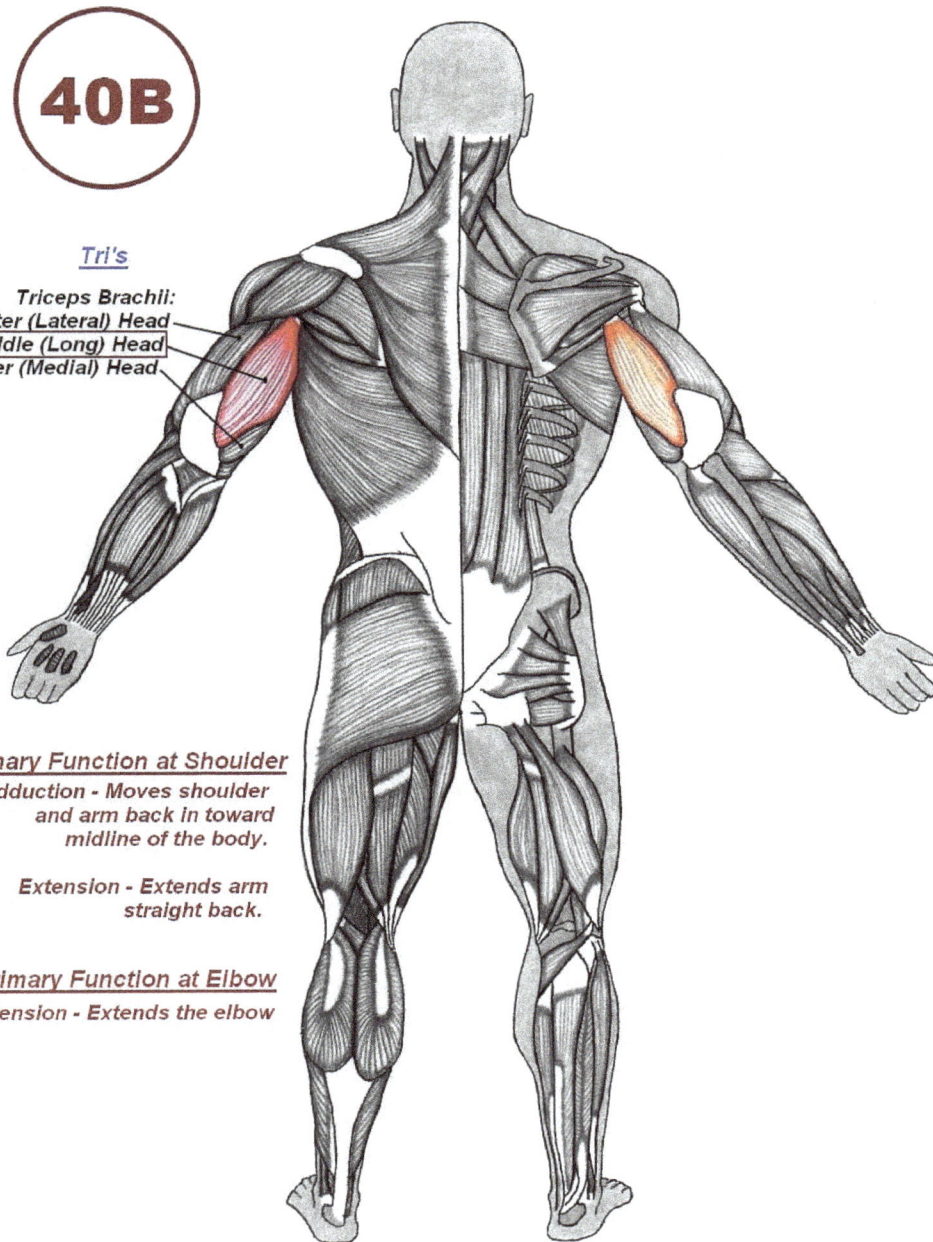

Primary Function at Shoulder

Adduction - Moves shoulder and arm back in toward midline of the body.

Extension - Extends arm straight back.

Primary Function at Elbow

Extension - Extends the elbow

Tri's - Triceps Inner (Medial) Head

40C

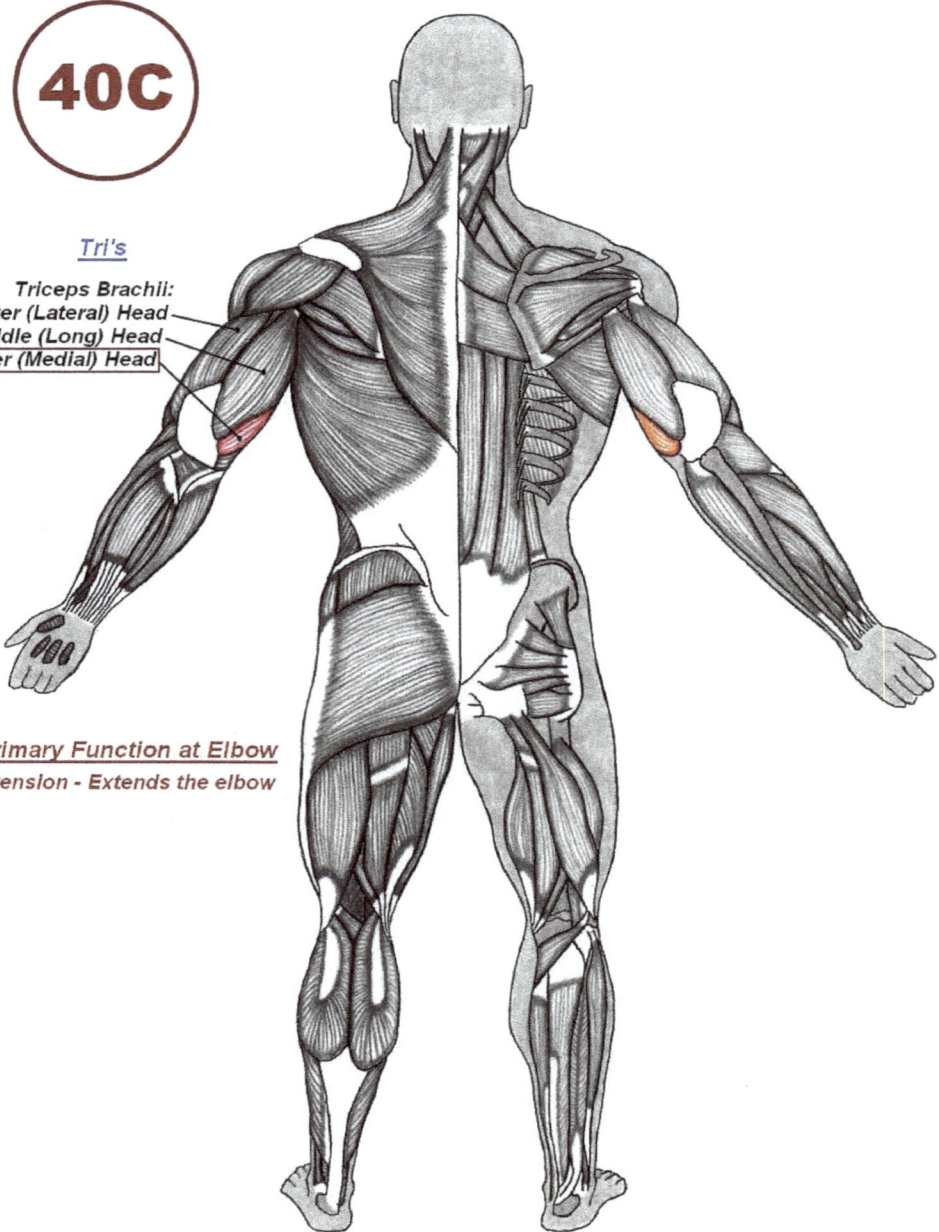

Tri's

Triceps Brachii:
Outer (Lateral) Head
Middle (Long) Head
Inner (Medial) Head

Primary Function at Elbow
Extension - Extends the elbow

146

Anconeus

40D

Anconeus
(Assists Triceps)

Primary Function at Elbow

Extension - Extends elbow.

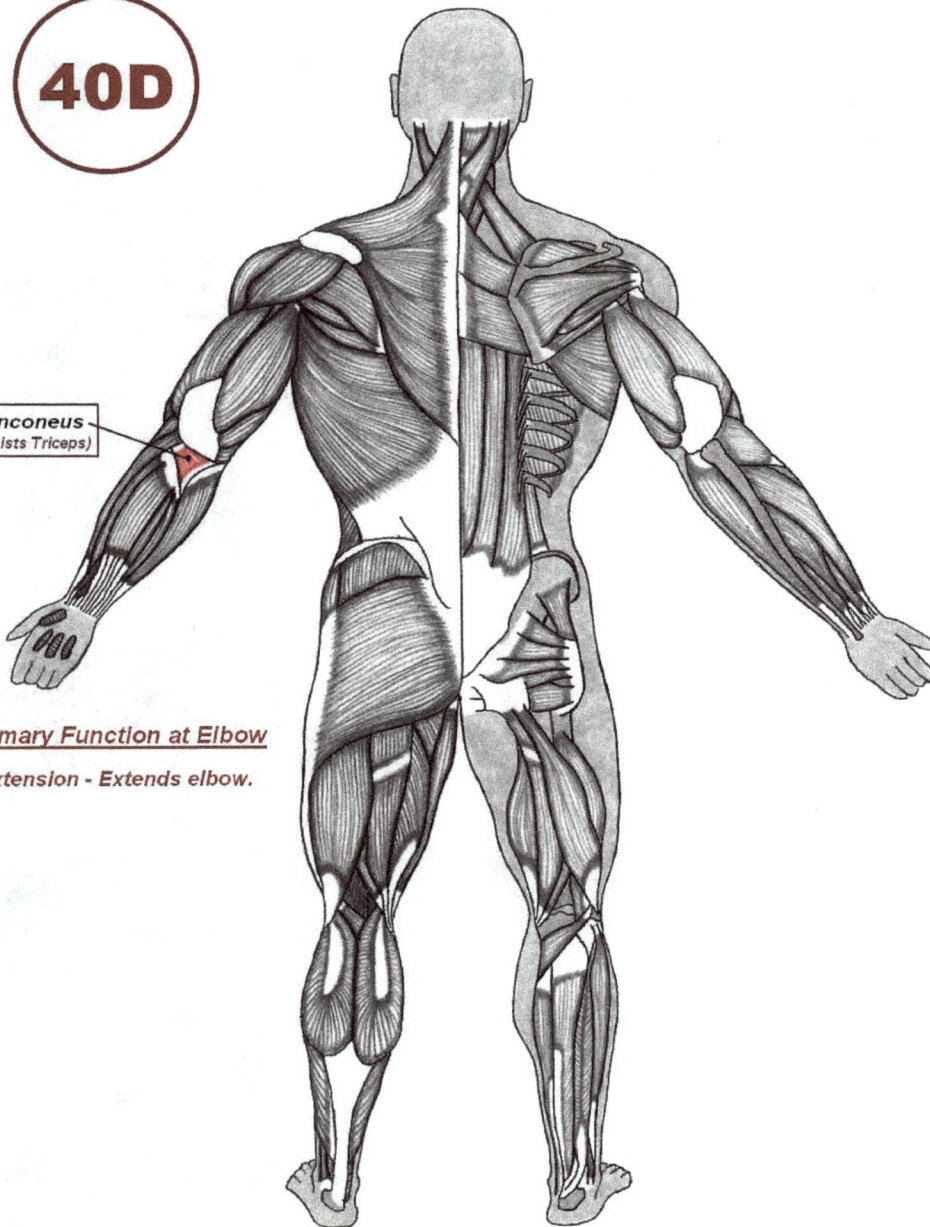

40 A,B, C and D - Exercises

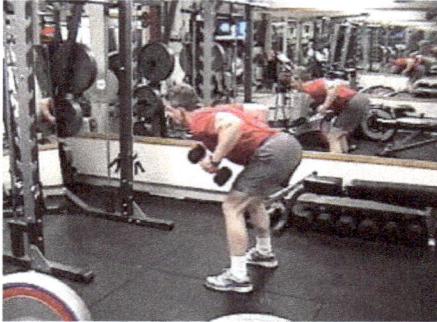

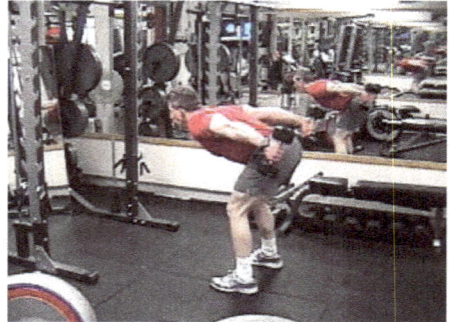

Triceps Standing Bent Dumbbell Extension (1-3 Sets 7-10 Reps)

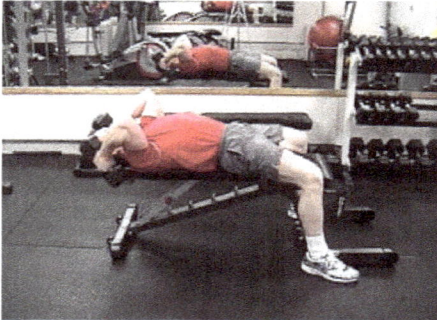

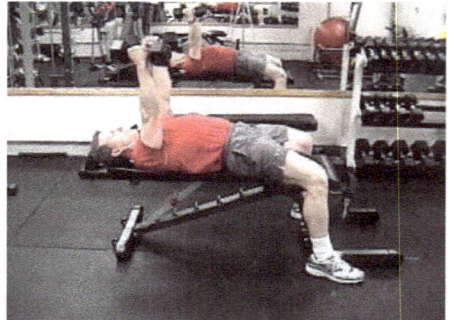

Triceps Lying Double Dumbbell Extension (1-3 Sets 7-15 Reps)

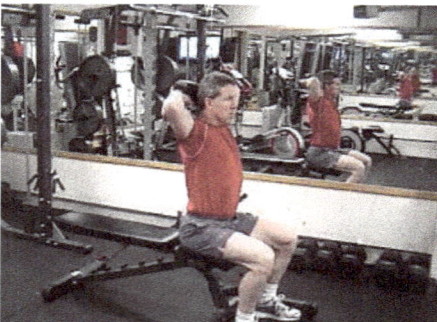

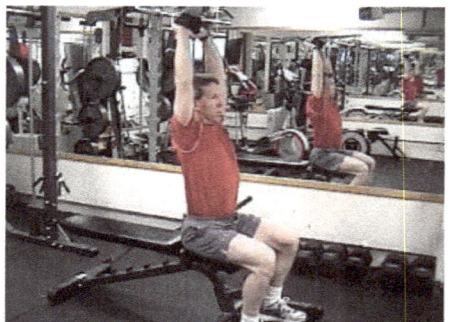

Triceps Seated Single Dumbbell Extension (1-3 Sets 7-15 Reps)

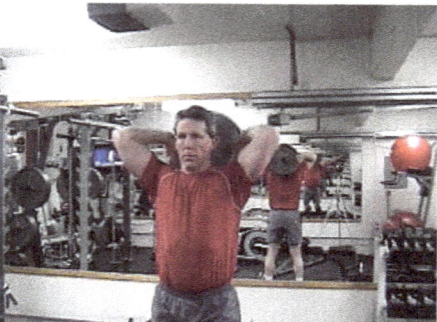

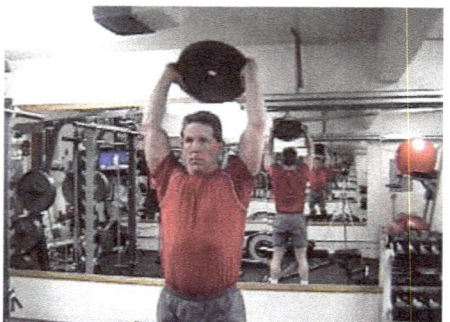

Triceps Standing Plate Extension (1-3 Sets 7-10 Reps)

40 A,B, C and D - Exercises

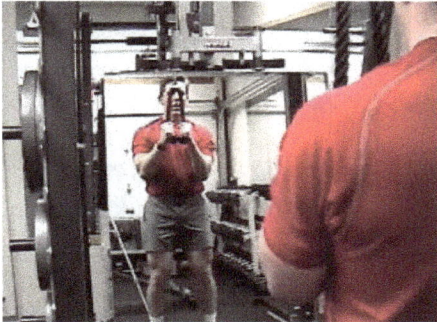

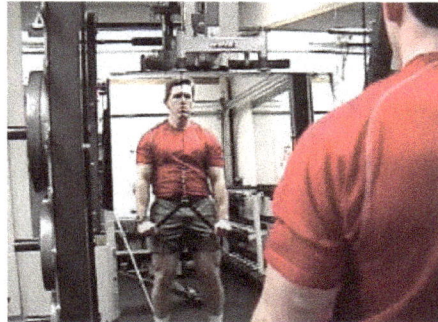

Triceps Cable Push Down (1-3 Sets 7-15 Reps)

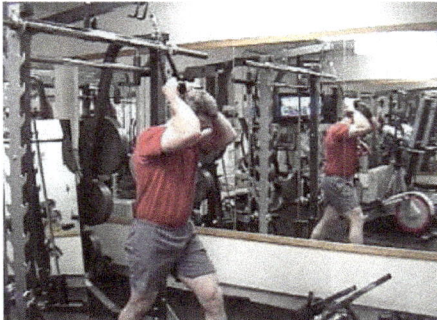

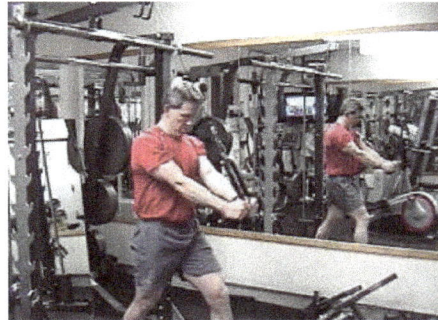

Triceps Standing Cable Extension (1-3 Sets 7-15 Reps)

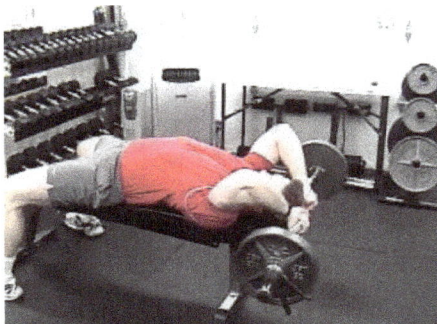

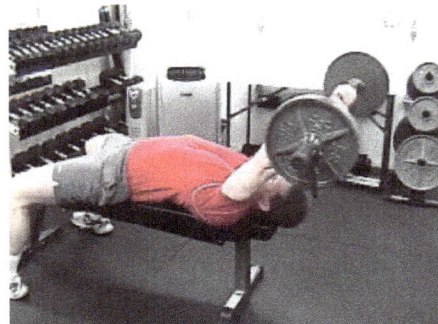

Tricpeps Lying EZ-Bar Extension (1-3 Sets 7-15 Reps)

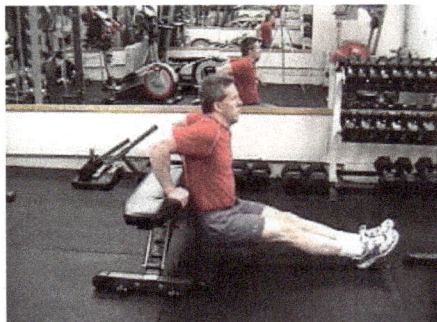

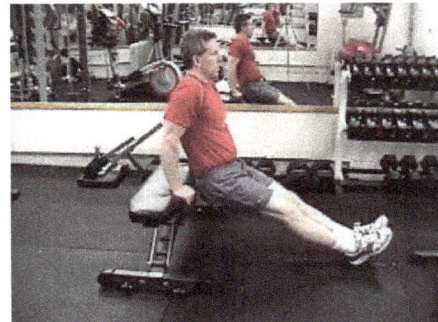

Bench Dips (1-3 Sets 7-10 Reps)

40 A,B, C and D - Exercises

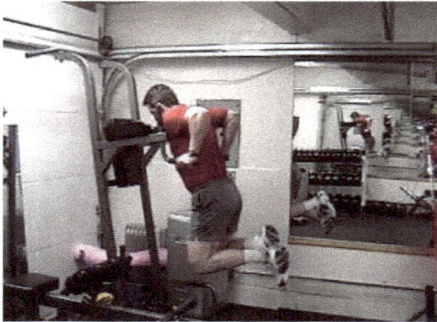

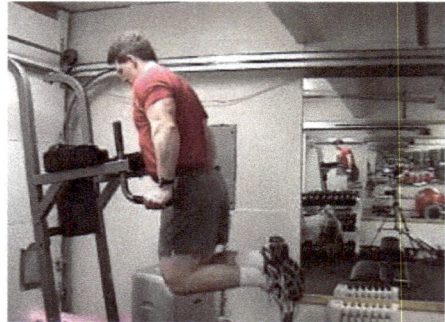

Parallel Bar Dips (1-3 Sets 7-15 Reps)

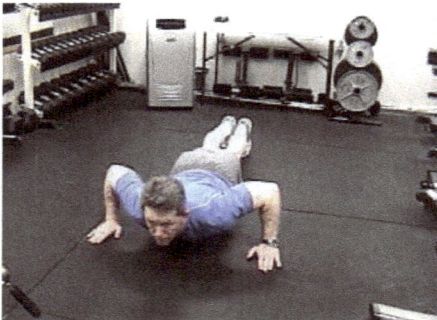

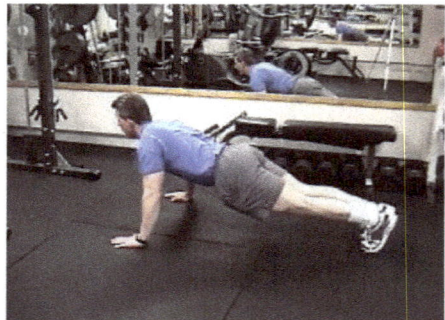

Push Ups (1-3 Sets 10-50 Reps)

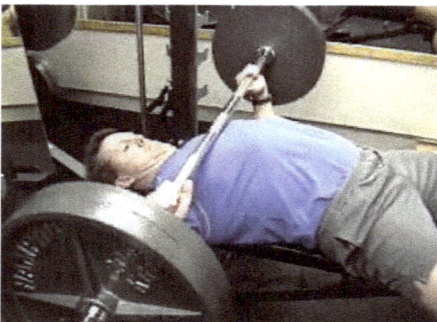

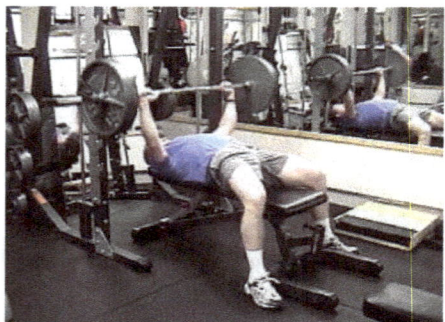

Chest Flat Bar Press "Bench Press" (1-3 Sets 7-15 Reps)

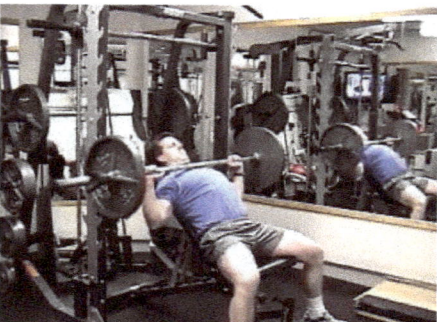

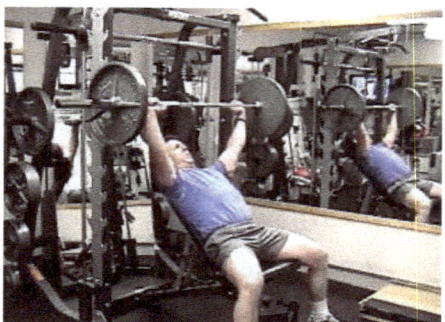

Chest Incline Bar Press (1-3 Sets 7-10 Reps)

40 A, B, C and D - Exercises

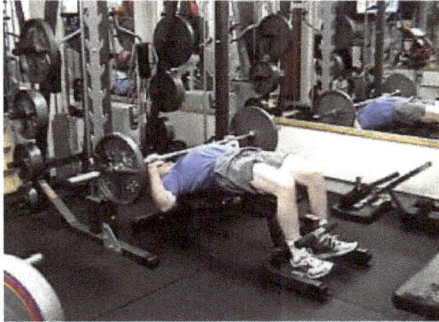

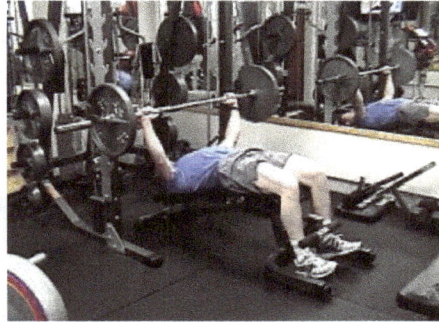

Chest Decline Bar Press (1-3 Sets 7-10 Reps)

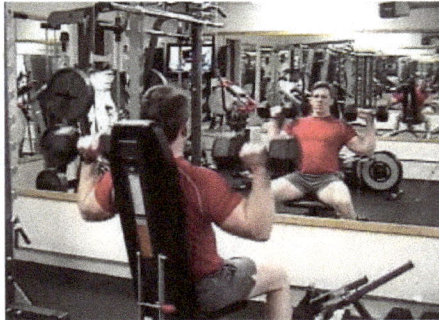

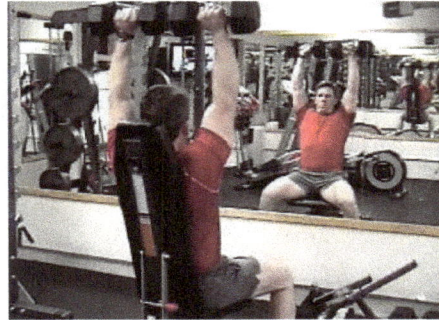

Shoulder Seated Dumbbell Press (1-5 Sets 7-10 Reps)

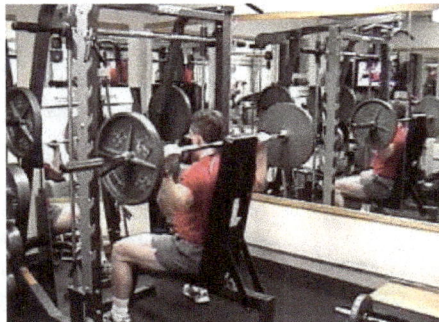

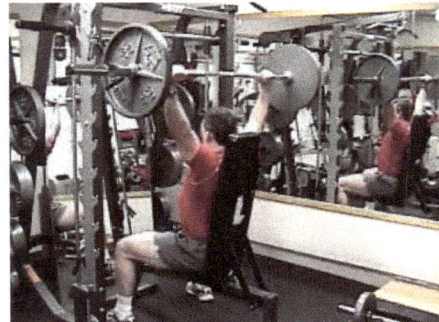

Shoulder Seated Bar Press "Military Press" (1-5 Sets 7-10 Reps)

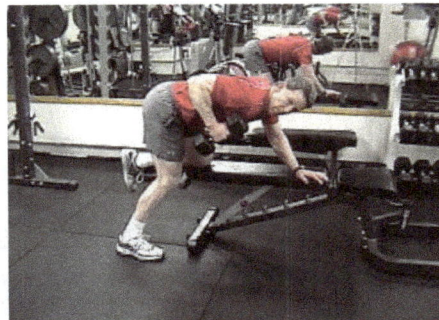

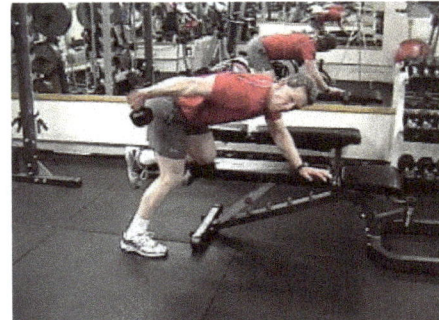

Triceps Kneeling Dumbbell Extension (1-3 Sets 7-15 Reps)

Wrist Extensors

41

Radius (Under)

Ulna

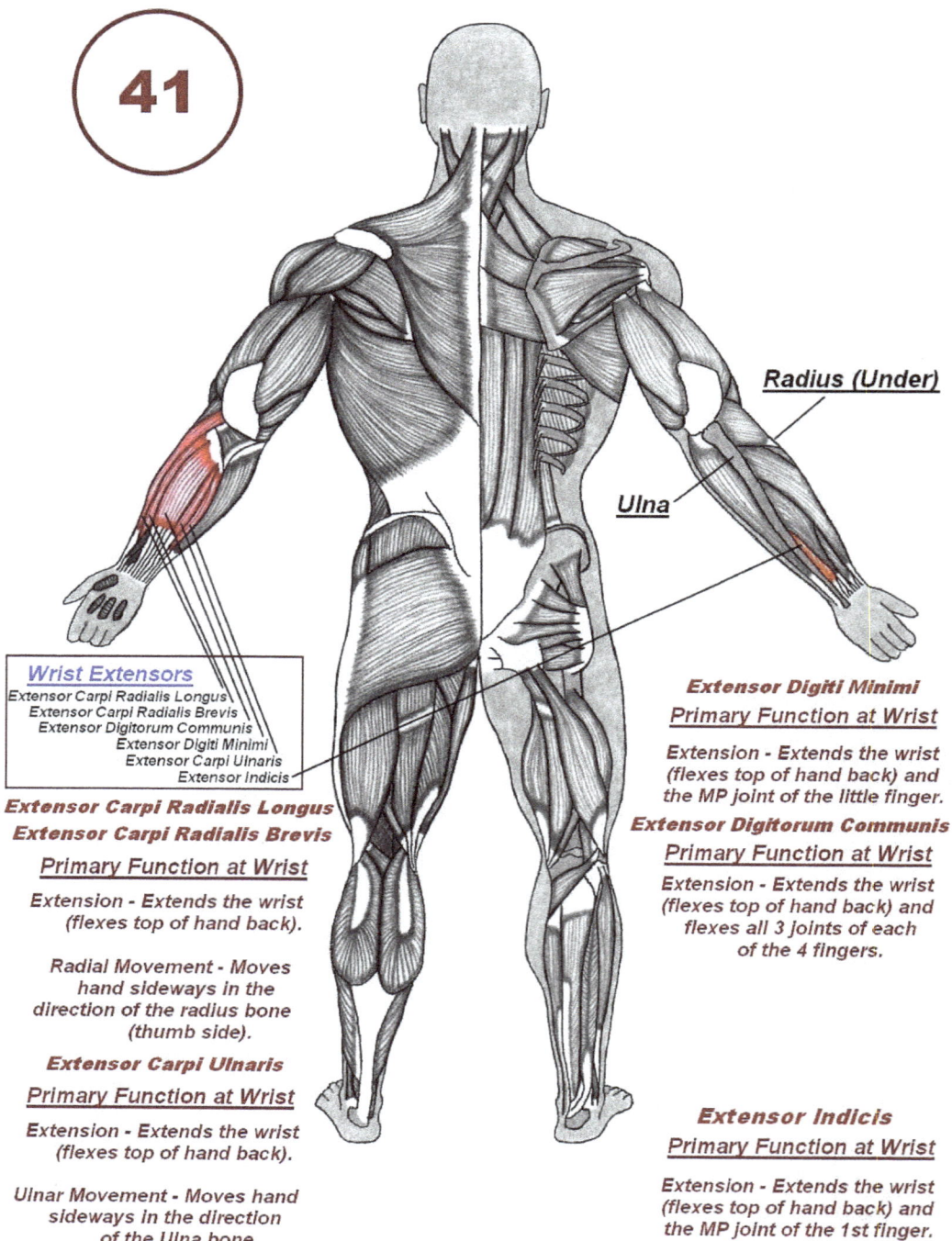

Wrist Extensors
Extensor Carpi Radialis Longus
Extensor Carpi Radialis Brevis
Extensor Digitorum Communis
Extensor Digiti Minimi
Extensor Carpi Ulnaris
Extensor Indicis

Extensor Carpi Radialis Longus
Extensor Carpi Radialis Brevis

Primary Function at Wrist

Extension - Extends the wrist (flexes top of hand back).

Radial Movement - Moves hand sideways in the direction of the radius bone (thumb side).

Extensor Carpi Ulnaris

Primary Function at Wrist

Extension - Extends the wrist (flexes top of hand back).

Ulnar Movement - Moves hand sideways in the direction of the Ulna bone.

Extensor Digiti Minimi
Primary Function at Wrist

Extension - Extends the wrist (flexes top of hand back) and the MP joint of the little finger.

Extensor Digitorum Communis
Primary Function at Wrist

Extension - Extends the wrist (flexes top of hand back) and flexes all 3 joints of each of the 4 fingers.

Extensor Indicis
Primary Function at Wrist

Extension - Extends the wrist (flexes top of hand back) and the MP joint of the 1st finger.

41 - Exercises

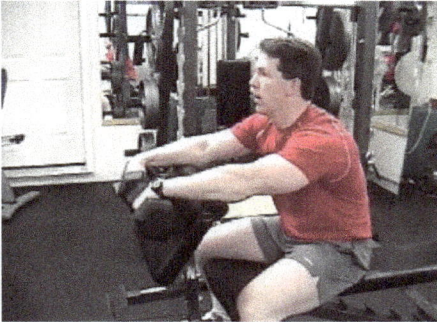

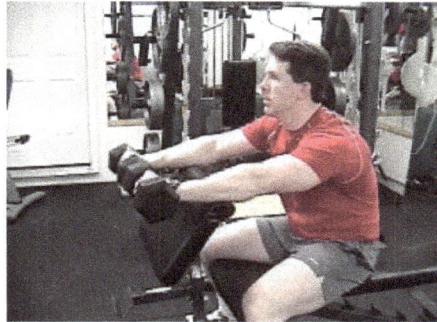

Forearm Extension "Reverse Wrist Curl"(1-3 Sets 7-10 Reps)

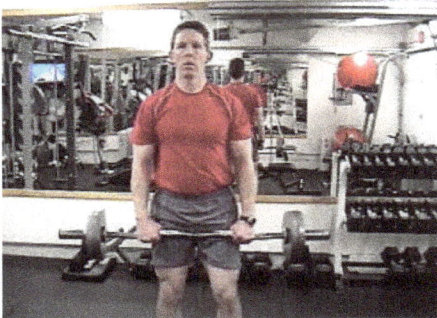

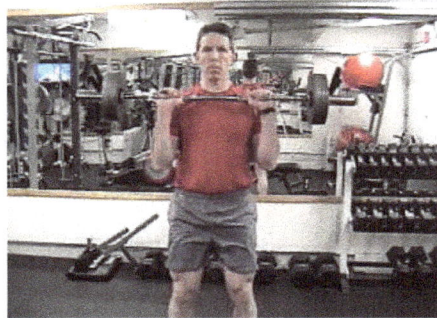

Biceps Standing Reverse EZ-Bar Curl (1-3 Sets 7-10 Reps)

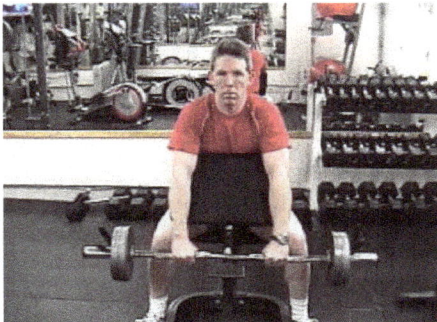

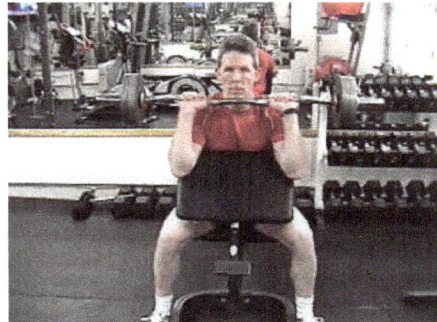

Biceps Seated Reverse EZ-Bar Preacher Curl (1-3 Sets 7-10 Reps)

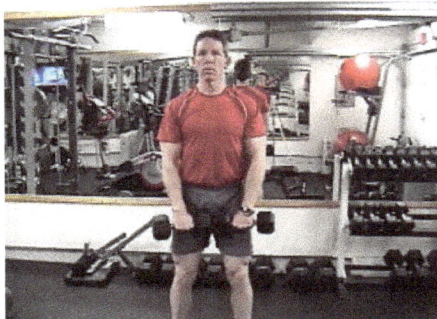

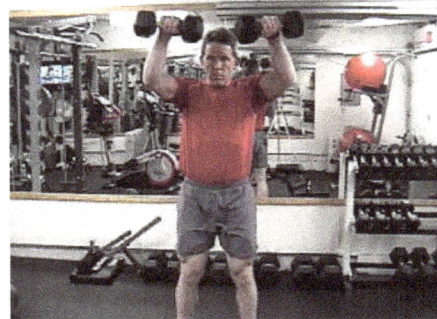

Shoulder Front Double Dumbbell Raise (1-3 Sets 7-10 Reps)

41 - Exercises

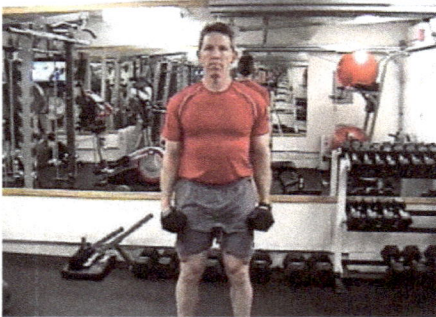

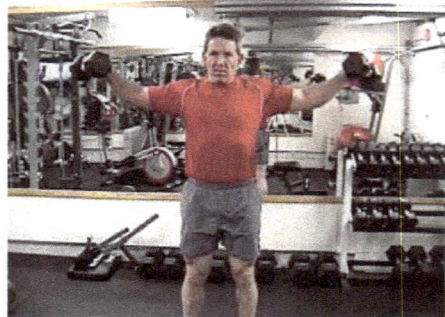

Shoulder Upright Lateral Raise (Side Start Position: 1-3 Sets 7-10 Reps)

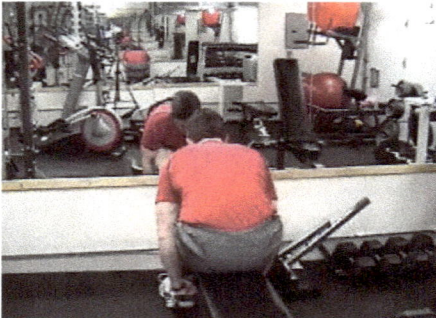

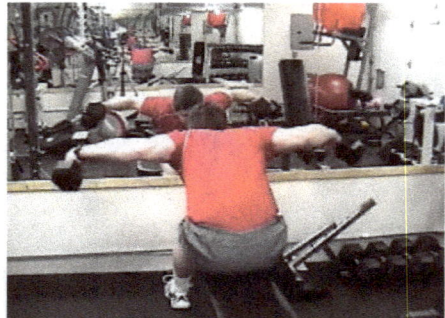

Shoulder Seated Bent Dumbbell Lateral Raise (1-3 Sets 7-10 Reps)

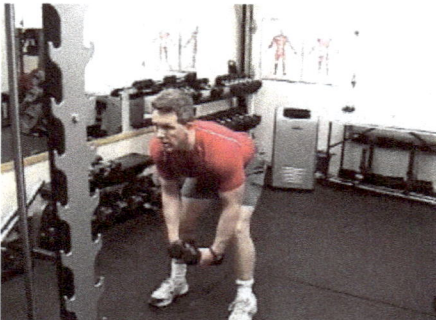

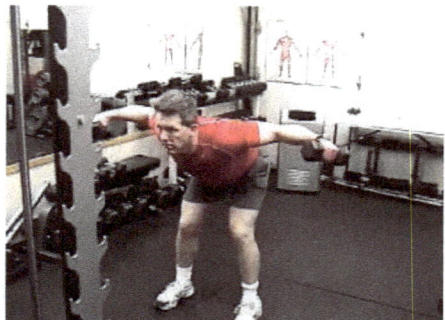

Shoulder Standing Bent Dumbbell Lateral Raise (1-3 Sets 7-10 Reps)

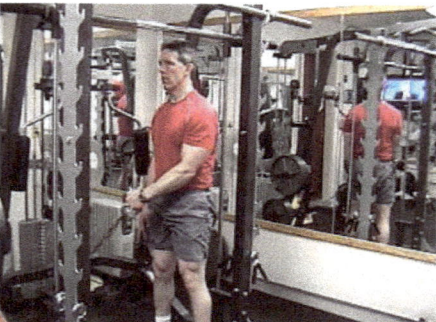

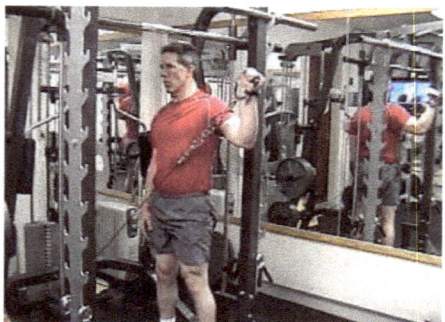

Shoulder Standing Cable External Rotation (1-3 Sets 7-10 Reps)

Forearm - Supinator

42

Supinator

Thumb Abductors
Abductor Pollicis Brevis
Abductor Pollicis Longus

Thumb Extensors
Extensor Pollicis Brevis
Extensor Pollicis Longus

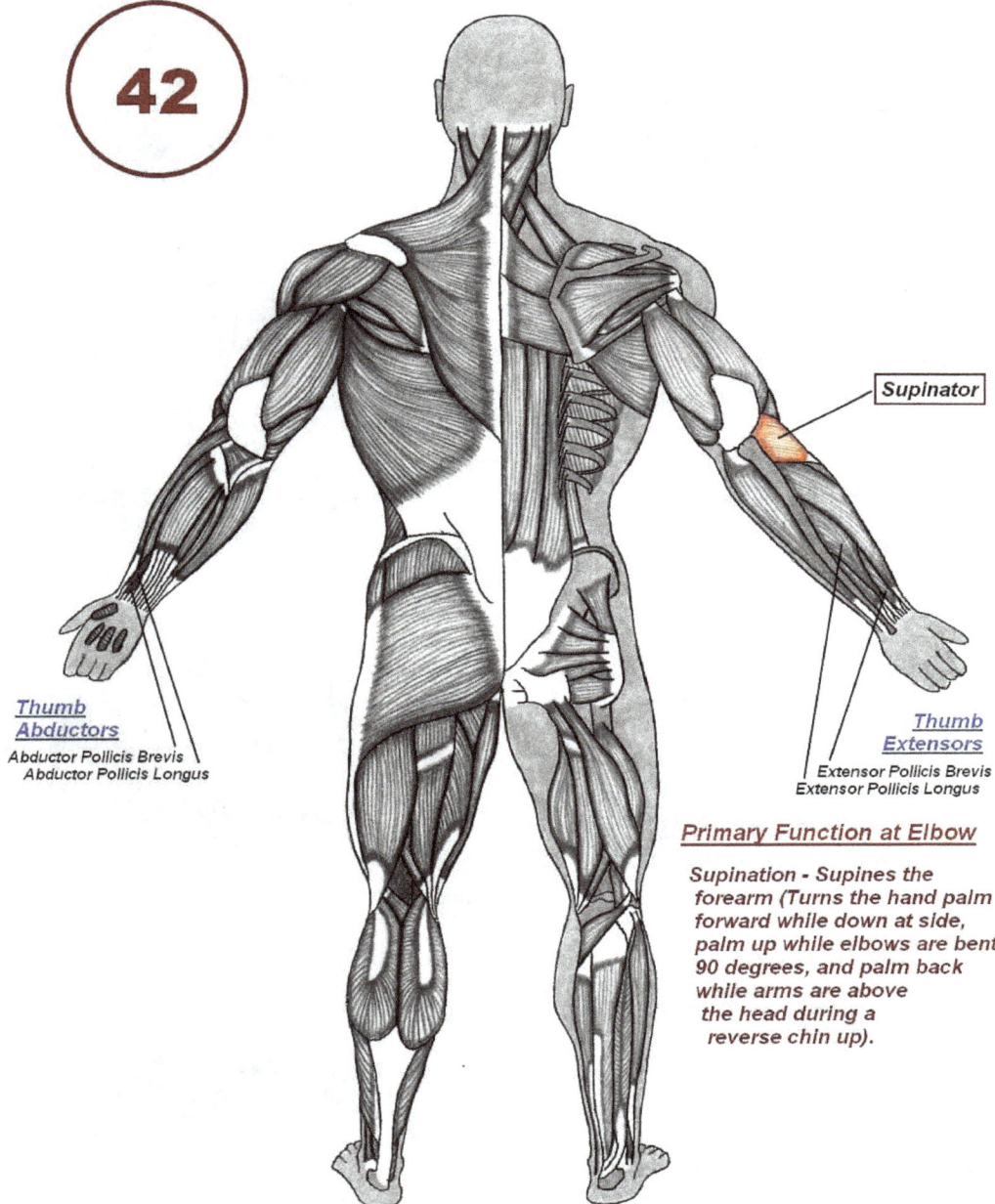

Primary Function at Elbow

Supination - Supines the forearm (Turns the hand palm forward while down at side, palm up while elbows are bent 90 degrees, and palm back while arms are above the head during a reverse chin up).

155

42 - Exercises

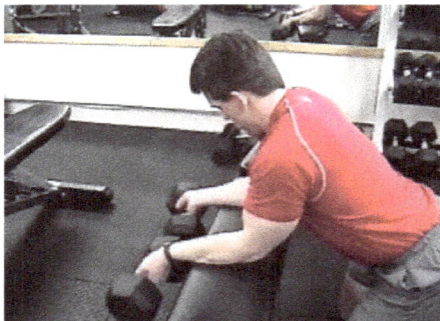

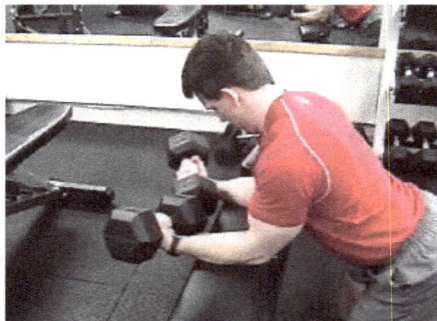

Wrist Curls on Bench (Turns Hands Palms Up: 1-3 Sets 7-10 Reps)

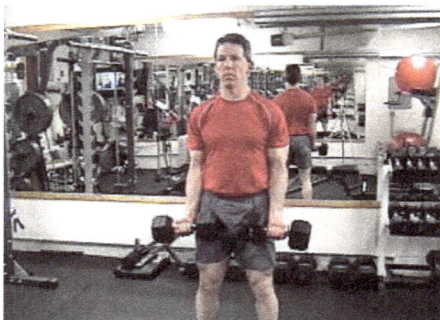

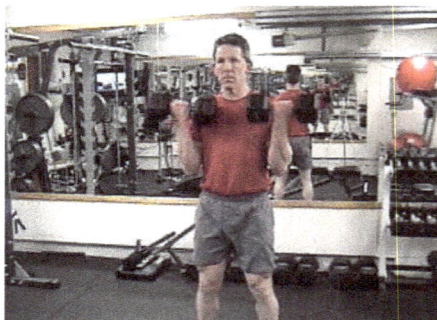

Biceps Standing Dumbbell Curl (Turns Hands Palms Up: 1-3 Sets 7-15 Reps)

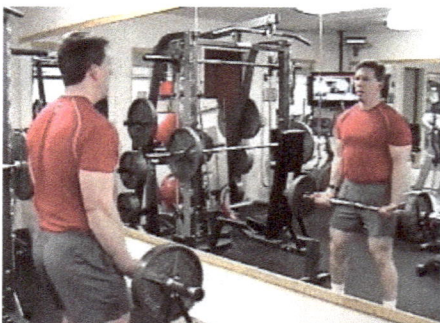

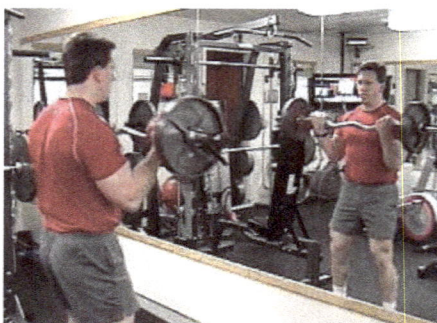

Biceps Standing EZ-Bar Curl (Turns Hands Palms Up: 1-3 Sets 7-15 Reps)

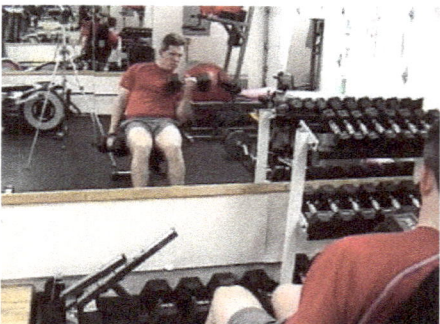

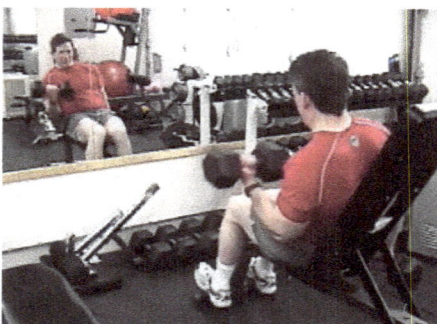

Biceps Seated Incline Dumbbell Curl (Turns Hands Palms Up: 1-3 Sets 7-10 Reps)

42 - Exercises

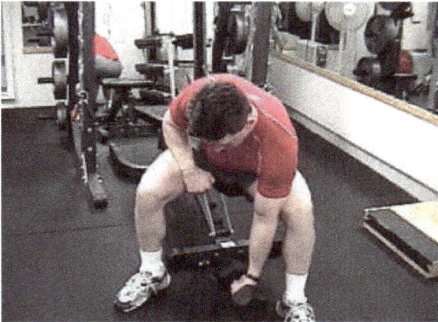

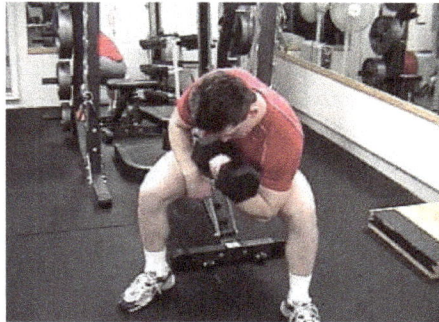

Biceps Seated Concentration Curl (Turns Hands Palms Up: 1-3 Sets 7-15 Reps)

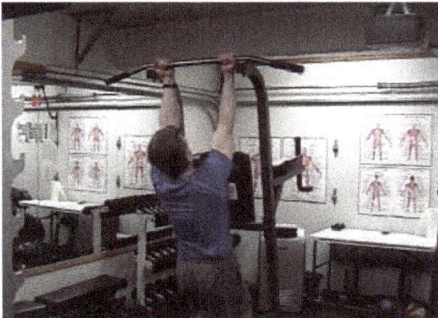

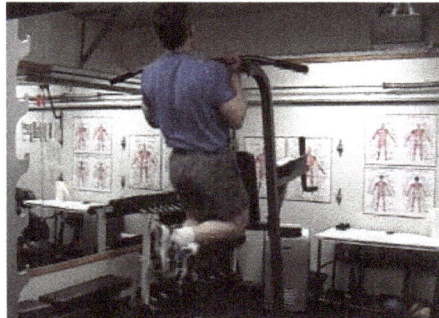

Reverse Chin Ups (Turns Hands Palms Back: 1-3 Sets 7-15 Reps)

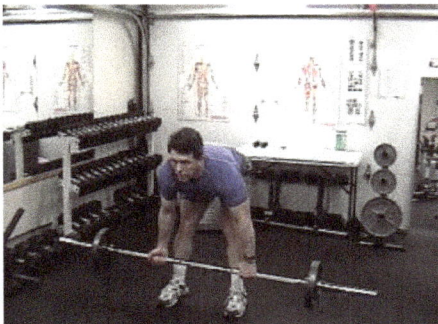

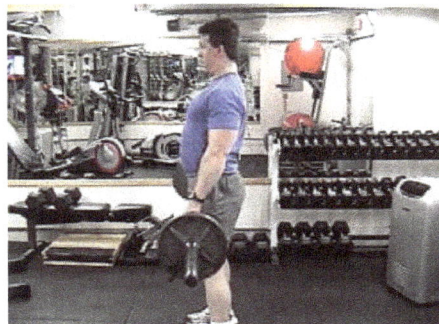

Straight Leg Bar Dead-Lift (Turns One Hand Palm Forward: 1-3 Sets 7-10 Reps)

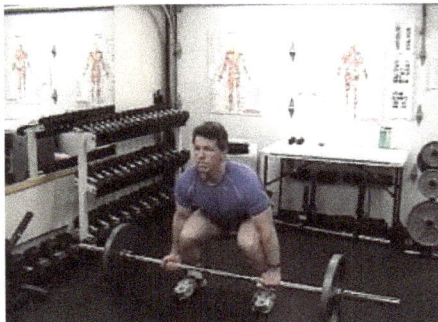

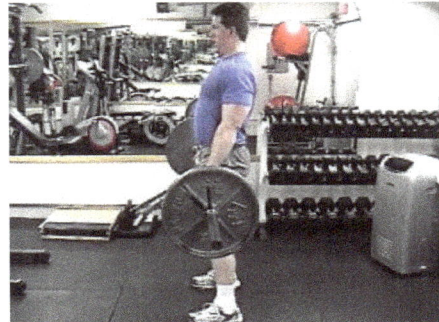

Dead-Lift (Turns One Hand Palm Forward: 1-3 Sets 7-10 Reps)

Forearm - Flexor Carpi Ulnaris

43

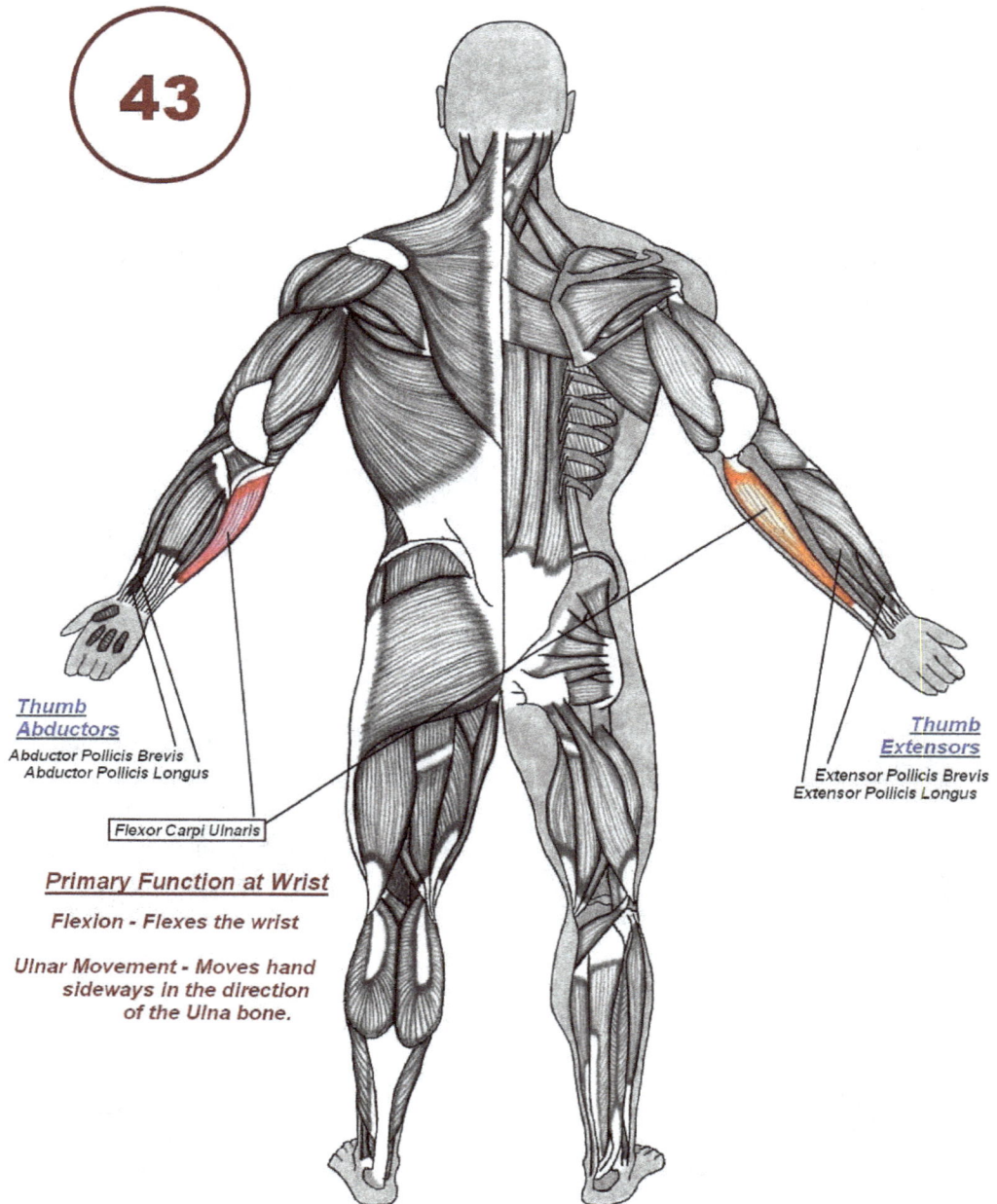

Thumb Abductors
Abductor Pollicis Brevis
Abductor Pollicis Longus

Flexor Carpi Ulnaris

Thumb Extensors
Extensor Pollicis Brevis
Extensor Pollicis Longus

Primary Function at Wrist

Flexion - Flexes the wrist

Ulnar Movement - Moves hand sideways in the direction of the Ulna bone.

43 - Exercises

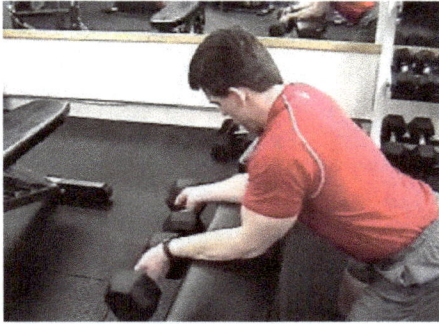

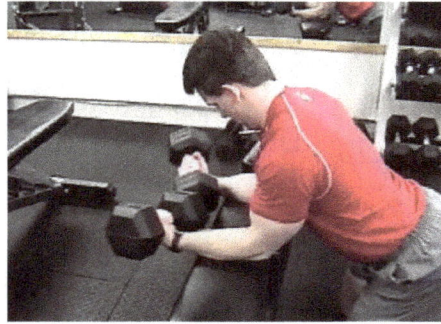

Wrist Curl on Bench (1-3 Sets 7-10 Reps)

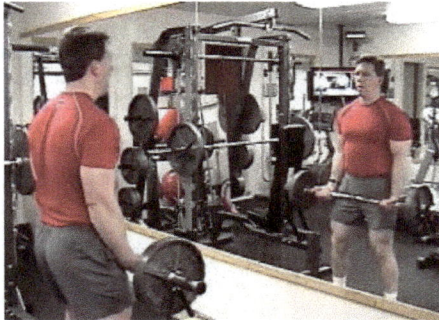

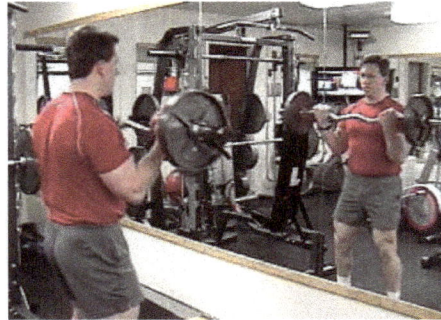

Biceps Standing EZ-Bar Curl (1-3 Sets 7-15 Reps)

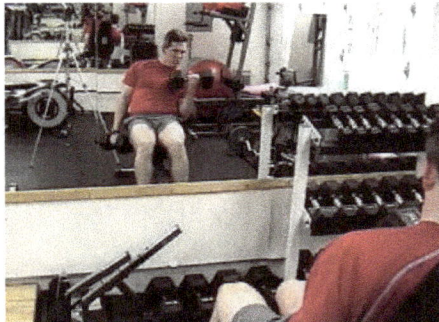

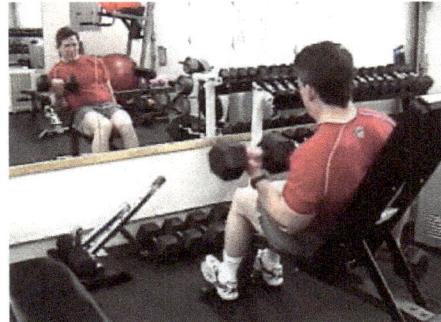

Biceps Seated Incline Dumbbell Curl (1-3 Sets 7-10 Reps)

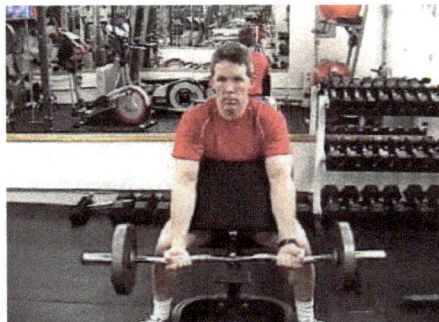

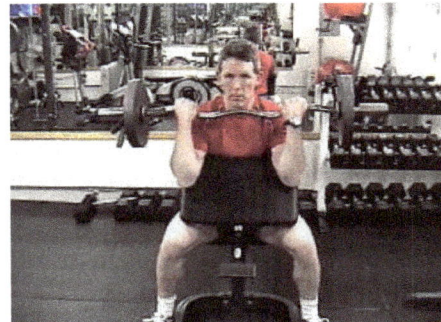

Biceps Seated EZ-Bar Preacher Curl (1-3 Sets 7-15 Reps)

43 - Exercises

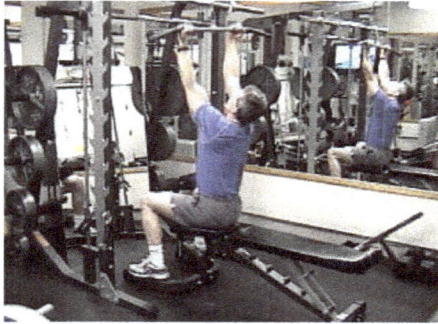

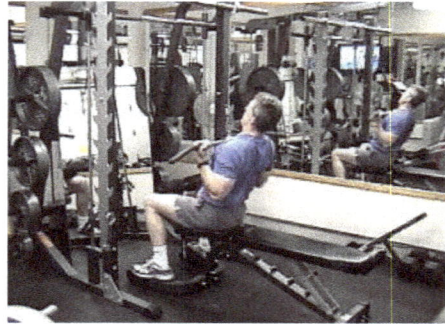

Lat Reverse Grip Pull Down (1-3 Sets 7-15 Reps)

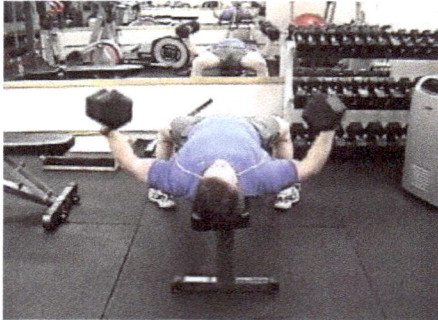

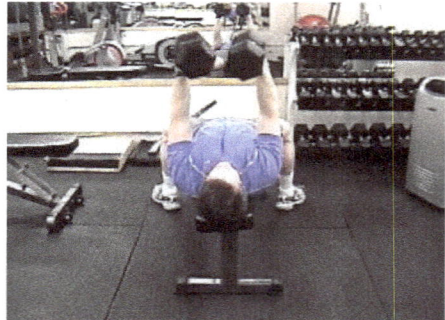

Chest Flat Flye (1-3 Sets 7-15 Reps)

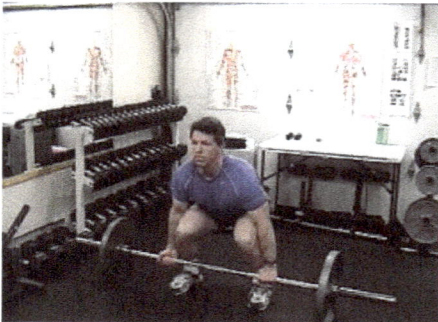

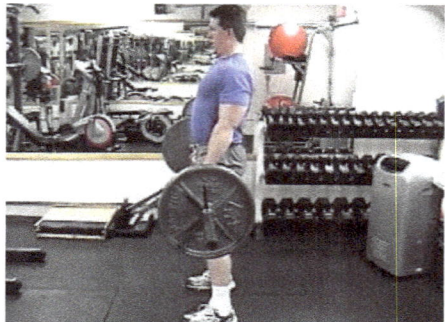

Dead-Lift (1-3 Sets 7-10 Reps)

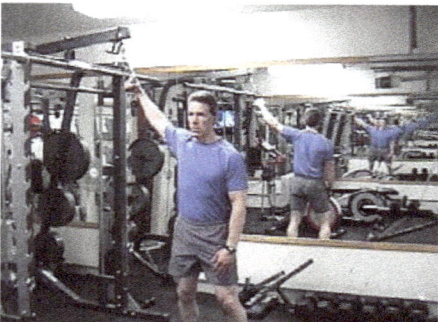

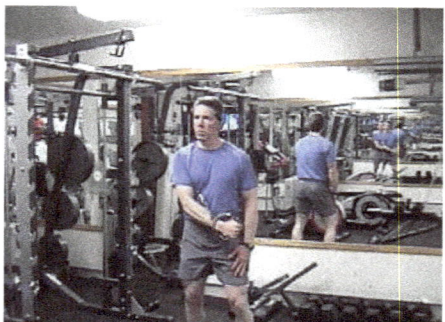

Cable Cross-Over (1-3 Sets 7-15 Reps)

Thumb Abductor - Abductor Pollicis Brevis

44A

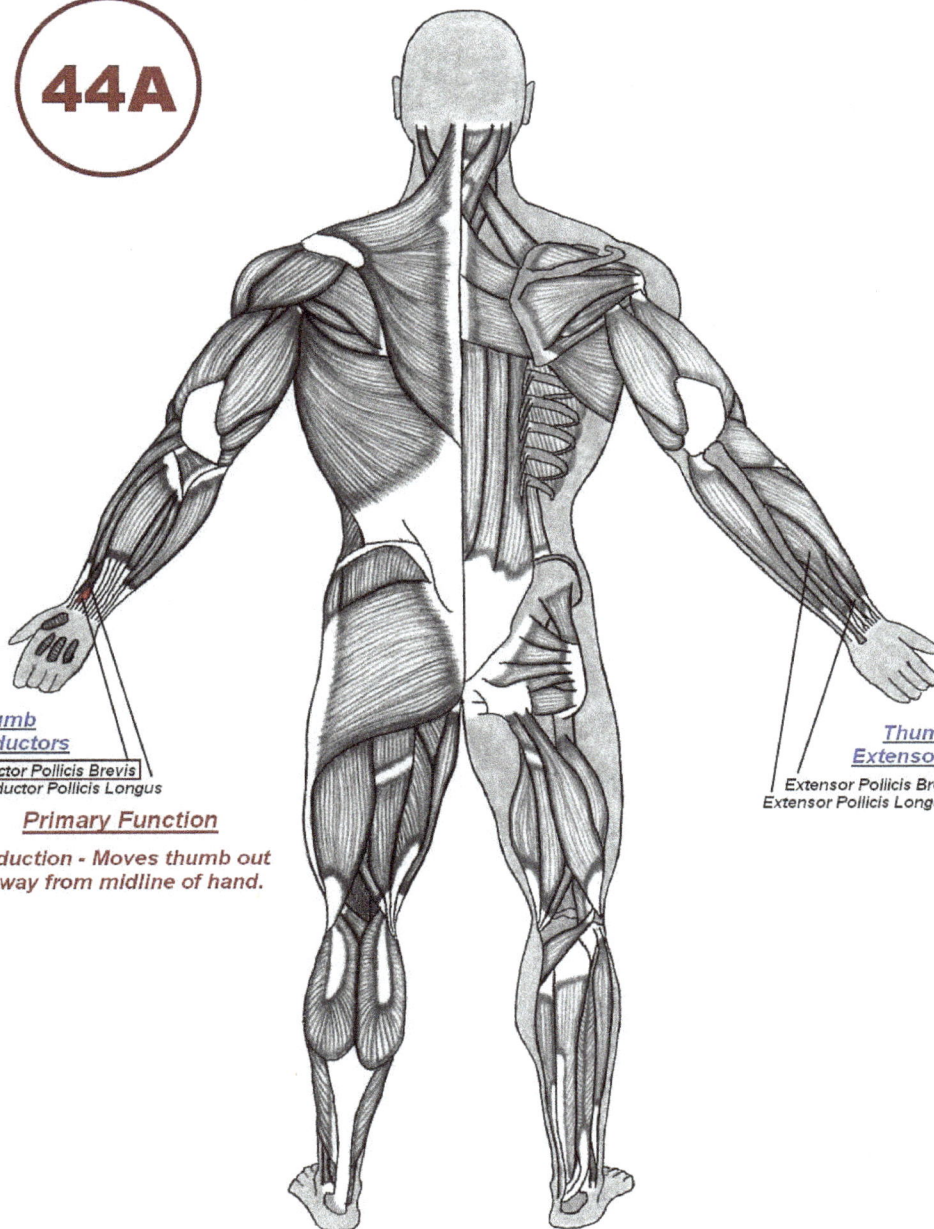

Thumb Abductors
Abductor Pollicis Brevis
Abductor Pollicis Longus

Primary Function

Abduction - Moves thumb out away from midline of hand.

Thumb Extensors
Extensor Pollicis Brevis
Extensor Pollicis Longus

Thumb Abductor - Abductor Pollicis Longus

44B

Radius (Under)

Ulna

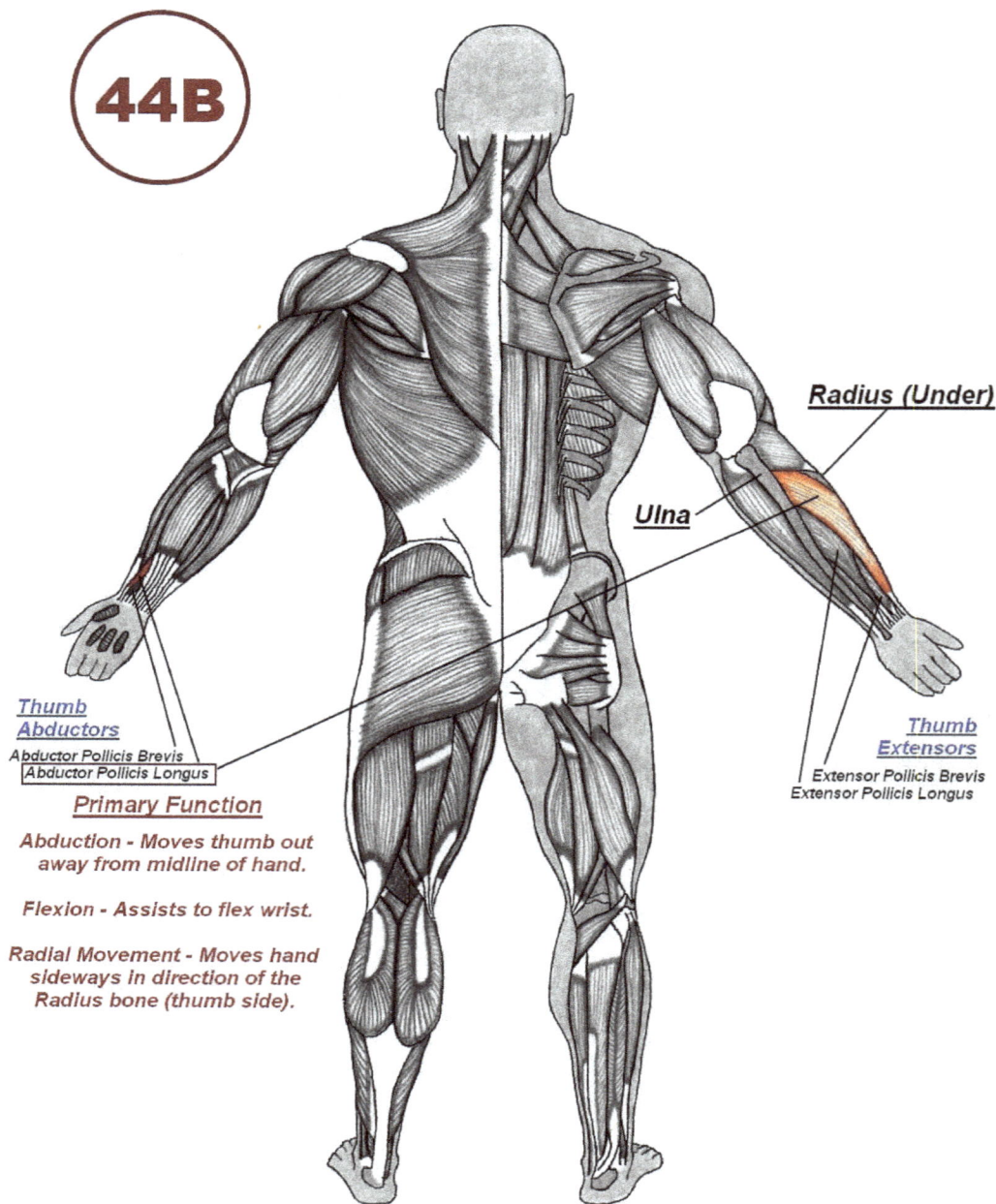

Thumb
Abductors
Abductor Pollicis Brevis
Abductor Pollicis Longus

Thumb
Extensors
Extensor Pollicis Brevis
Extensor Pollicis Longus

Primary Function

Abduction - Moves thumb out
away from midline of hand.

Flexion - Assists to flex wrist.

Radial Movement - Moves hand
sideways in direction of the
Radius bone (thumb side).

Thumb Extensor - Extensor Pollicis Brevis

45A

Radius (Under)

Ulna

Thumb Abductors

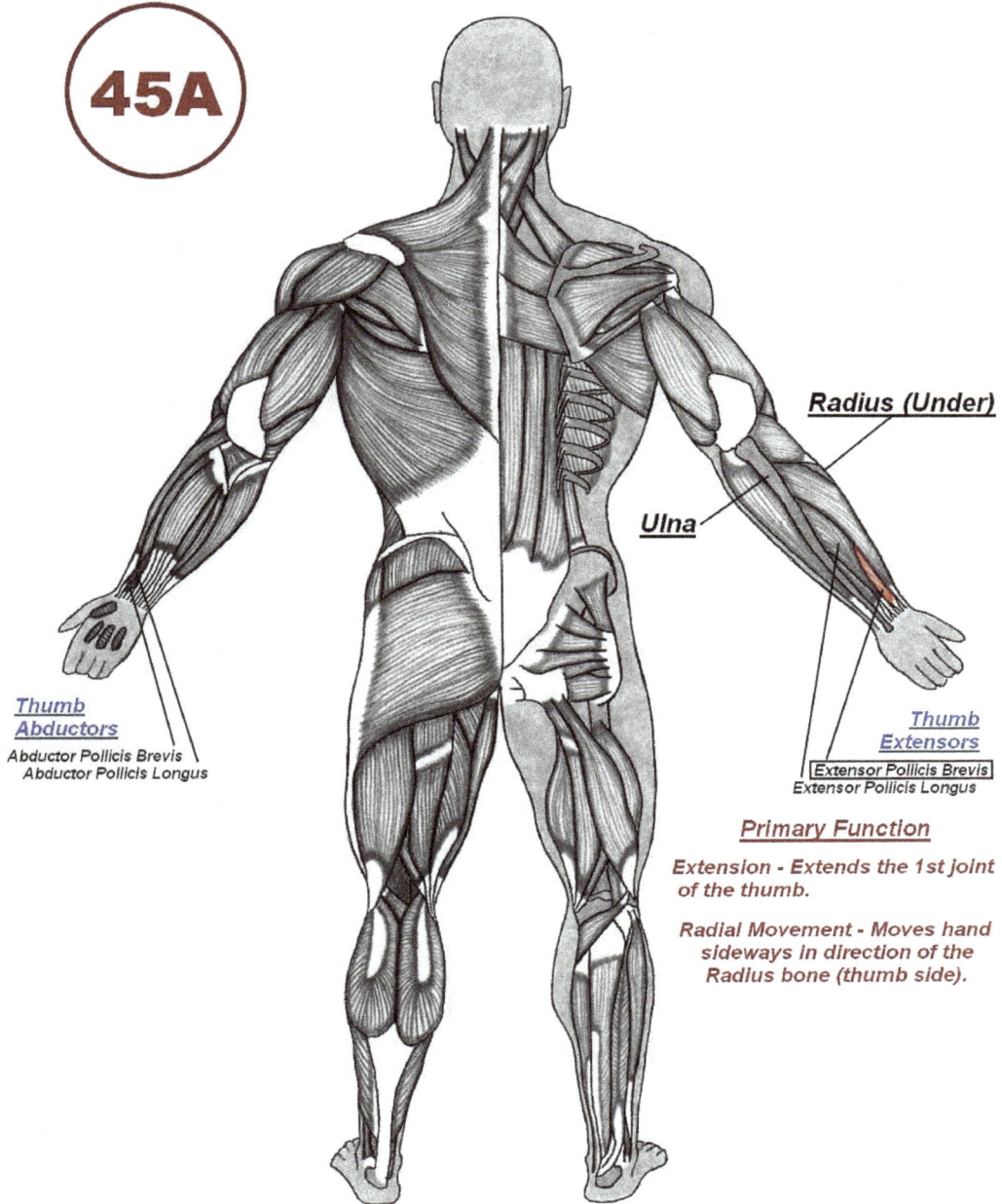

Abductor Pollicis Brevis
Abductor Pollicis Longus

Thumb Extensors

Extensor Pollicis Brevis
Extensor Pollicis Longus

Primary Function

Extension - Extends the 1st joint of the thumb.

Radial Movement - Moves hand sideways in direction of the Radius bone (thumb side).

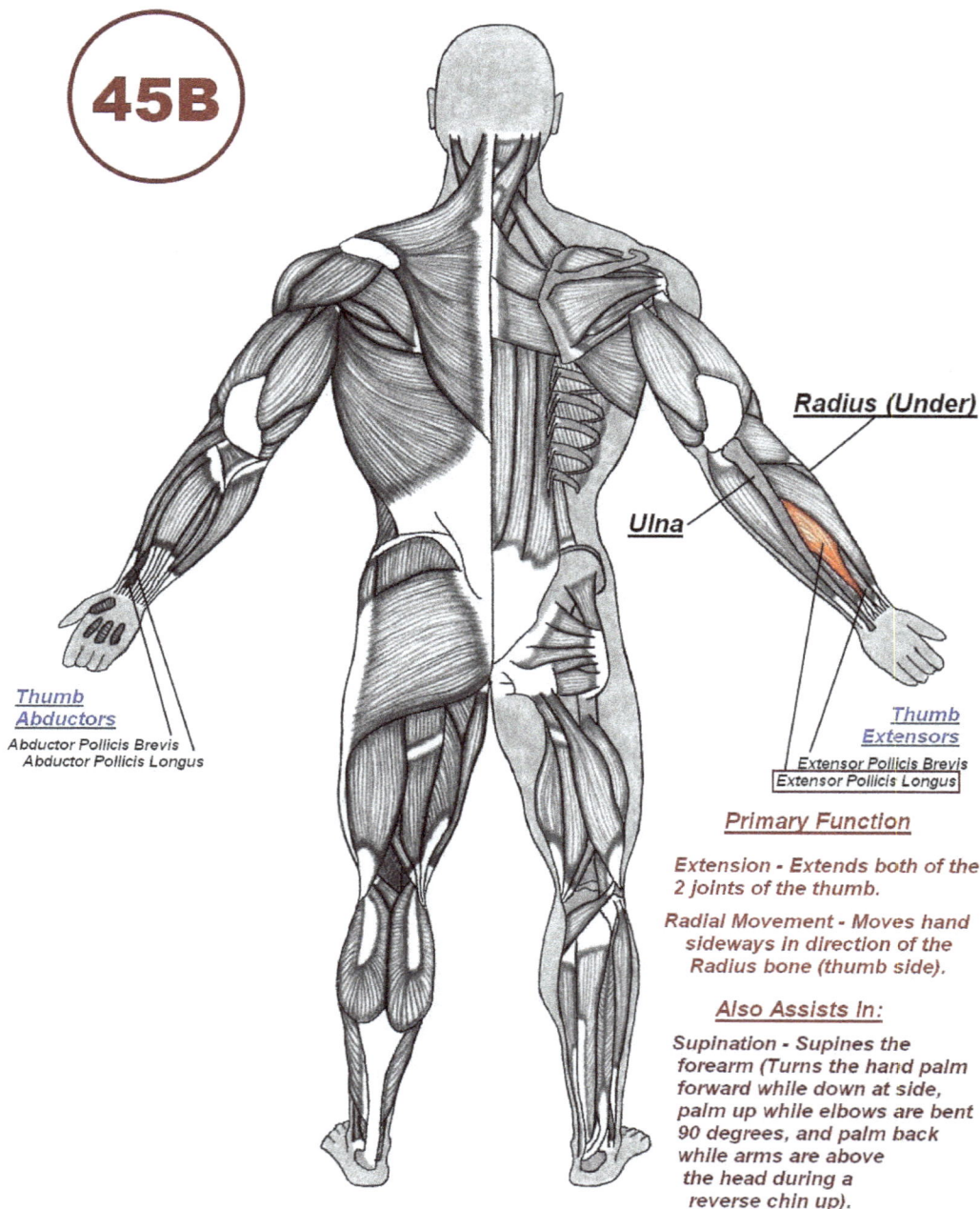

Thumb Extensor - Extensor Pollicis Longus

45B

Radius (Under)

Ulna

Thumb Abductors
Abductor Pollicis Brevis
Abductor Pollicis Longus

Thumb Extensors
Extensor Pollicis Brevis
Extensor Pollicis Longus

Primary Function

Extension - Extends both of the 2 joints of the thumb.

Radial Movement - Moves hand sideways in direction of the Radius bone (thumb side).

Also Assists In:

Supination - Supines the forearm (Turns the hand palm forward while down at side, palm up while elbows are bent 90 degrees, and palm back while arms are above the head during a reverse chin up).

Glute Muscles

46

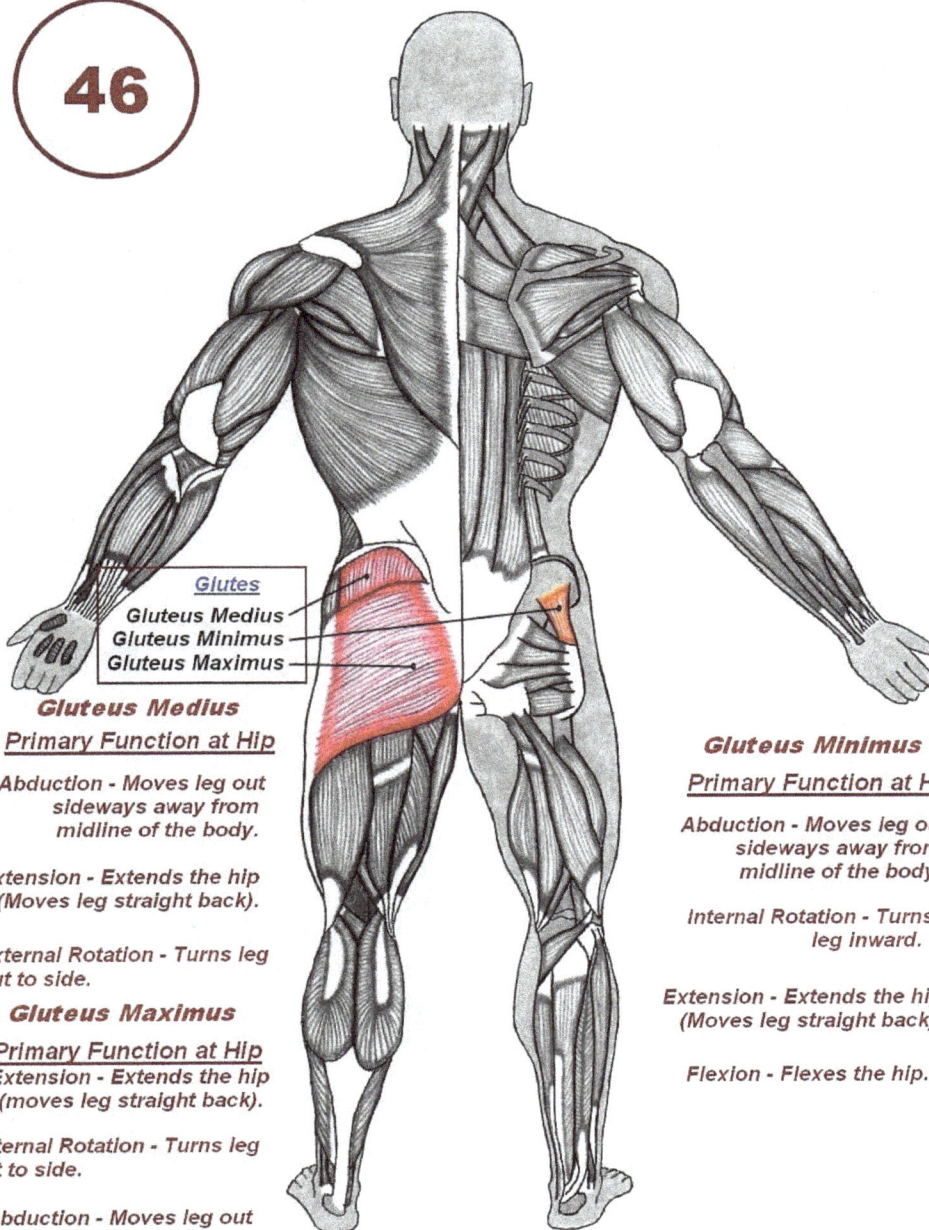

Glutes
Gluteus Medius
Gluteus Minimus
Gluteus Maximus

Gluteus Medius

Primary Function at Hip

Abduction - Moves leg out sideways away from midline of the body.

Extension - Extends the hip (Moves leg straight back).

External Rotation - Turns leg out to side.

Gluteus Maximus

Primary Function at Hip
Extension - Extends the hip (moves leg straight back).

External Rotation - Turns leg out to side.

Abduction - Moves leg out sideways away from midline of the body.

Adduction - Moves leg in toward midline of the body.

Gluteus Minimus

Primary Function at Hip

Abduction - Moves leg out sideways away from midline of the body.

Internal Rotation - Turns leg inward.

Extension - Extends the hip (Moves leg straight back).

Flexion - Flexes the hip.

46 - Exercises

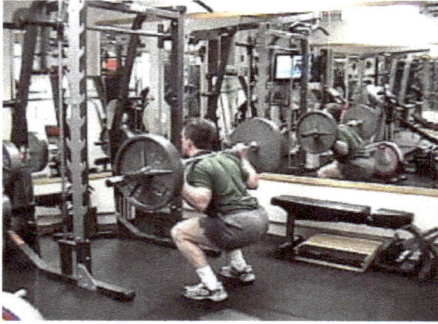

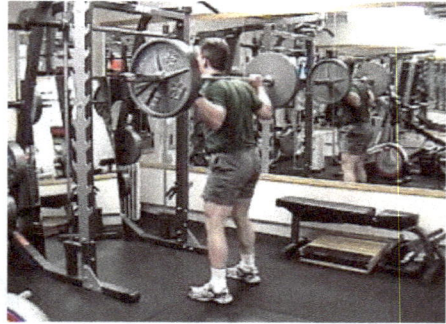

Free Weight Bar Squat (1-5 Sets 7-10 Reps)

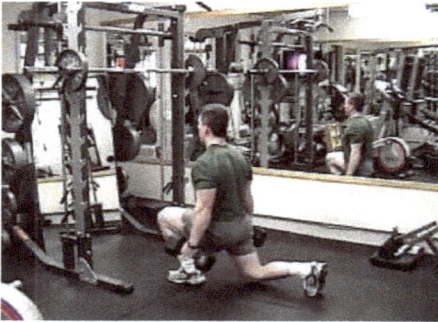

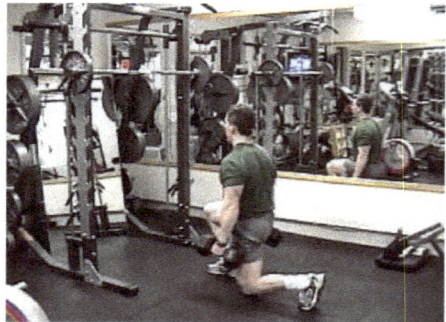

Alternating Dumbbell Lunge (1-3 Sets 7-10 Reps)

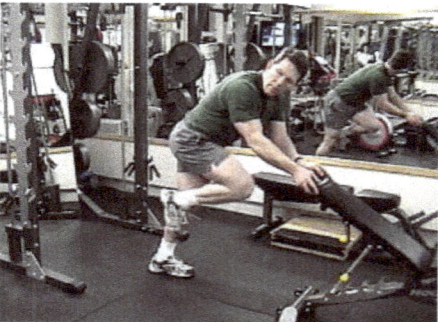

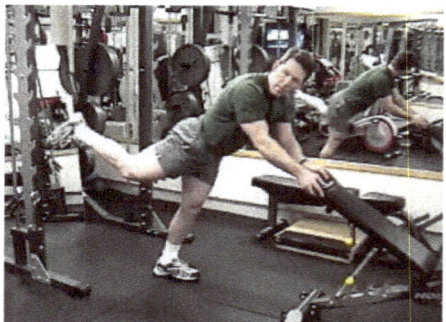

Standing Glute Curl (1-3 Sets 7-15 Reps)

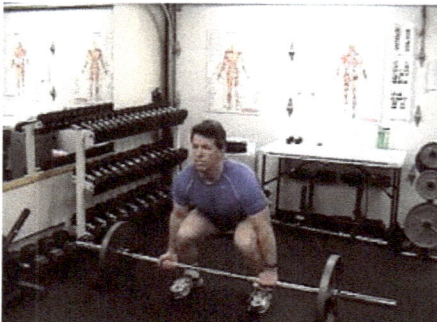

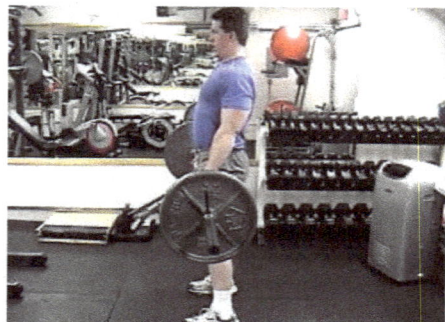

Dead-Lift (1-3 Sets 7-10 Reps)

Hip External Rotators

47

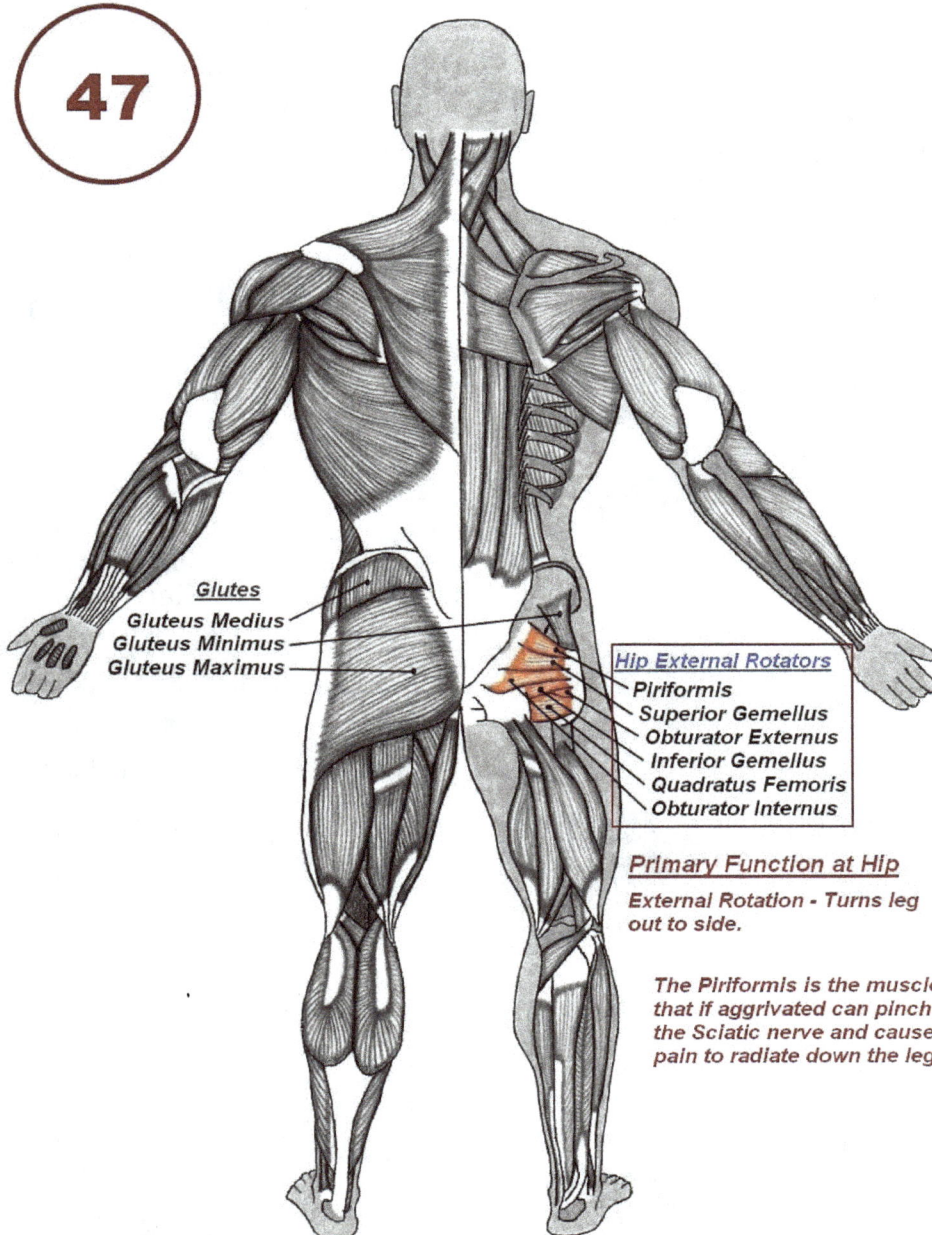

Glutes
Gluteus Medius
Gluteus Minimus
Gluteus Maximus

Hip External Rotators
Piriformis
Superior Gemellus
Obturator Externus
Inferior Gemellus
Quadratus Femoris
Obturator Internus

Primary Function at Hip

External Rotation - Turns leg out to side.

The Piriformis is the muscle that if aggrivated can pinch the Sciatic nerve and cause pain to radiate down the leg.

47 - Exercises

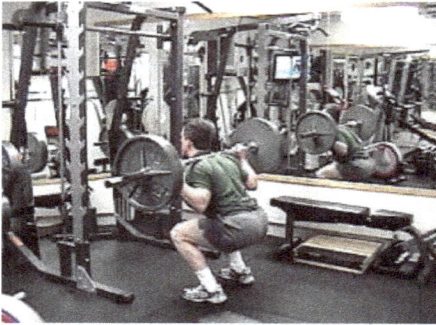

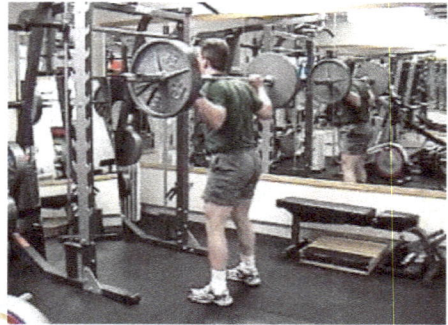

Free Weight Bar Squat (1-5 Sets 7-10 Reps)

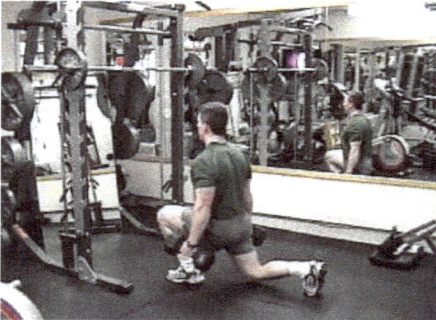

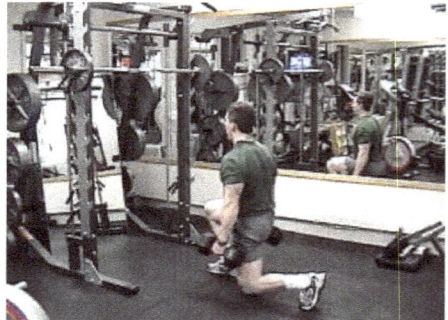

Alternating Dumbbell Lunge (1-3 Sets 7-10 Reps)

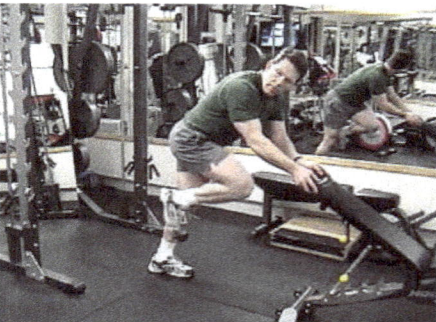

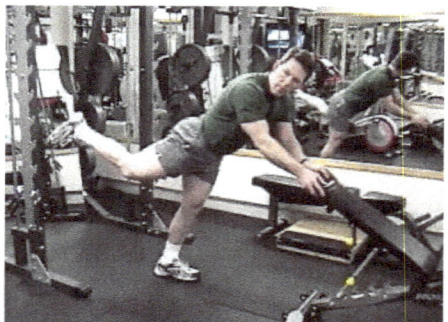

Standing Glute Curl (1-3 Sets 7-15 Reps)

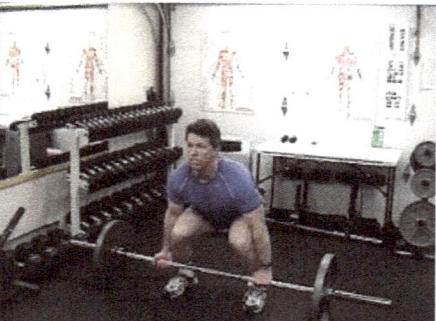

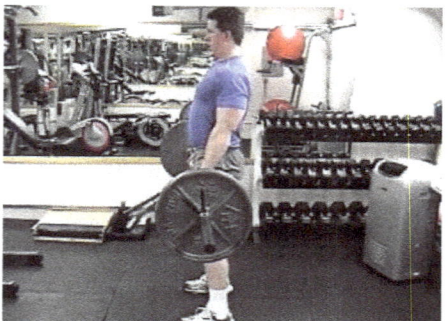

Dead-Lift (1-3 Sets 7-10 Reps)

Hamstring Muscles

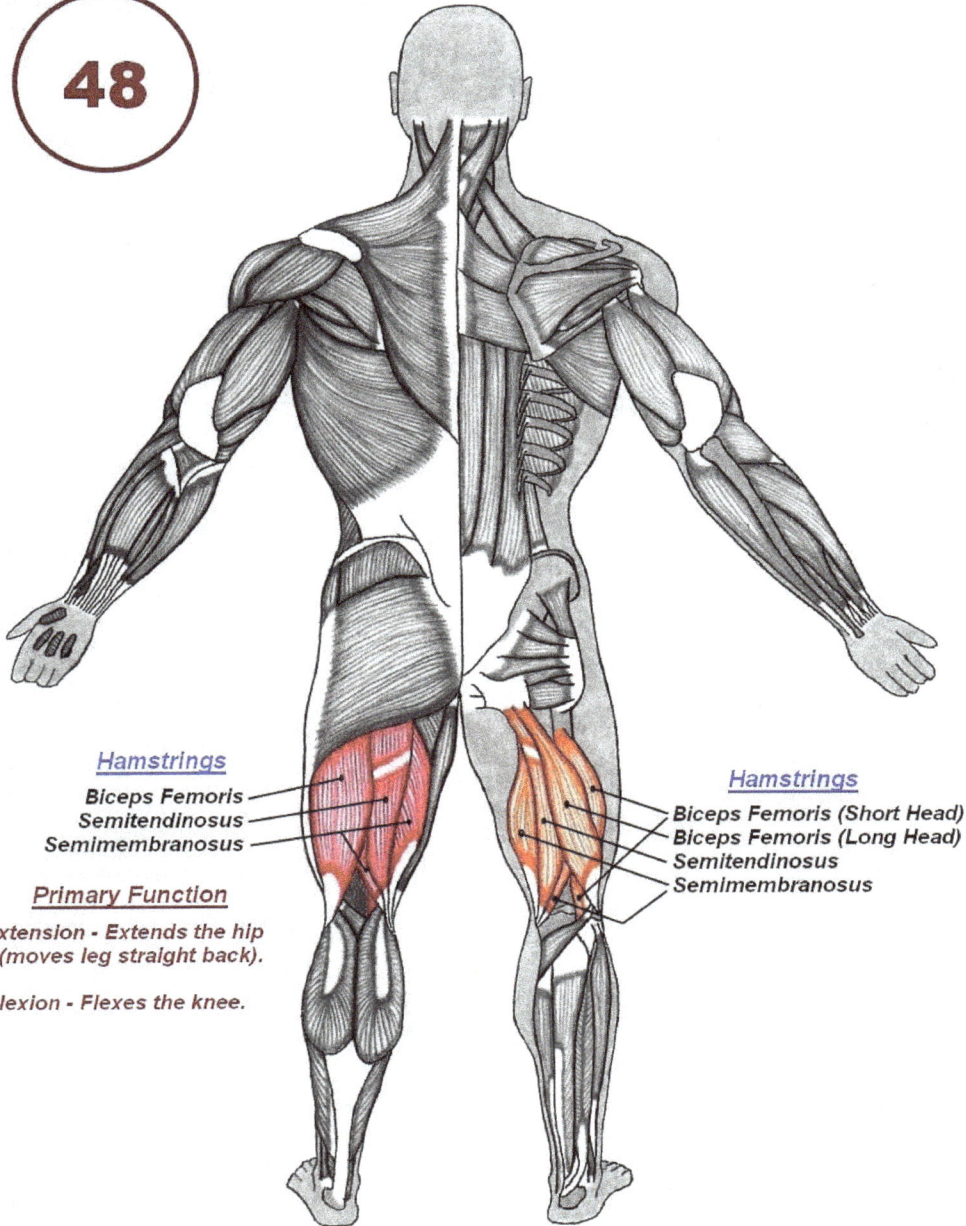

48

Hamstrings
Biceps Femoris
Semitendinosus
Semimembranosus

Primary Function
Extension - Extends the hip (moves leg straight back).

Flexion - Flexes the knee.

Hamstrings
Biceps Femoris (Short Head)
Biceps Femoris (Long Head)
Semitendinosus
Semimembranosus

48 - Exercises

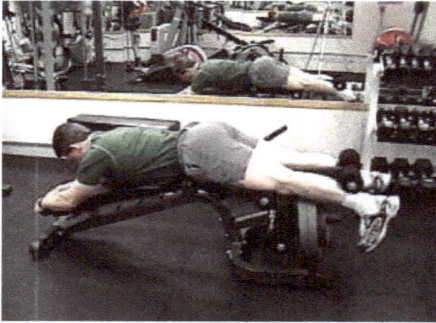

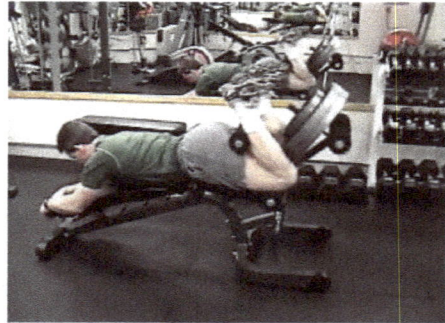

Lying Prone Leg Curl (1-3 Sets 7-10 Reps)

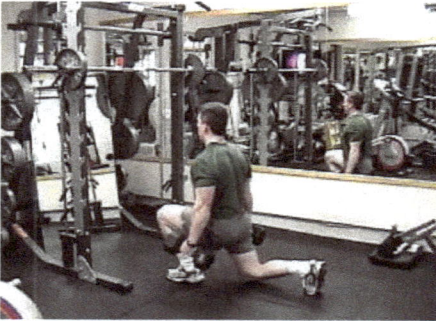

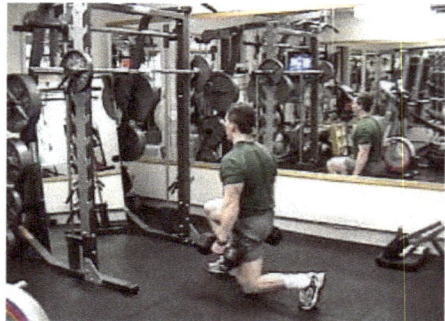

Alternating Dumbbell Lunge (1-3 Sets 7-10 Reps)

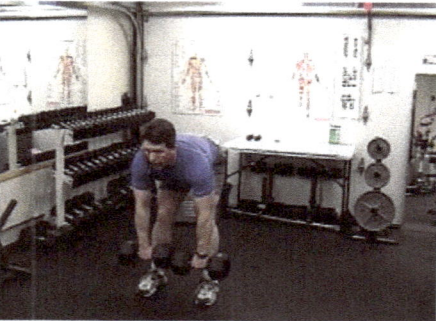

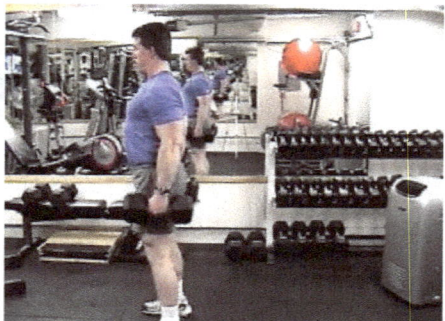

Straight Leg Dumbbell Dead-Lift (1-3 Sets 7-10 Reps)

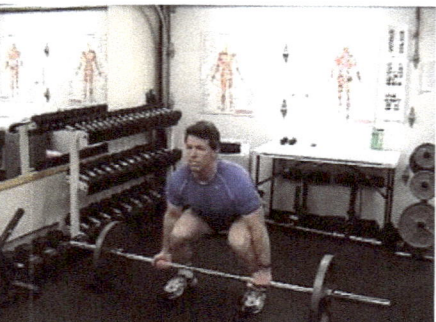

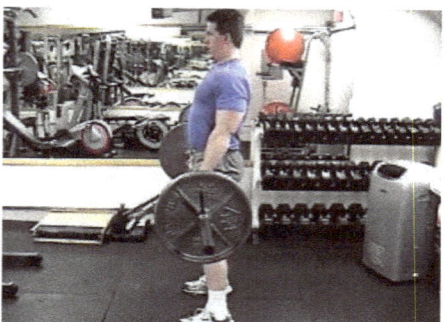

Dead-Lift (1-3 Sets 7-10 Reps)

Plantaris

49

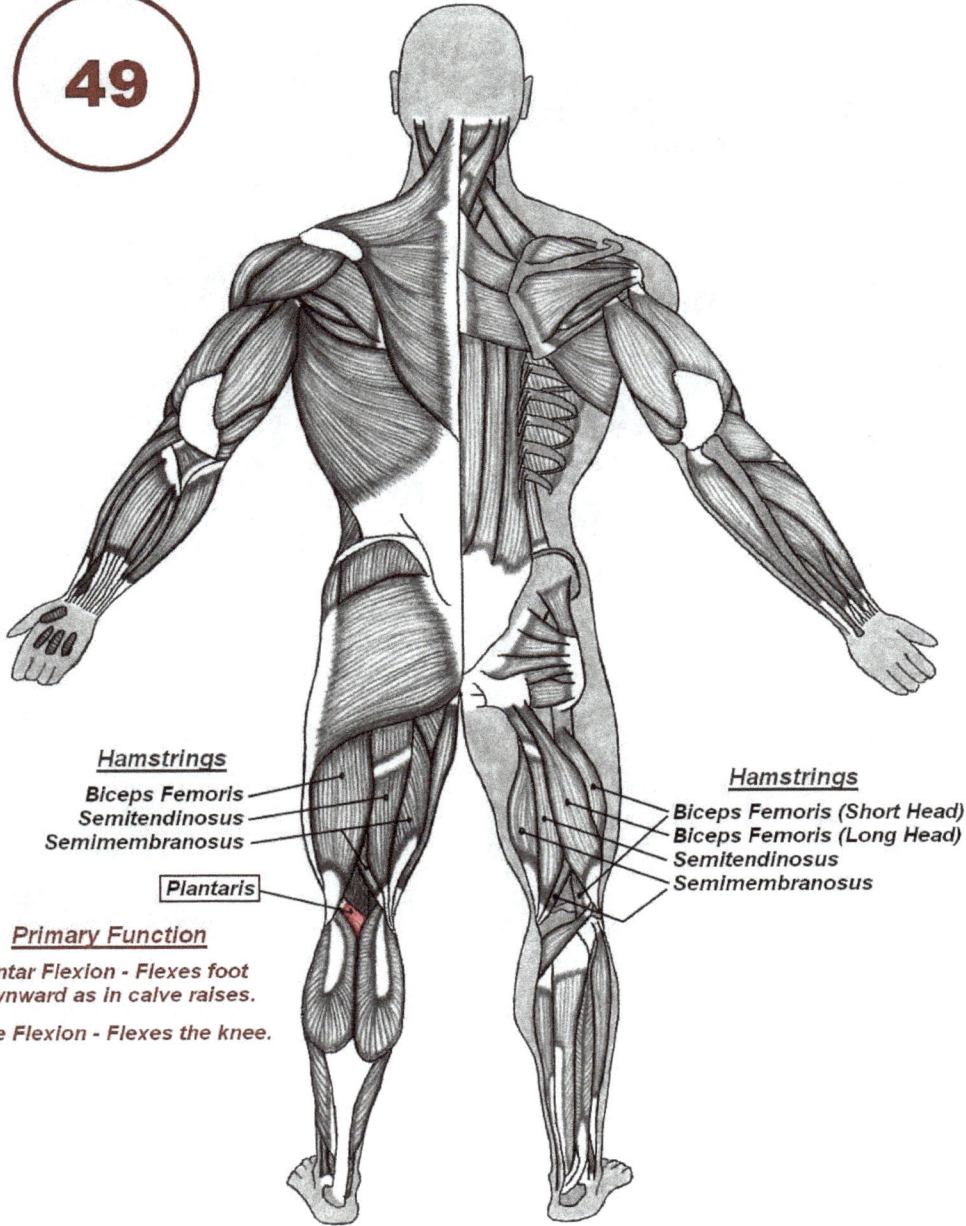

Hamstrings
Biceps Femoris
Semitendinosus
Semimembranosus

Plantaris

Hamstrings
Biceps Femoris (Short Head)
Biceps Femoris (Long Head)
Semitendinosus
Semimembranosus

Primary Function

Plantar Flexion - Flexes foot
downward as in calve raises.

Knee Flexion - Flexes the knee.

49 - Exercises

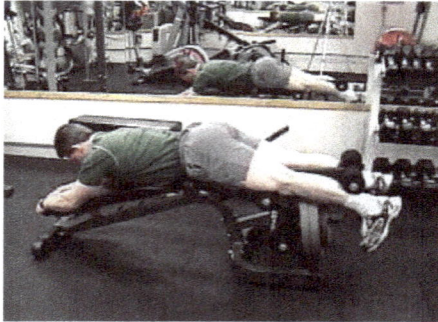

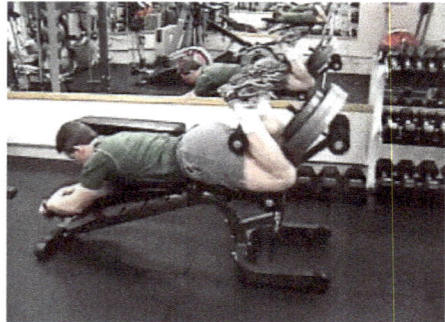

Lying Prone Leg Curl (1-3 Sets 7-10 Reps)

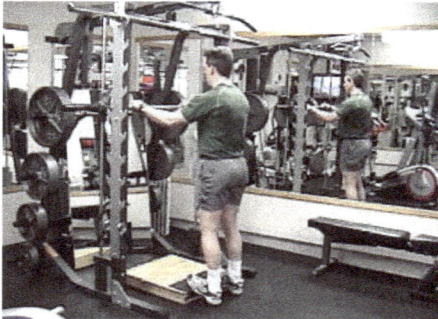

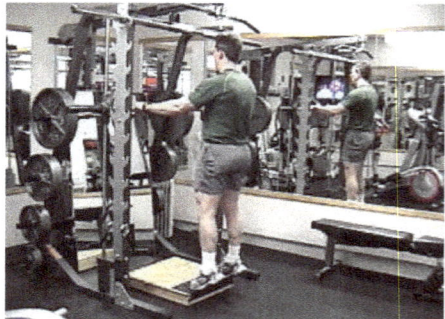

Standing Calve Raise - No Weight, High Rep (1-3 Sets 10-30 Reps)

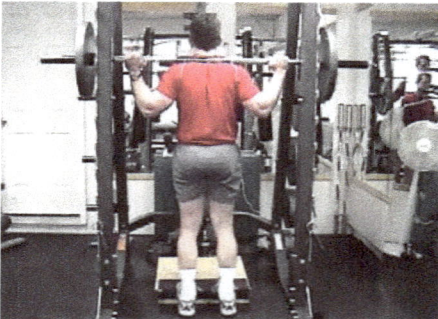

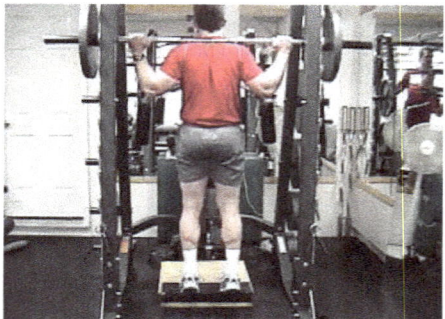

Standing Calve Raise - Weighted (1-3 Sets 10-15 Reps)

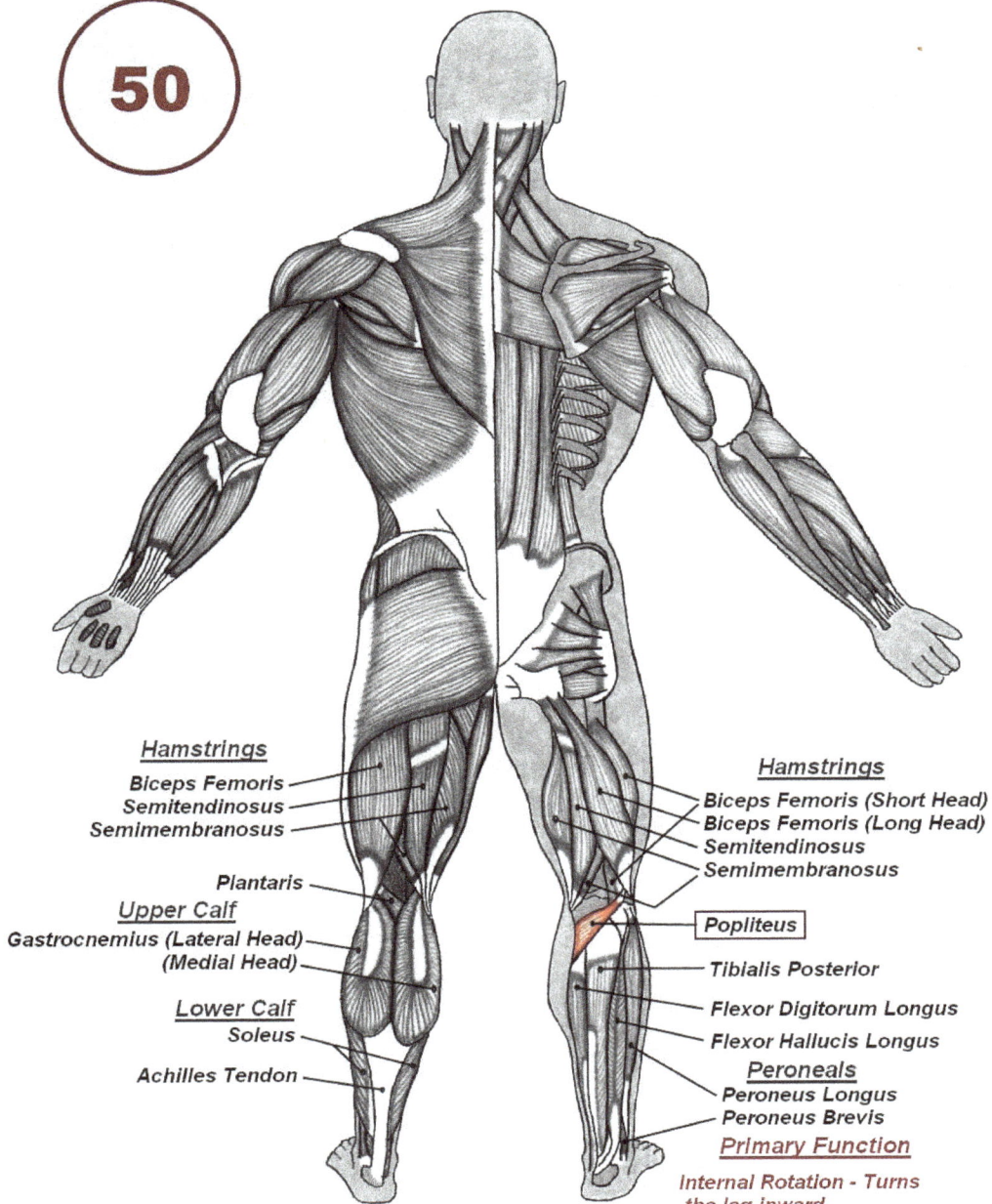

Popliteus

50

Hamstrings
Biceps Femoris
Semitendinosus
Semimembranosus

Plantaris
Upper Calf
Gastrocnemius (Lateral Head)
(Medial Head)

Lower Calf
Soleus

Achilles Tendon

Hamstrings
Biceps Femoris (Short Head)
Biceps Femoris (Long Head)
Semitendinosus
Semimembranosus

Popliteus

Tibialis Posterior

Flexor Digitorum Longus

Flexor Hallucis Longus
Peroneals
Peroneus Longus
Peroneus Brevis
Primary Function

Internal Rotation - Turns
the leg inward.

Knee Flexion - Flexes the knee.

50 - Exercises

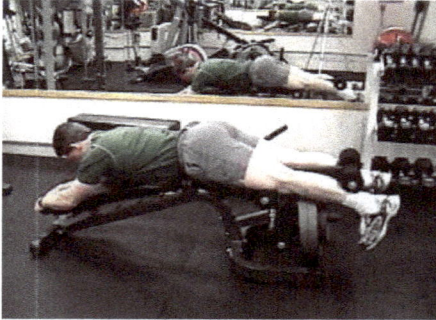
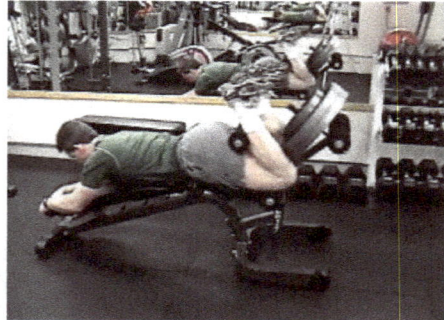

Lying Prone Leg Curl (1-3 Sets 7-10 Reps)

Gastrocnemius (Lateral & Medial Head)

51

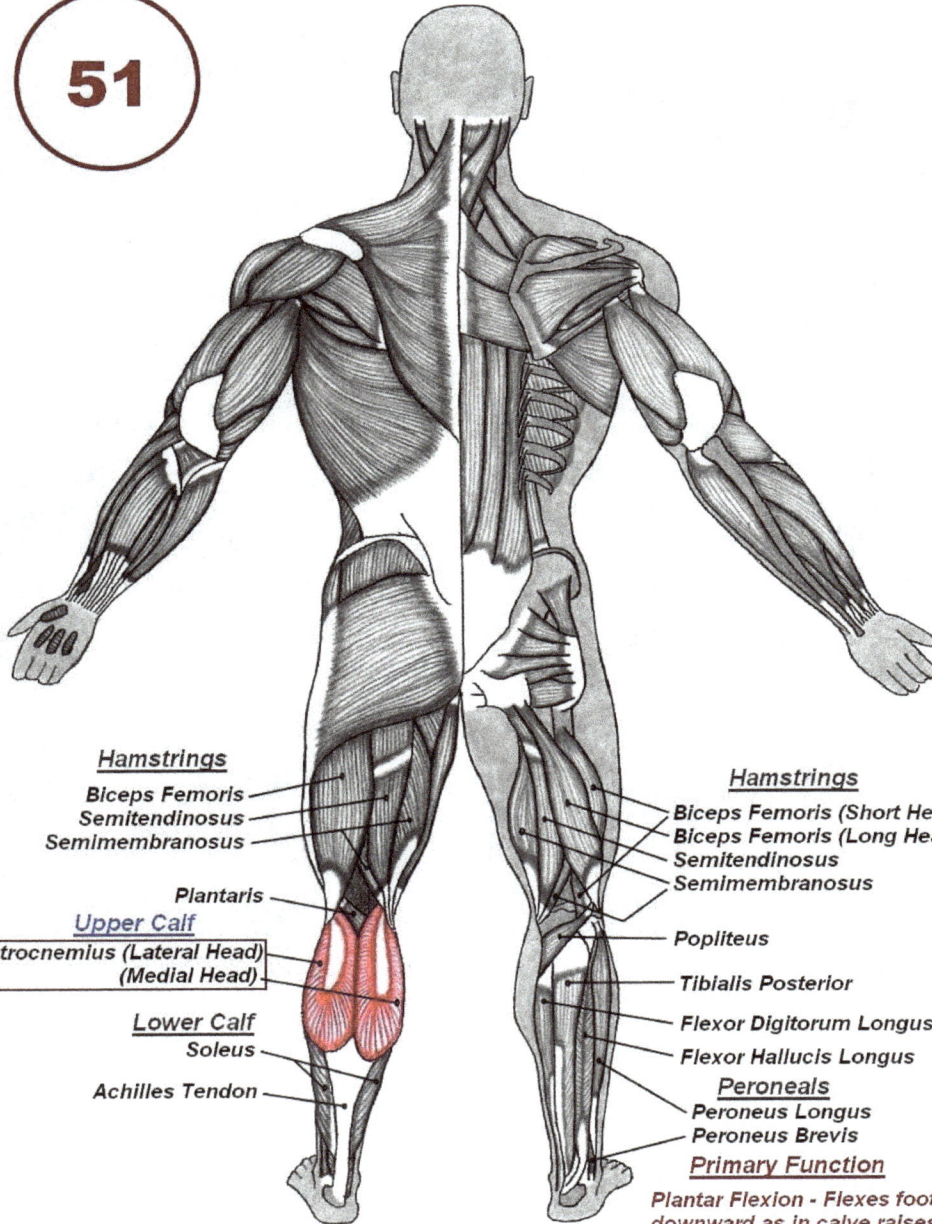

<u>Hamstrings</u>
Biceps Femoris
Semitendinosus
Semimembranosus

Plantaris

<u>Upper Calf</u>
Gastrocnemius (Lateral Head)
        (Medial Head)

<u>Lower Calf</u>
Soleus

Achilles Tendon

<u>Hamstrings</u>
Biceps Femoris (Short Head)
Biceps Femoris (Long Head)
Semitendinosus
Semimembranosus

Popliteus

Tibialis Posterior

Flexor Digitorum Longus

Flexor Hallucis Longus

<u>Peroneals</u>
Peroneus Longus
Peroneus Brevis

<u>Primary Function</u>

*Plantar Flexion - Flexes foot
downward as in calve raises.*

Knee Flexion - Flexes the knee.

51 - Exercises

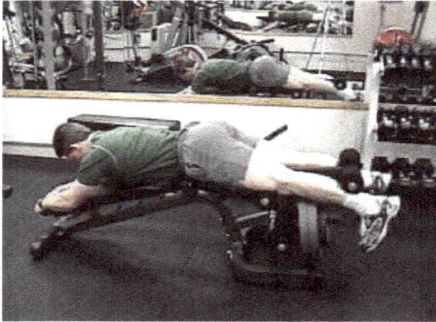

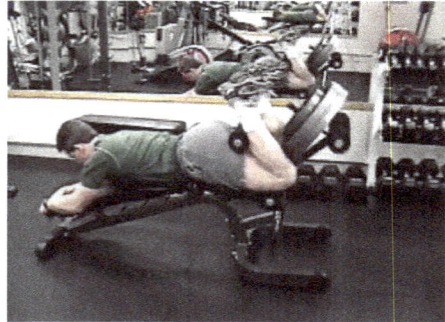

Lying Prone Leg Curl (1-3 Sets 7-10 Reps)

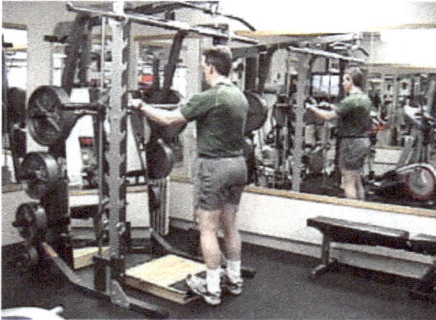

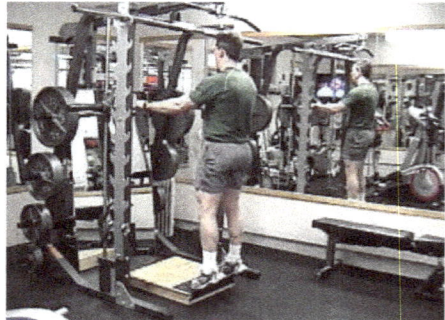

Standing Calve Raise - No Weight, High Rep (1-3 Sets 10-30 Reps)

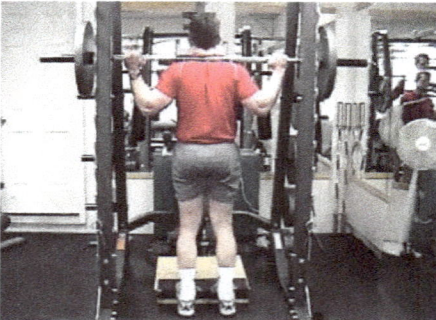

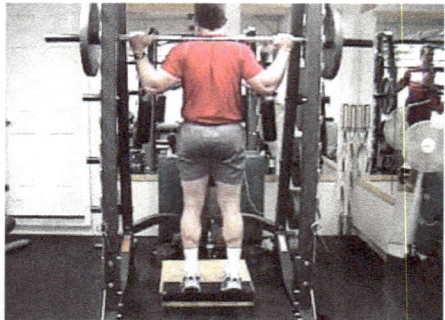

Standing Calve Raise - Weighted (1-3 Sets 10-15 Reps)

Lower Calf - Soleus

52

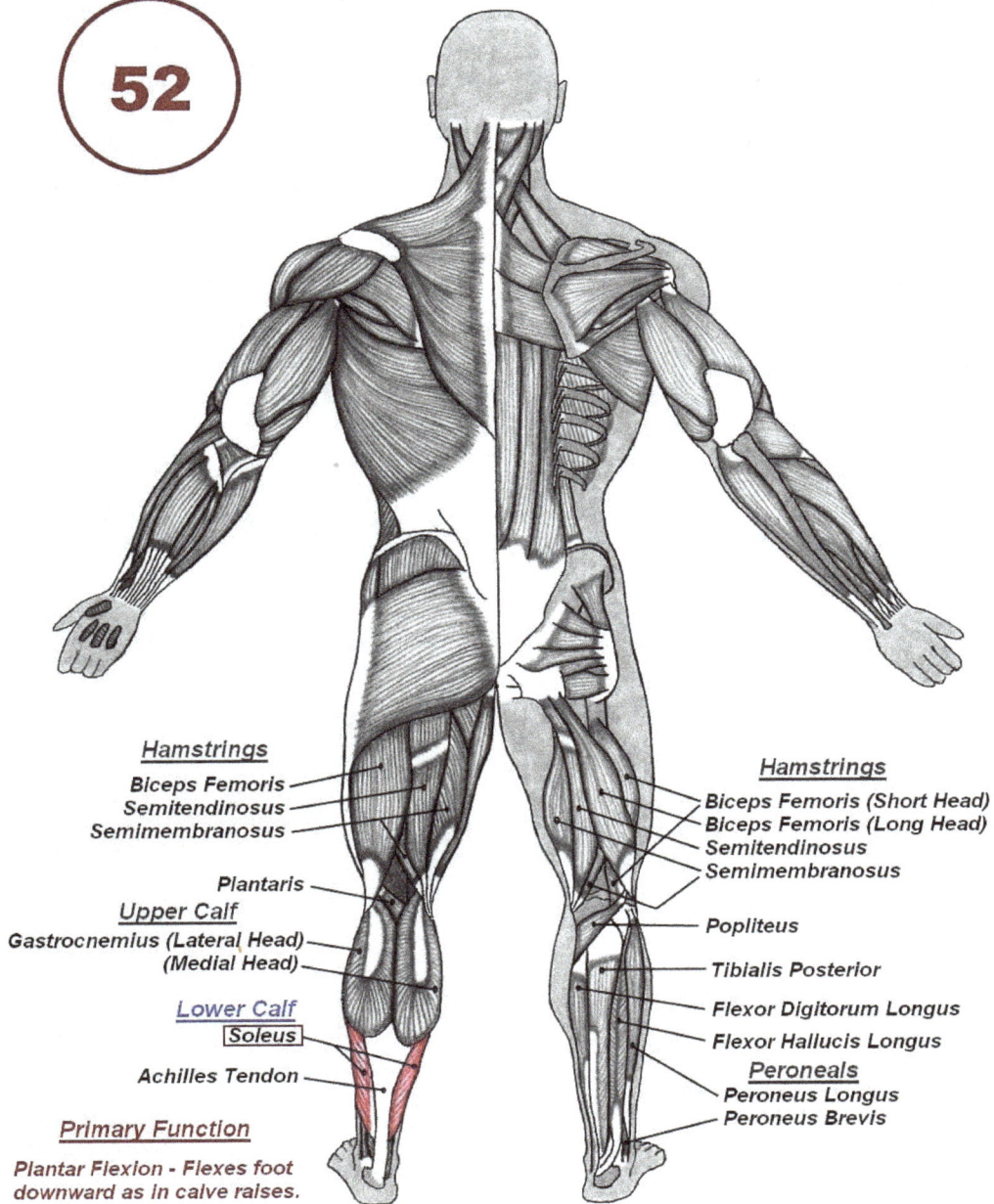

Hamstrings
Biceps Femoris
Semitendinosus
Semimembranosus

Plantaris

Upper Calf
Gastrocnemius (Lateral Head)
(Medial Head)

Lower Calf
Soleus

Achilles Tendon

Primary Function

Plantar Flexion - Flexes foot downward as in calve raises.

Hamstrings
Biceps Femoris (Short Head)
Biceps Femoris (Long Head)
Semitendinosus
Semimembranosus

Popliteus

Tibialis Posterior

Flexor Digitorum Longus

Flexor Hallucis Longus

Peroneals
Peroneus Longus
Peroneus Brevis

52 - Exercises

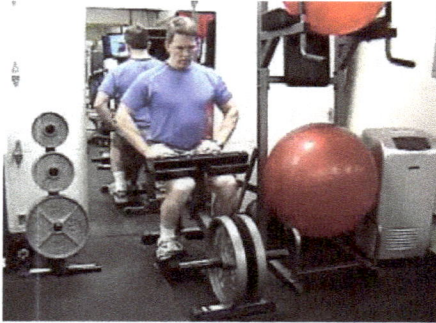

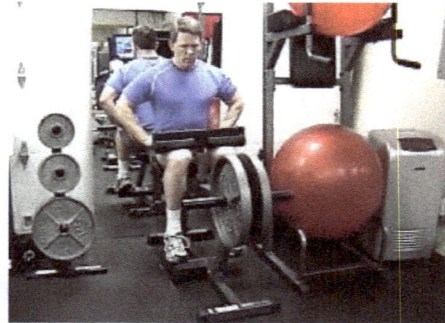

Seated Calve Raise (90 Degree Knee Isolates Soleus: 1-3 Sets 7-15 Reps)

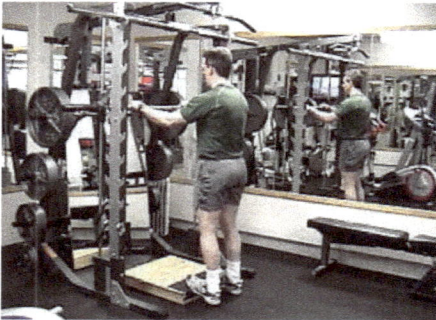

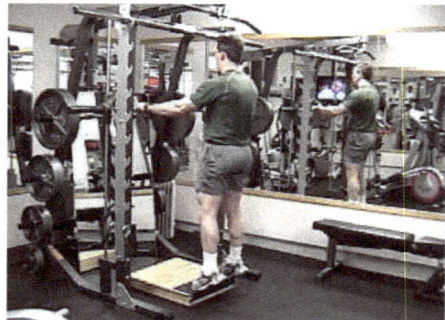

Standing Calve Raise - No Weight, High Rep (1-3 Sets 10-30 Reps)

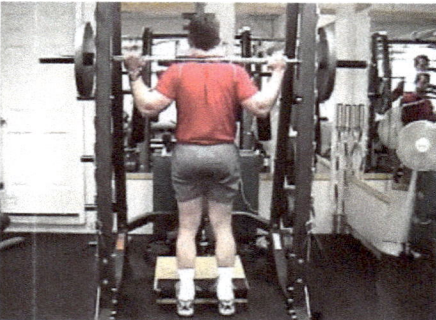

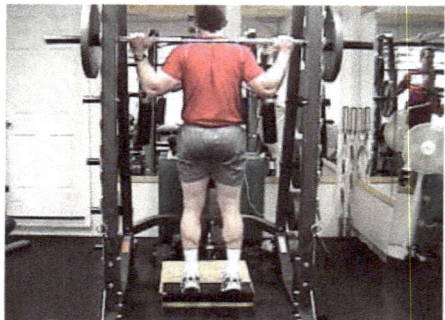

Standing Calve Raise - Weighted (1-3 Sets 10-15 Reps)

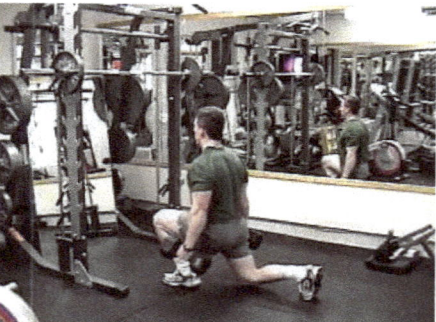

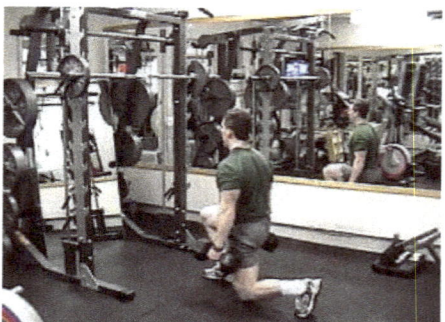

Alternating Dumbbell Lunge (Push Back Up: 1-3 Sets 7-10 Reps)

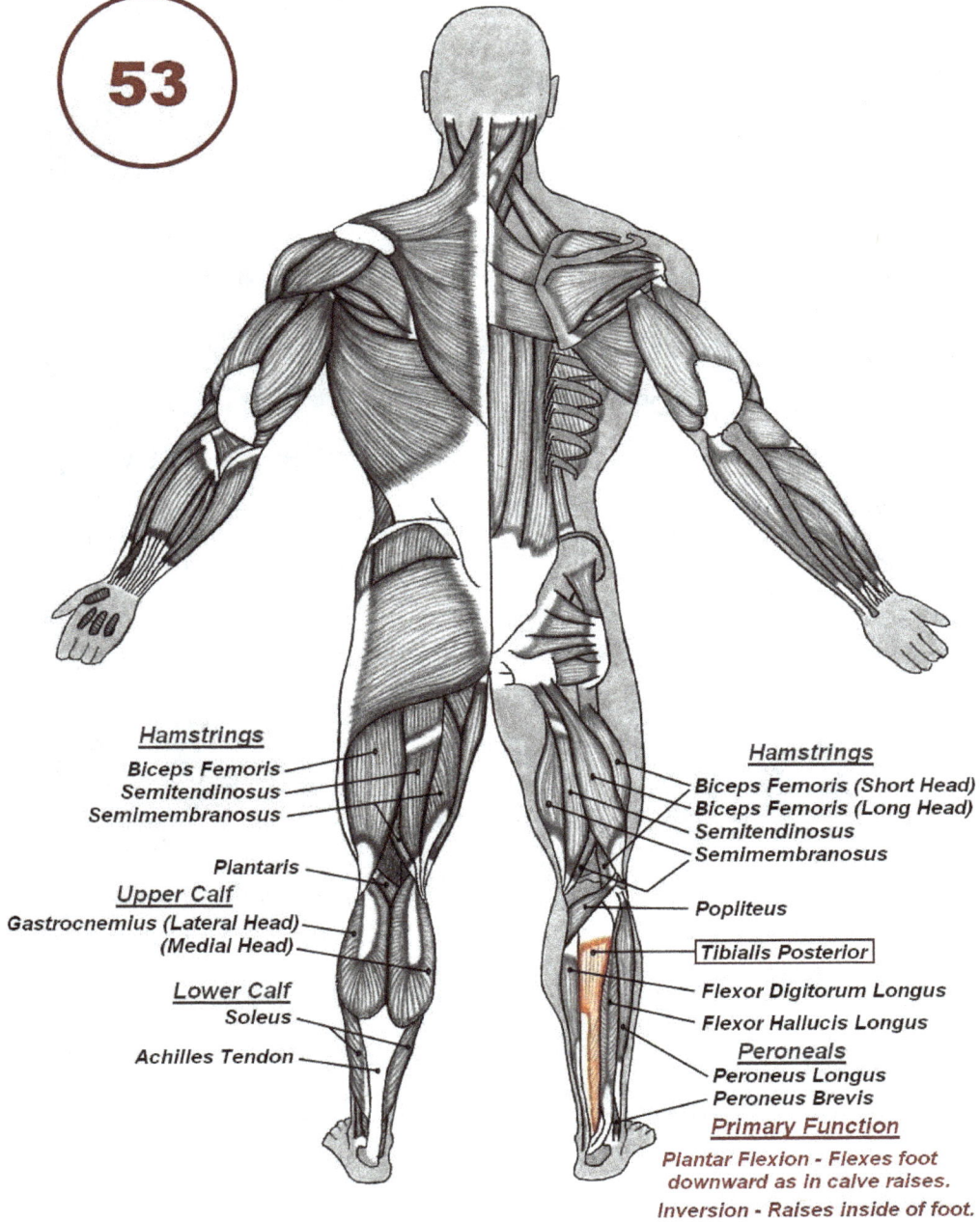

Lower Leg - Tibialis Posterior

53

Hamstrings
Biceps Femoris
Semitendinosus
Semimembranosus

Plantaris
Upper Calf
Gastrocnemius (Lateral Head)
(Medial Head)

Lower Calf
Soleus

Achilles Tendon

Hamstrings
Biceps Femoris (Short Head)
Biceps Femoris (Long Head)
Semitendinosus
Semimembranosus

Popliteus

Tibialis Posterior
Flexor Digitorum Longus
Flexor Hallucis Longus
Peroneals
Peroneus Longus
Peroneus Brevis
Primary Function
Plantar Flexion - Flexes foot
downward as in calve raises.
Inversion - Raises inside of foot.

53 - Exercises

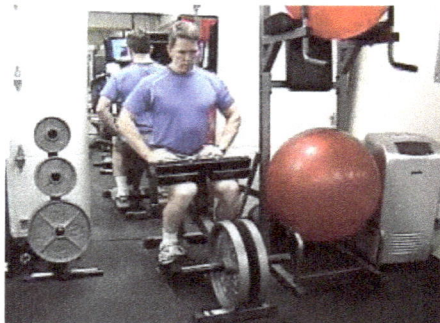

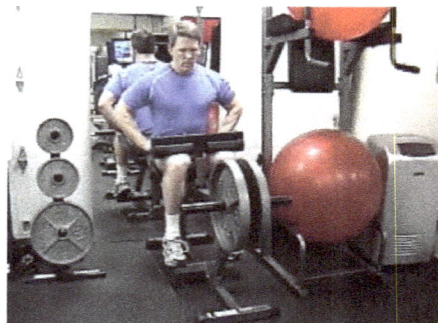

Seated Calve Raise (1-3 Sets 7-15 Reps)

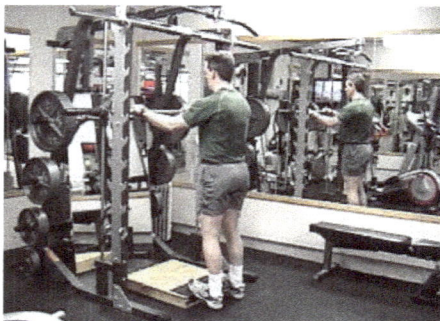

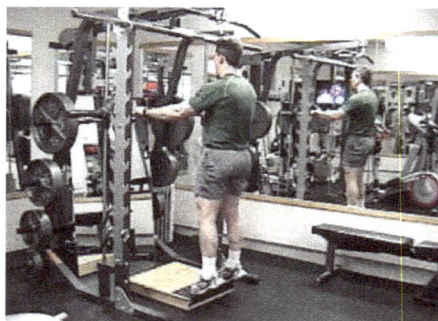

Standing Calve Raise - No Weight, High Rep (1-3 Sets 10-30 Reps)

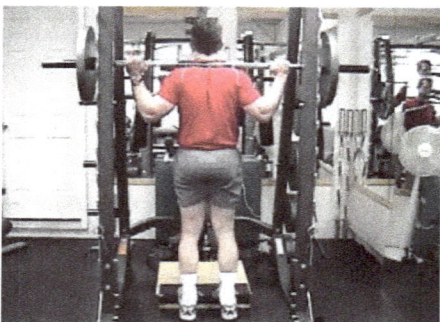

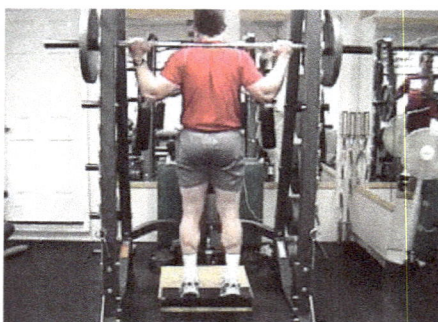

Standing Calve Raise - Weighted (1-3 Sets 10-15 Reps)

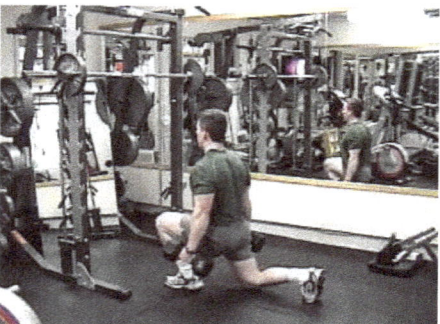

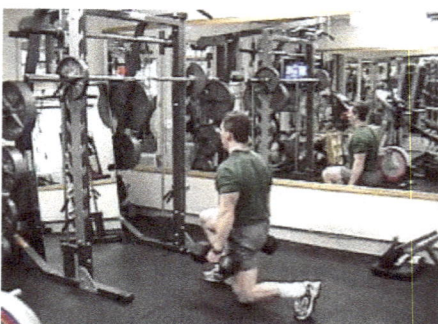

Alternating Dumbbell Lunge (Push Back Up: 1-3 Sets 7-10 Reps)

Lower Leg - Flexor Digitorum Longus

54A

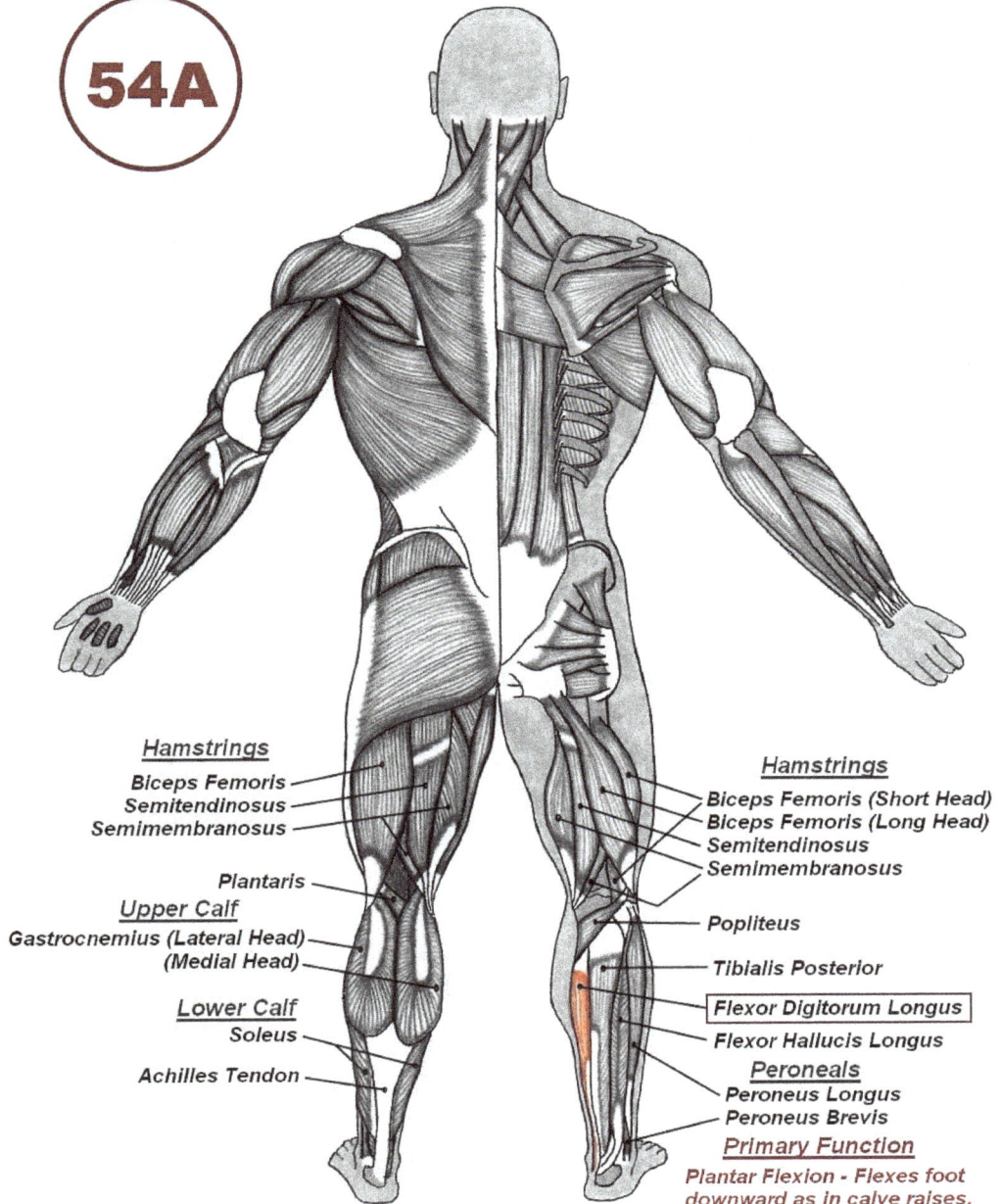

Hamstrings
Biceps Femoris
Semitendinosus
Semimembranosus

Plantaris
Upper Calf
Gastrocnemius (Lateral Head)
(Medial Head)

Lower Calf
Soleus

Achilles Tendon

Hamstrings
Biceps Femoris (Short Head)
Biceps Femoris (Long Head)
Semitendinosus
Semimembranosus

Popliteus

Tibialis Posterior

Flexor Digitorum Longus

Flexor Hallucis Longus
Peroneals
Peroneus Longus
Peroneus Brevis
Primary Function
Plantar Flexion - Flexes foot downward as in calve raises.

Inversion - Raises inside of foot.

Flexion - Flexes all 3 joints of each of the 4 toes.

Lower Leg - Flexor Hallucis Longus

54B

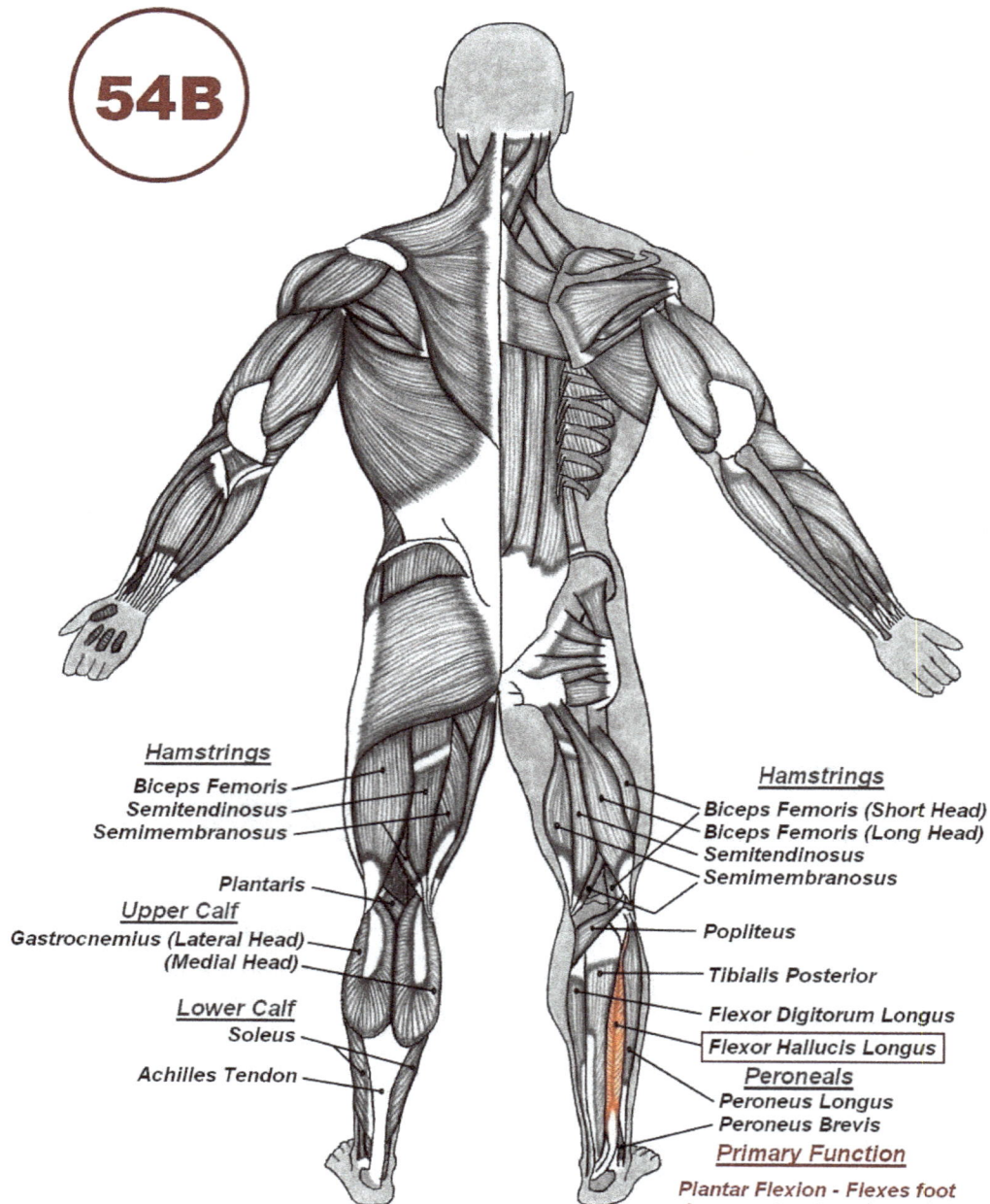

Hamstrings
Biceps Femoris
Semitendinosus
Semimembranosus

Plantaris
Upper Calf
Gastrocnemius (Lateral Head)
(Medial Head)

Lower Calf
Soleus

Achilles Tendon

Hamstrings
Biceps Femoris (Short Head)
Biceps Femoris (Long Head)
Semitendinosus
Semimembranosus

Popliteus

Tibialis Posterior

Flexor Digitorum Longus

Flexor Hallucis Longus

Peroneals
Peroneus Longus
Peroneus Brevis

Primary Function
Plantar Flexion - Flexes foot
downward as in calve raises.

Inversion - Raises inside of foot.

Flexion - Flexes both joints
of the big toe.

54A and B - Exercises

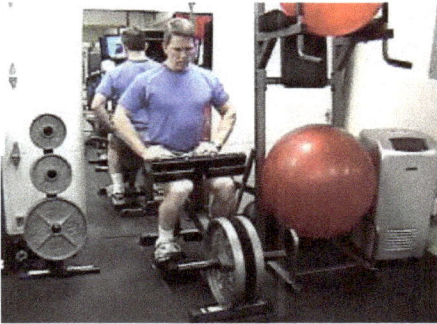

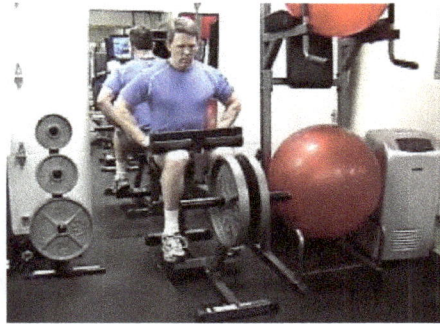

Seated Calve Raise (1-3 Sets 7-15 Reps)

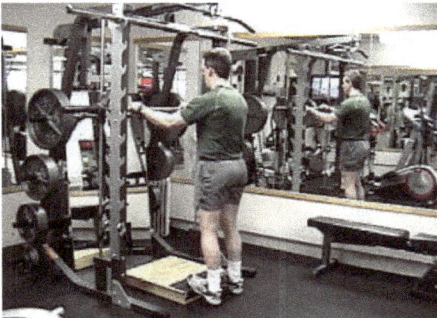

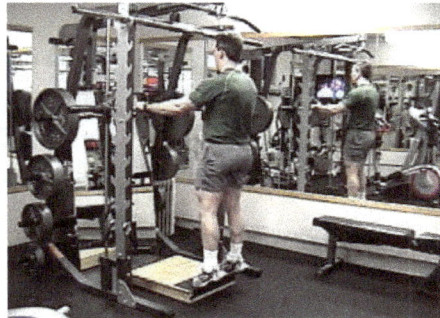

Standing Calve Raise - No Weight, High Rep (1-3 Sets 10-30 Reps)

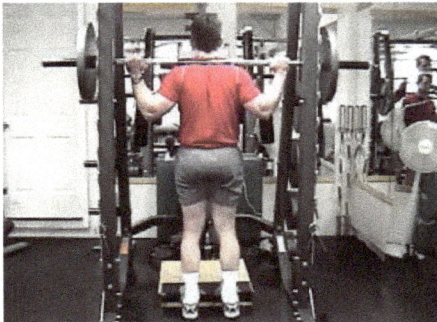

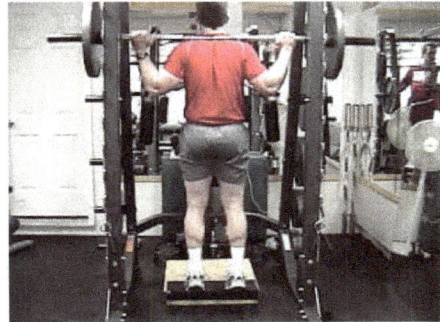

Standing Calve Raise - Weighted (1-3 Sets 10-15 Reps)

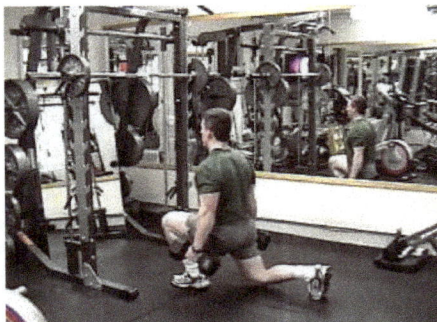

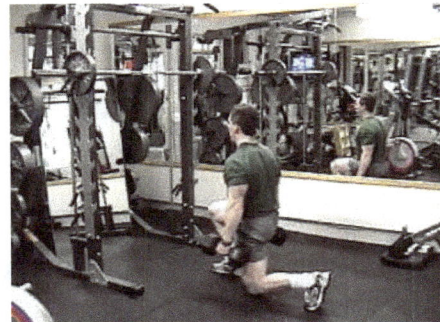

Alternating Dumbbell Lunge (Push Back Up: 1-3 Sets 7-10 Reps)

Lower Leg - Peroneals

55

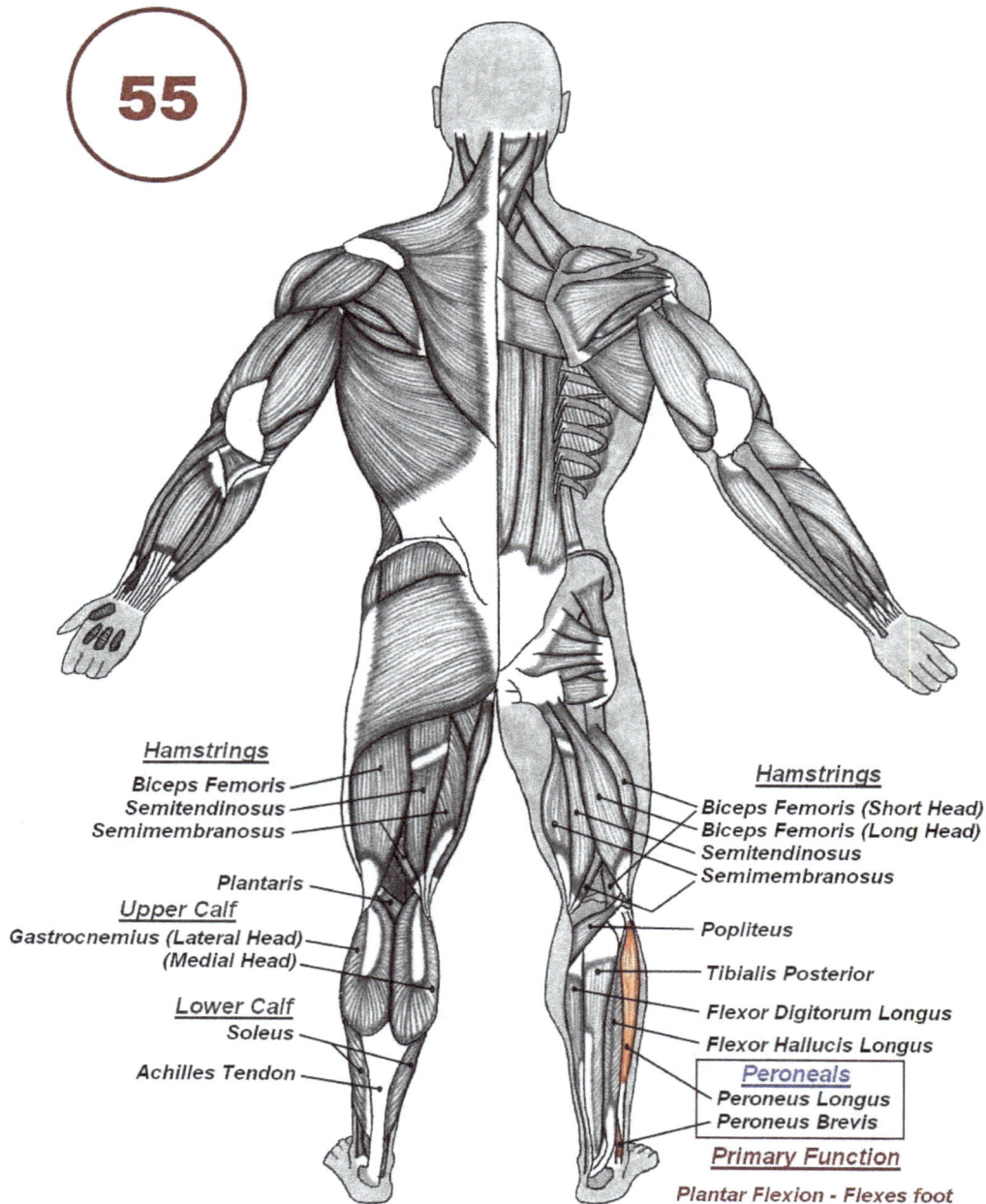

Hamstrings
Biceps Femoris
Semitendinosus
Semimembranosus

Plantaris

Upper Calf
Gastrocnemius (Lateral Head)
(Medial Head)

Lower Calf
Soleus

Achilles Tendon

Hamstrings
Biceps Femoris (Short Head)
Biceps Femoris (Long Head)
Semitendinosus
Semimembranosus

Popliteus

Tibialis Posterior

Flexor Digitorum Longus

Flexor Hallucis Longus

Peroneals
Peroneus Longus
Peroneus Brevis

Primary Function

*Plantar Flexion - Flexes foot
downward as in calve raises.*

Eversion - Raises outside of foot.

55 - Exercises

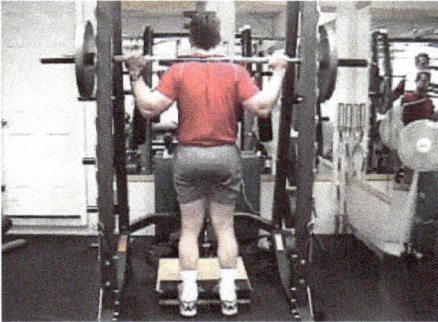

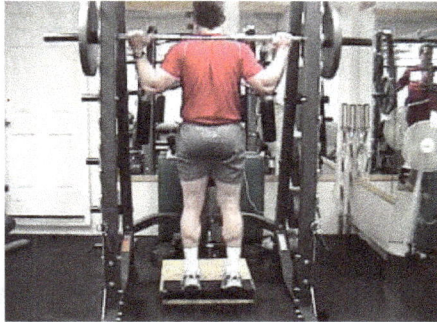

Standing Weighted Calve Raise (Flex Foot Down: 1-3 Sets 10-15 Reps)

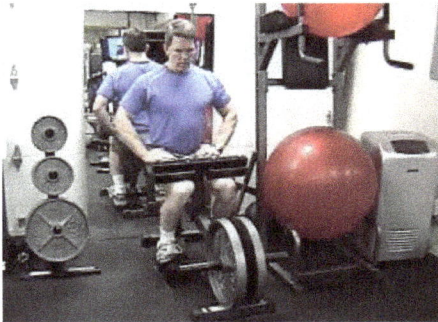

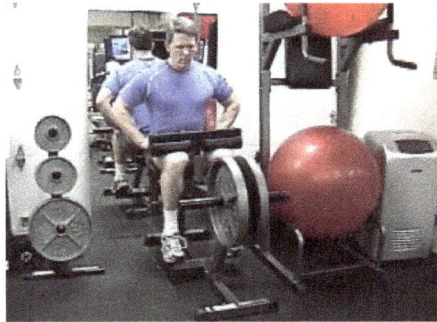

Seated Calve Raise (Flex Foot Down: 1-3 Sets 7-15 Reps)

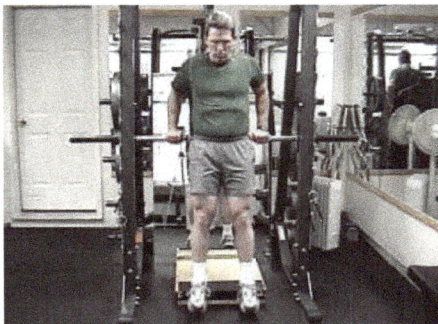

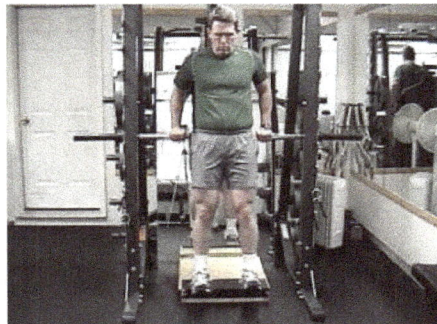

Tibialis Crunch (Evert Foot at Top - See Anterior View: 1-3 Sets 10-20 Reps)

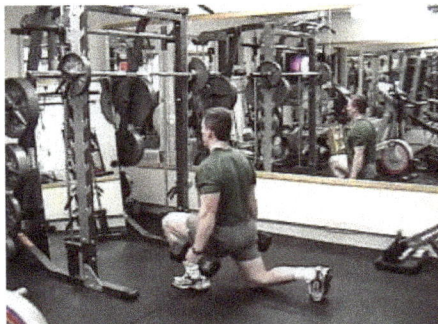

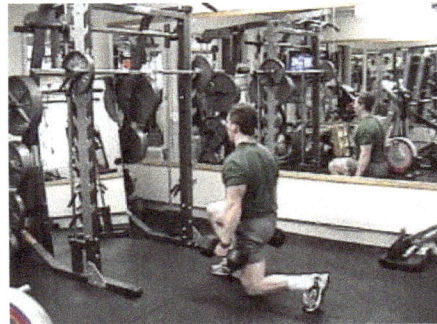

Alternating Dumbbell Lunge (Involved in Balancing: 1-3 Sets 7-10 Reps)

Posterior Muscles of Neck

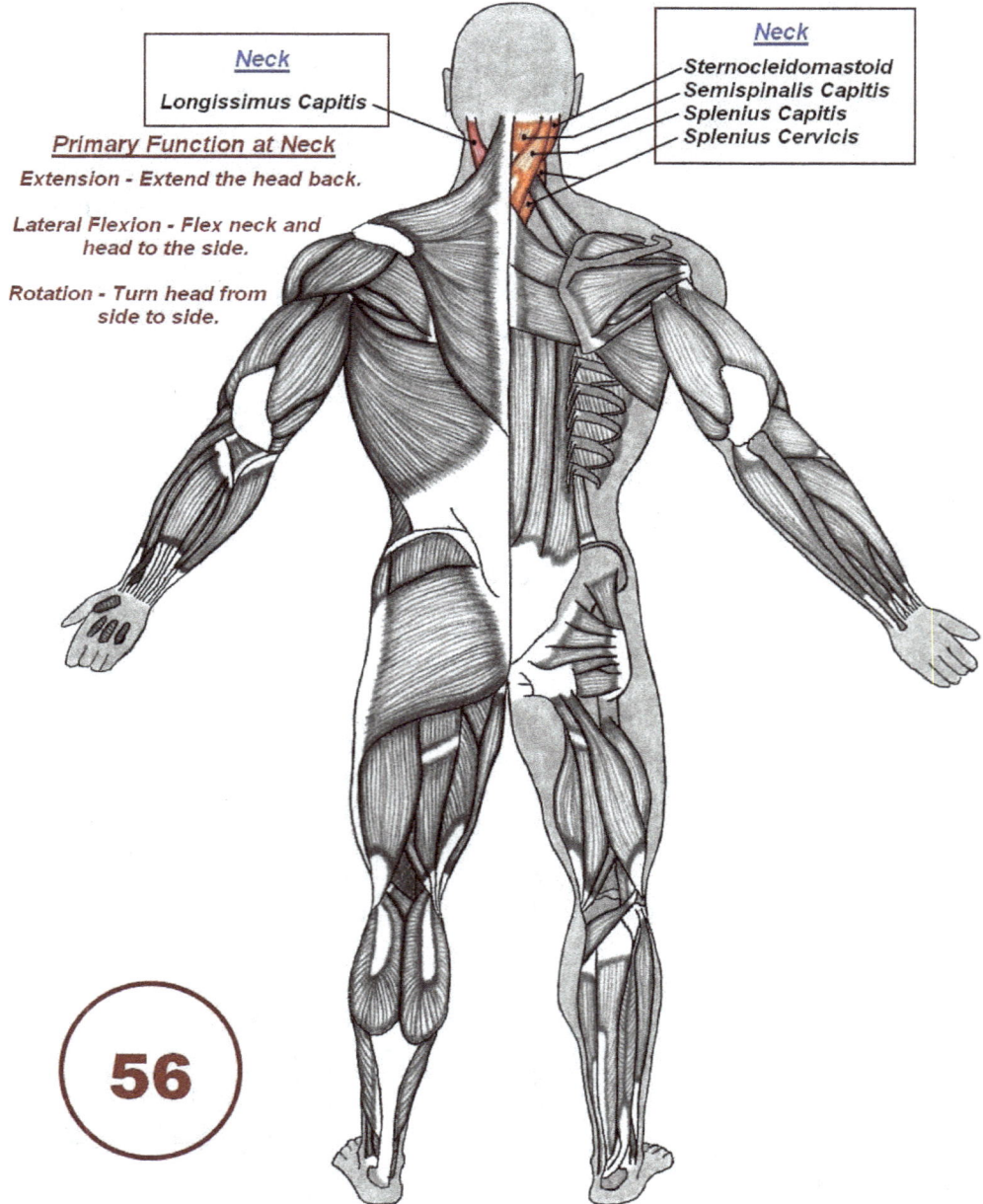

Neck

Longissimus Capitis

Neck
- Sternocleidomastoid
- Semispinalis Capitis
- Splenius Capitis
- Splenius Cervicis

Primary Function at Neck

Extension - Extend the head back.

Lateral Flexion - Flex neck and head to the side.

Rotation - Turn head from side to side.

56

56 - Exercises

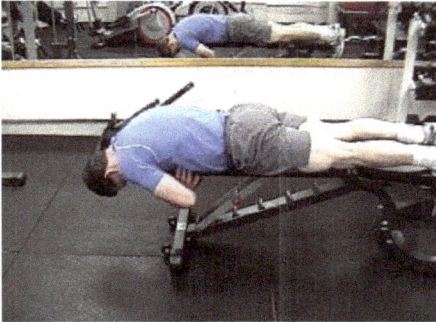
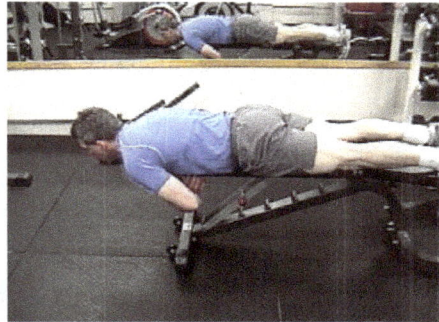

Lying Prone Neck Extension (Weighted/No Weight: 1 Set 7-10 Reps)

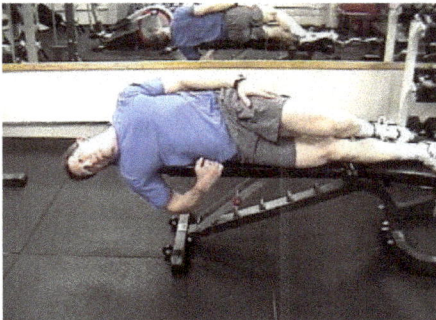
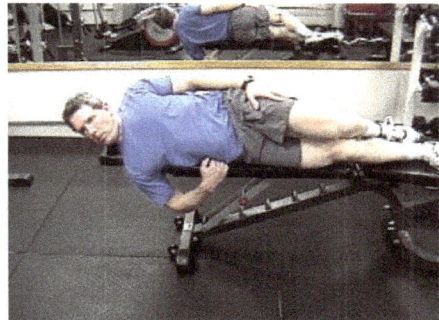

Side-Lying Lateral Neck Flex (1 Set 7-10 Reps Each Side)

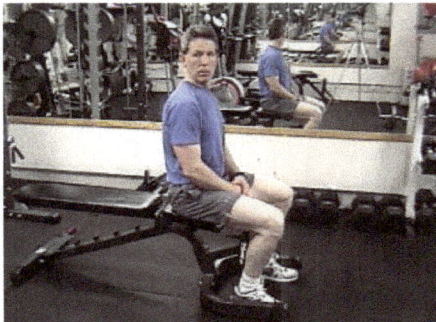
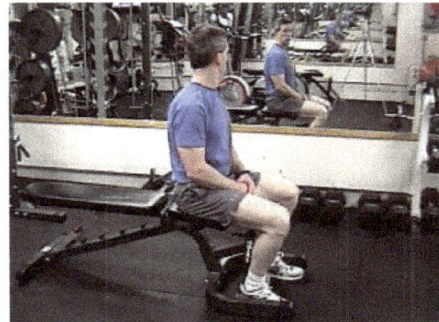

Head Rotation (1 Set 7-10 Reps Each Side)

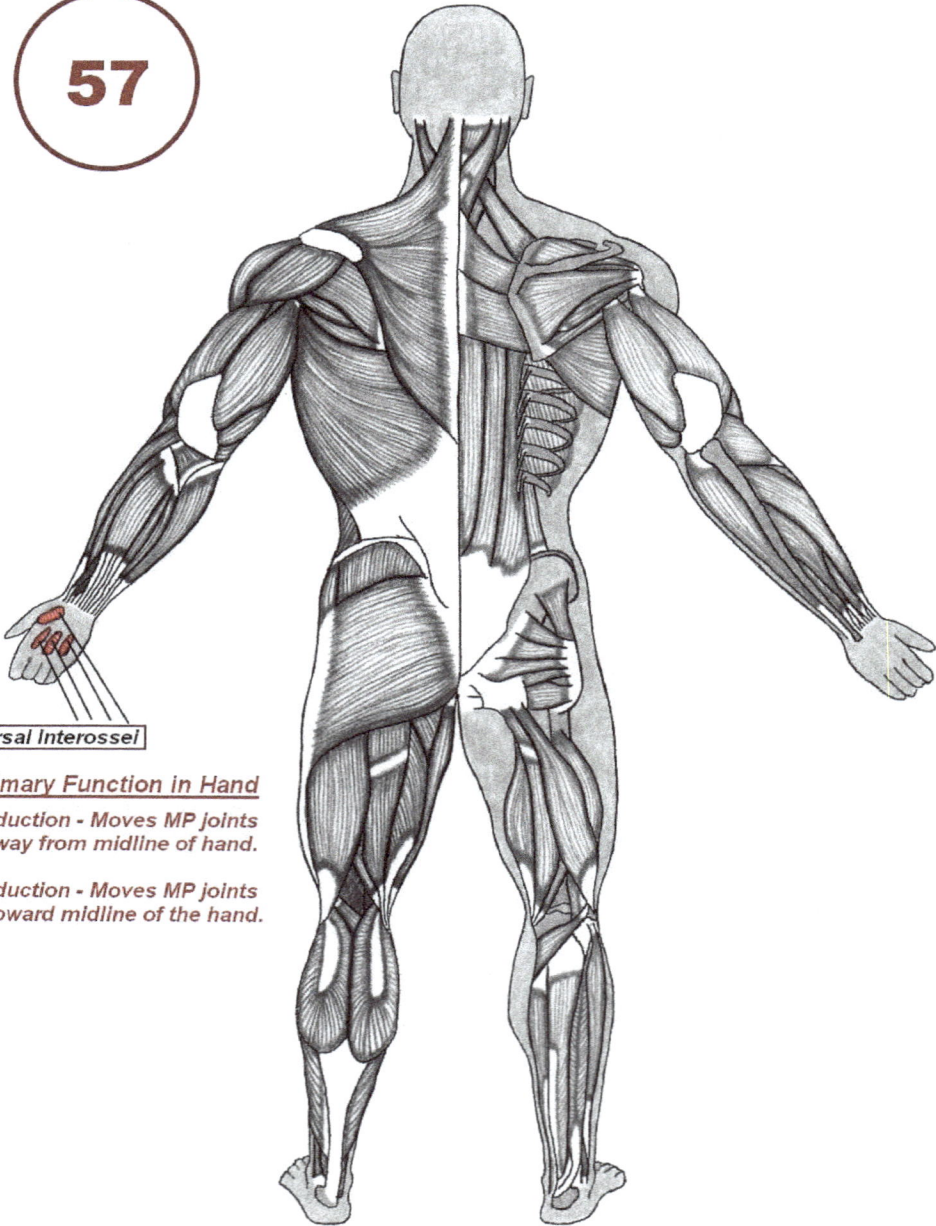

Hand - Dorsal Interossei

57

Dorsal Interossei

Primary Function in Hand

Abduction - Moves MP joints away from midline of hand.

Adduction - Moves MP joints in toward midline of the hand.

57 - Exercises

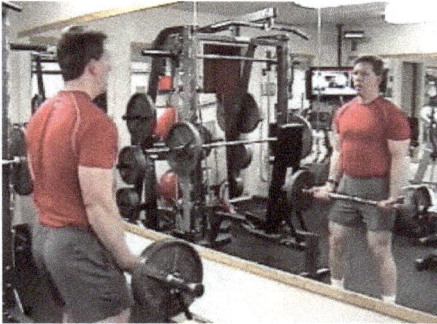

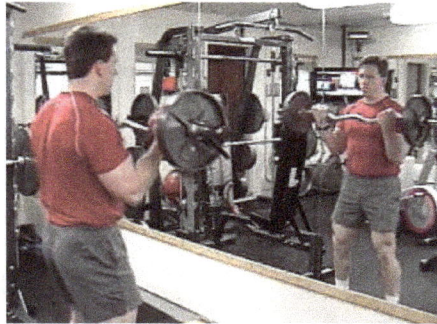

Biceps Standing EZ-Bar Curl (Hand Grip: 1-3 Sets 7-15 Reps)

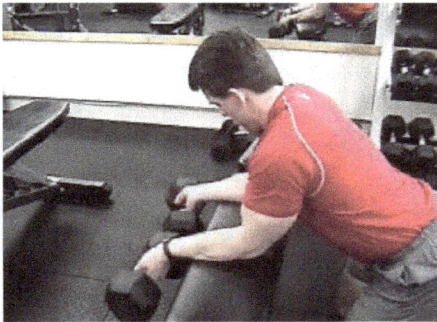

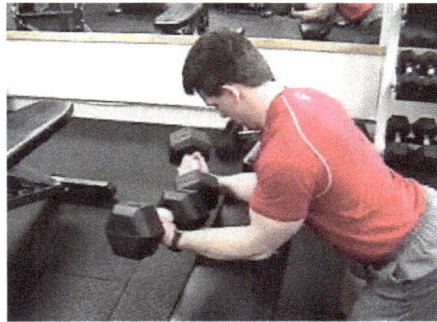

Wrist Curl on Bench (Hand Grip: 1-3 Sets 7-10 Reps)

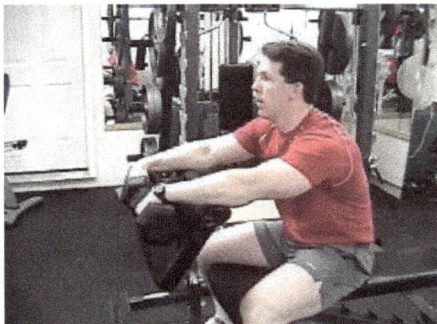

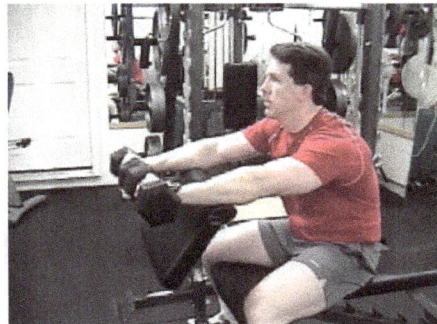

Forearm Extension "Reverse Wrist Curl" (Hand Grip: 1-3 Sets 7-10 Reps)

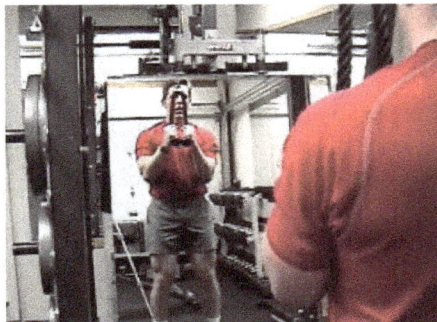

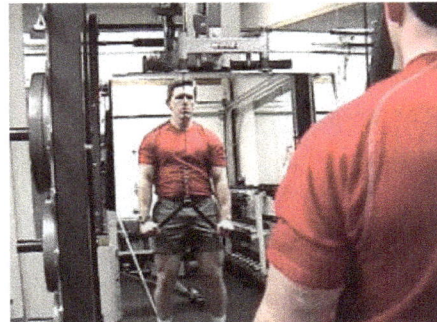

Triceps Cable Push Down (Hand Grip: 1-3 Sets 7-15 Reps)

57 - Exercises

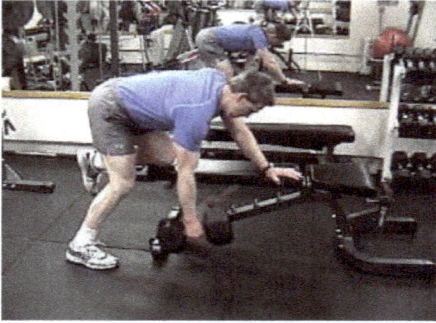

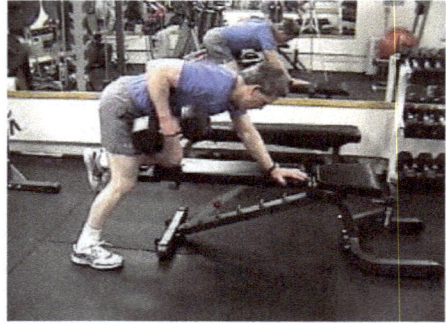

Kneeling Dumbbell Row (Hand Grip: 1-3 Sets 7-15 Reps)

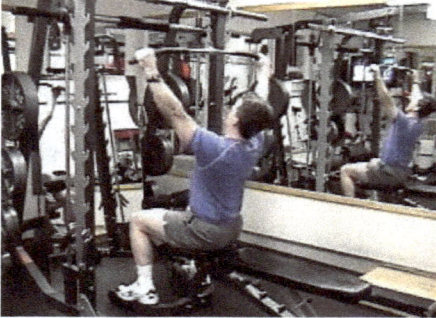

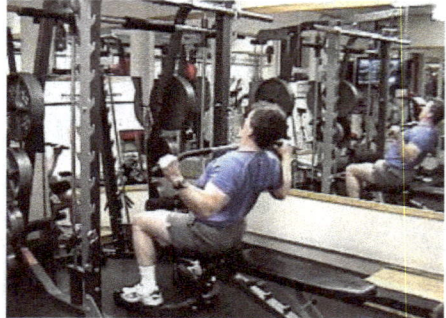

Lat Wide Grip Front Pull Down (Hand Grip: 1-3 Sets 7-15 Reps)

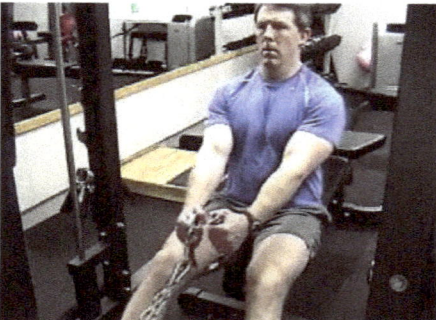

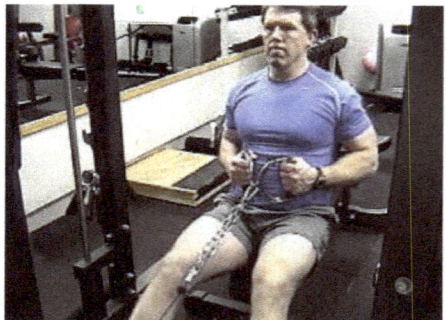

Seated Close Grip Cable Row (Hand Grip: 1-3 Sets 7-15 Reps)

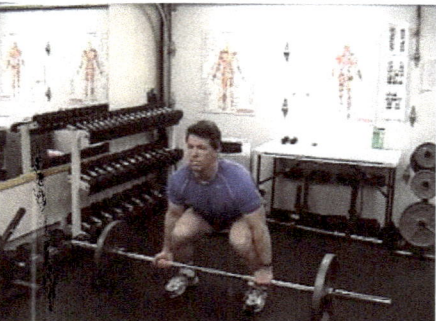

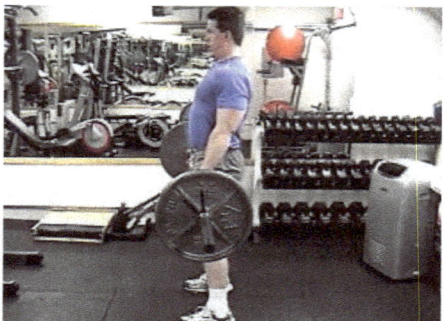

Dead-Lift (Hand Grip: 1-3 Sets 7-10 Reps)

Beginner Level 1 - Full Body Workout

On the following pages I provide a good beggining full body exercise routine with anatomy images and exercise pictures. This is a routine that healthy individuals cleared to exercise can perform at home, to begin to get into shape (with or without weights). This routine can be used in conjunction with the anatomy and exercise pictures throughout the book, as I also provide the page number of the exercise picture for the muscles being exercised.

Exercise	Page
Squats (No weight)	61
Push Ups (On toes or modified on knees)	4
Straight Leg Deadlift	122
Ab Crunch (On floor)	42
Row (Standing Bent Double Dumbbell)	116
Calve Raise (Standing on stairs)	176
Shoulder Upright Lateral Raise	24
Biceps Curls	30
Glute Curls	166
Triceps Extension	148
Leg Curls	170
Twists (Standing)	46

Begin with 1 set of 7-15 repetitions for each of the 12 exercises that work all of the major muscle groups (chest, back muscles, shoulder deltoids, arm biceps and triceps, glutes or buttocks, upper leg quadriceps and hamstrings, lower leg calves, abs and obliques). Perform the routine 2-3 days per week with 1 day of rest between workouts.

As the body conditions, increase to 2-3 sets of 7-12 reps per set, and 20-30 reps per set for abs and calves. I have split the routine into 3 rounds of 4 exercises, where a person can perform the additional sets for one round and then move to the next round of 4 exercises.

Use light weights initially for conditioning and practising the proper form for each exercise, and then increase weights as the body adapts.

I recommend walking a half mile to a mile after each workout 2-6 days per week for cardio exercise, and for weight loss.

Beginner Level 1 - Full Body Workout (Round 1)

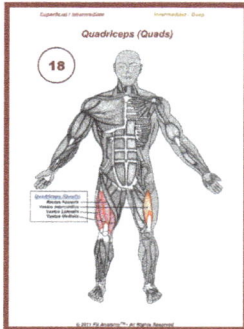

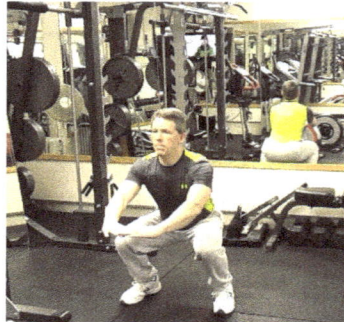

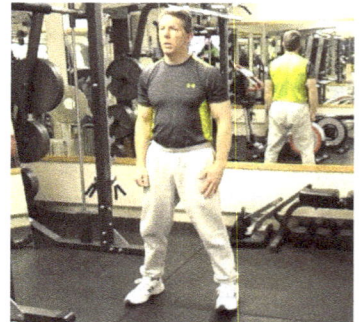

Quadriceps: Squats (1-3 Sets 10-25 Reps)

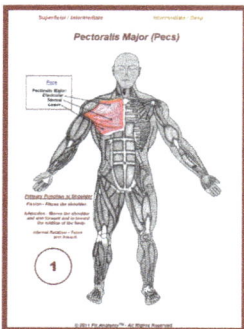

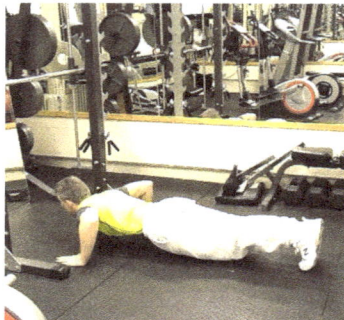

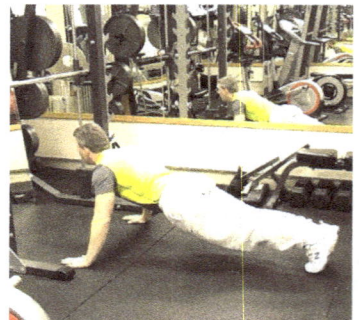

Pectoralis Major: Push Ups (1-3 Sets 10-50 Reps)

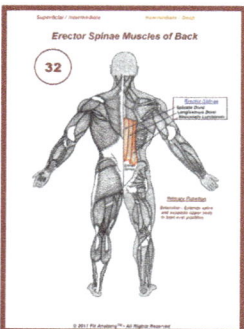

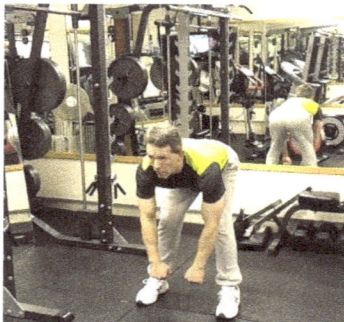

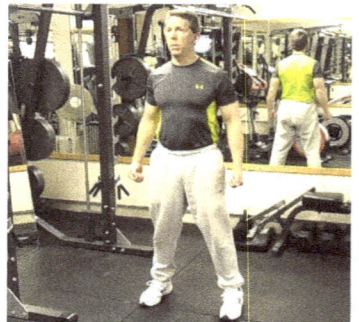

Erector Spinae: Back Extension (1-3 Sets 7-10 Reps)

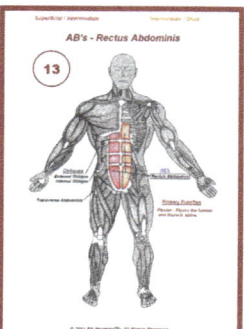

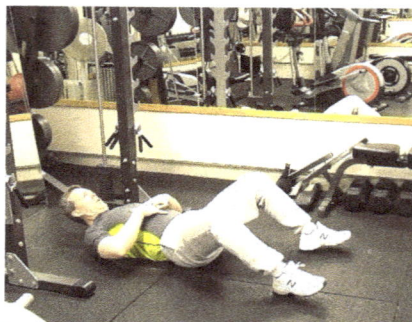

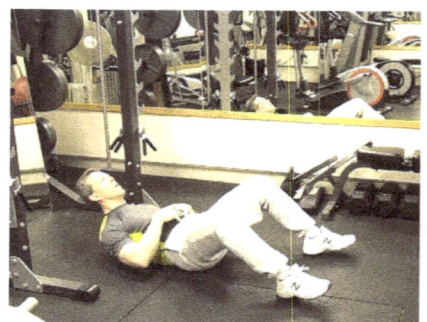

Rectus Abdominis: Crunches (1-3 Sets 10-30 Reps)

Beginner Level 1 - Full Body Workout (Round 2)

Latissimus Dorsi: Standing Bent Row (1-3 Sets 7-10 Reps)

Gastrocnemius: Calve Raises (1-3 Sets 10-30 Reps)

Middle Deltoid: Shoulder Upright Lateral Raise (1-3 Sets 7-10 Reps)

Biceps Brachii: Biceps Curl (1-3 Sets 7-10 Reps)

Beginner Level 1 - Full Body Workout (Round 3)

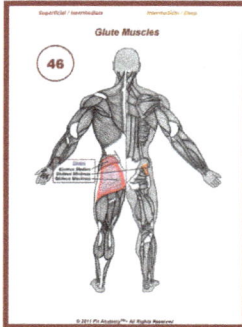

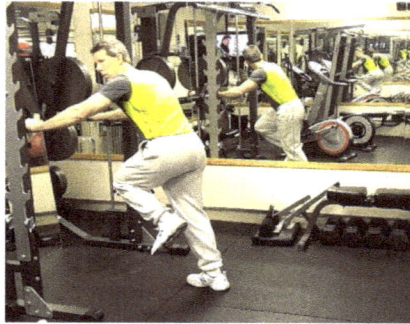

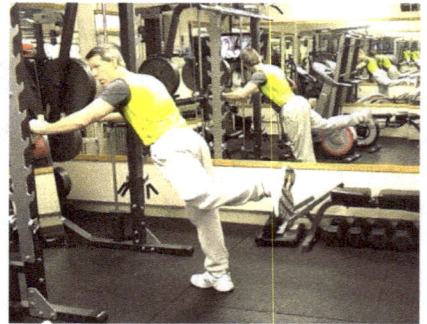

Glutes: Glute Curls (1-3 Sets 7-15 Reps Each Side)

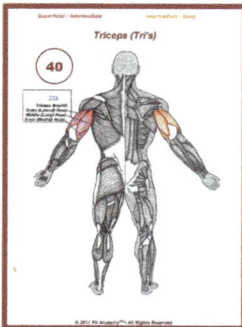

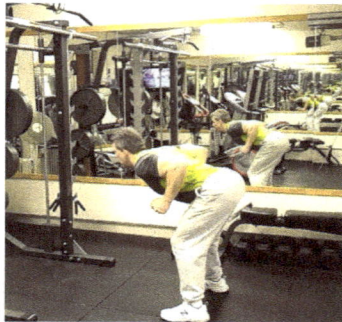

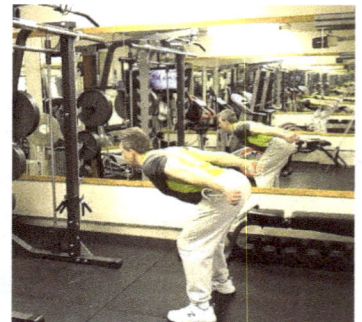

Triceps: Triceps Standing Bent Extension (1-3 Sets 7-10 Reps)

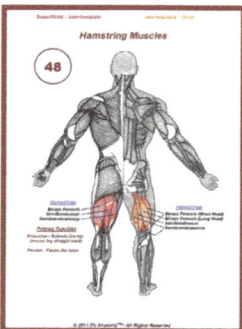

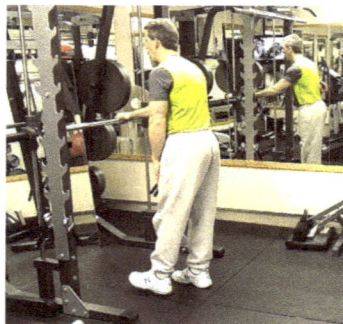

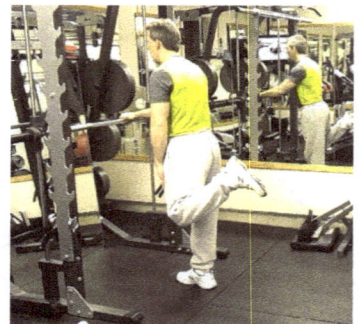

Hamstrings: Leg Curls (1-3 Sets 7-10 Reps Each Side)

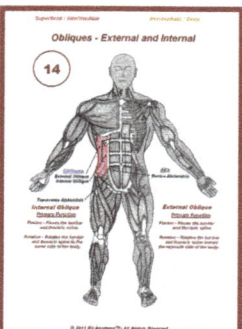

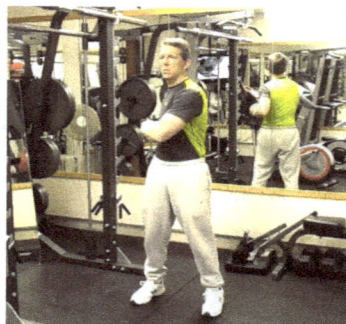

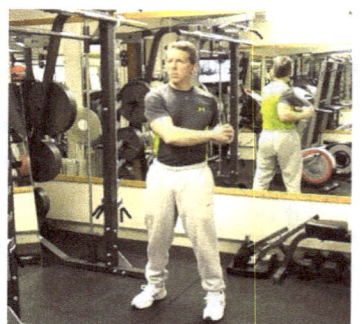

Obliques: Twists Standing (1-3 Sets 7-15 Reps Each Side)

References and Suggested Reading

Behnke, Robert S. (2006) Kinetic Anatomy. 4th ed. Champaign, IL: Human Kinetics.

Delavier, Frederic (2006) Strength Training Anatomy. 2nd ed. Champaign, IL: Human Kinetics.

Brooks, Douglas (2001) Effective Strength Training. Champaign, IL: Human Kinetics

www.ingramcontent.com/pod-product-compliance
Lightning Source LLC
Chambersburg PA
CBHW080330270326
41927CB00014B/3161